MedEd1
to Drug Food
Interactions

Author:
Eric Christianson, Pharm.D., BCPS, BCGP

Edited by:
Jennifer Salling, Pharm.D.

INTRODUCTION

I've learned a great deal from the hundreds of thousands healthcare professionals and students who've listened to the Real Life Pharmacology Podcast or have read the MedEd101.com blog. One of the important principles I've learned is that many don't understand the clinical significance of drug food interactions. As an expert in clinical pharmacology, the importance of the interplay between food and medicine cannot be understated. Food can significantly alter the effectiveness of some medications. Alternatively, medications can contribute to nutritional deficiencies that negatively impact our patients. In this reference book, we lay out over 500 of the most commonly used medications and how they impact diet or how diet can alter the effects of drugs.

This guide is a perfect resource for any student or young healthcare professional doing clinicals. In addition to highlighting potential food medication interactions, we have also laid out common adverse effects, indications, clinical pearls, mechanisms of action and monitoring parameters that are critical for each medication.

The MedEd101 Guide to Drug Food Interactions is meant to be a quick reference for healthcare professionals and students who work as dietitians, pharmacists, nurses, nurse practitioners, physicians, physician assistants, and many more.

ABOUT THE AUTHOR

Eric Christianson, Pharm.D., BCPS, BCGP is a clinical pharmacist who is passionate about patient safety. Eric is the founder of meded101.com, a website dedicated to providing quality, real world medication education for healthcare professionals.

He is also the creator of the Real Life Pharmacology podcast. This podcast geared toward healthcare professionals has been downloaded over 700,000 times in over 150 different countries.

He has been acknowledged by The Wall Street Journal, American Journal of Nursing, National Association Directors of Nursing, Pharmacy Podcast, Pharmacy Today, and Pharmacy Times.

Please take the time to check out the free resources provided through the Real Life Pharmacology and MedEd101 websites.

If you have comments or suggestions regarding the content of this book, feel free to reach out to Eric on LinkedIn: Eric Christianson, Pharm.D., BCPS, BCGP or at: mededucation101@gmail.com

Table of Contents

5

14

15

16

17

18

20

24

Abacavir (Ziagen, ABC)

- Class: Antiretroviral, Nucleoside Reverse Transcriptase Inhibitor (NRTI)
- Mechanism of Action: Converted to active triphosphate forms which compete with natural substrates to inhibit reverse transcriptase; the HIV virus uses the enzyme reverse transcriptase to convert RNA into DNA
- Common Uses: Treatment of HIV
- Memorable Side Effects: Lactic acidosis/fatty liver warning, GI adverse effects, elevated cholesterol, fatigue, neuropathy, skin rash, hypersensitivity reaction
- Clinical Pearls:
  - Risk of hypersensitivity reaction – patients who have the HLA-B*5701 allele are at increased risk of this reaction
  - Abacavir is in many combination products such as Trizivir (abacavir, lamivudine, and zidovudine) and Epzicom (abacavir and lamivudine)
- Monitoring: CBC, liver function, HIV viral load, CD4 count, renal function, HLA-B*5701 allele testing, lipids
- Drug and Diet Considerations:
  - May be given with or without meals
  - Monitor cholesterol and implement cholesterol lowering diet in patients who have elevated levels due to the adverse effects of the drug

Acamprosate (Campral)

- Class: Alcoholism agent, GABA agonist, glutamate antagonist
- Mechanism of Action: Enhances the effects of GABA and can blunt the effects of glutamate in the central nervous system; unclear exactly how this reduces alcohol intake, but has been therapeutically shown to reduce intake
- Common Uses: Alcohol use disorder
- Memorable Side Effects: Diarrhea, insomnia, dizziness, anorexia
- Clinical Pearls:
  - Contraindicated in CrCl less than 30 mL/min
  - Improves alcohol abstinence
- Monitoring: Kidney function, weight
- Drug and Diet Considerations:
  - Patients with alcohol use disorder are likely at risk for many nutritional deficiencies such as folic acid, thiamine, B12, B6, and the fat soluble vitamins A, D, E, and K – assess diet for possible deficiencies and supplement as appropriate
  - If diarrhea is significant, monitor fluid and electrolyte status
  - May have to change agent if side effects are severe
  - Can be given with or without food
  - Begin the medication when the patient achieves abstinence; it may be continued if a patient has a relapse

Acarbose (Precose)

- Class: Antidiabetic, Alpha-glucosidase inhibitor
- Mechanism of Action: Prevents the breakdown of complex sugars in the gut thus reducing blood sugar
- Common Uses: Management of type 2 diabetes
- Memorable Side Effects: Use is limited by significant GI side effects (diarrhea, pain and flatulence), increase in LFTs (rare)

- Clinical Pearls:
    - Seldom used due to GI side effects and frequent dosing
    - If the patient has a hypoglycemic episode, you MUST use simple sugars (i.e. glucose tablets) to treat it. Complex sugars may not be broken down due to the drug's mechanism of action
    - When used alone, hypoglycemia risk is typically not an issue
- Monitoring: Blood sugar, A1C, LFTs as clinically indicated
- Drug and Diet Considerations:
    - Must be administered with meals to be effective
    - Targets post-prandial glucose lowering
    - Implementation of a diabetic diet would be recommended for any diabetes patient

Acetaminophen (Tylenol)

- Class: Analgesic, Antipyretic
- Mechanism of Action: Inhibits prostaglandins in the CNS and may also block pain impulses
- Common Uses: Pain reliever and fever reducer
- Memorable Side Effects: Pretty well tolerated; rash (rare), liver toxicity (rare)
- Clinical Pearls:
    - One of the safest oral medications in the elderly for pain
    - 4 gram/day max (possibly 3 gram in elderly/over the counter use)
    - Often found in combinations with over the counter and prescription medications; cough and cold products, Vicodin, Percocet, etc. (be sure patients are well educated on this to avoid accidental overdose)
    - Liver toxicity is extremely rare at recommended doses, but can occur after accidental or intentional overdose
    - Acetylcysteine is the antidote for acetaminophen overdose
- Monitoring: Liver function if signs of toxicity (i.e. jaundice), acetaminophen levels if worried about overdose
- Drug and Diet Considerations:
    - Be cautious in patients who have a history of alcoholism; it could exacerbate the risk for liver complications
    - The liquid formulation rarely causes diarrhea if larger doses are used
    - Can be taken with or without food; stomach upset isn't very common, but if it happens, taking the drug with food is appropriate

Acetaminophen, Aspirin, and Caffeine (Excedrin, Excedrin Migraine, Vanquish)

- See individual agents

Acetazolamide (Diamox)

- Class: Carbonic anhydrase inhibitor, antiglaucoma agent
- Mechanism of Action: Inhibits carbonic anhydrase which can result in an increase in hydrogen ion reabsorption through the kidney; this can also cause increased excretion of potassium, bicarbonate, sodium, and water (diuretic effect)
- Common Uses: Prevention of altitude sickness, treatment of glaucoma, edema and epilepsy

27

- Memorable Side Effects: Electrolyte abnormalities such as hypokalemia and hyponatremia, increased urination, weight loss, GI upset, rare skin reactions, alterations in glucose control, taste alterations (rare) and respiratory acidosis (rare)
- Clinical Pearls:
  - Elderly may be at risk for more complications and adverse effects
- Monitoring: Renal function, electrolytes, CBC, ocular pressure (glaucoma)
- Drug and Diet Considerations:
  - Ok to give with food
  - Noted to contribute to weight loss as well as taste alterations; assess changes in dietary intake, particularly if the patient is losing weight
  - May increase elimination of folic acid from the body

Aclidinium (Tudorza)
- Class: Inhaled anticholinergic
- Mechanism of Action: Inhaled anticholinergic can open up airways and decrease secretions
- Common Uses: Treatment of COPD
- Memorable Side Effects: Dry mouth, cough, irritation to the lungs; usually well tolerated due to minimal systemic absorption
- Clinical Pearls:
  - Aclidinium is primarily used for COPD, and because it has anticholinergic activity, it can help dry up the airways as well as open them up to allow for better breathing in patients who have thick mucus/sputum
  - It is long acting and meant to be used as a controller medication
  - It will not provide acute relief from respiratory distress, not meant to be a rescue inhalation product
  - Often by using this medication in COPD, our goal is likely to improve respiratory status, but also to reduce the amount of as needed albuterol and/or albuterol/ipratropium (Duoneb or Combivent)
  - With the delivery device, it is imperative to assess if patients are able to adequately coordinate how to use the device as well as if they are able to inhale quickly and forcefully enough to get the drug into their lungs
  - Systemic anticholinergic effects are usually not a concern as systemic absorption is low
- Monitoring: FEV1, peak flow
- Drug and Diet Considerations:
  - Inhaled, local medication
  - Dry mouth may impact dietary/fluid intake

Acyclovir (Zovirax)
- Class: Antiviral
- Mechanism of Action: Inhibits DNA synthesis and viral replication
- Common Uses: Treatment of shingles, genital herpes, cold sores and chicken pox
- Memorable Side Effects: GI adverse effects, CNS side effects (dizziness, sedation and confusion) more likely in elderly and/or patients with poor kidney function
- Clinical Pearls:

- o For most viral infections, treatment works best at the first sign of an outbreak
- o May need to reduce the dose and/or have a heightened awareness for potential adverse effects in patients with poor kidney function
- o Also comes in a topical form that can be used for cold sores (herpes labialis)
- Monitoring: Renal function, CBC, liver function (as clinically indicated and with long term therapy)
- Drug and Diet Considerations:
  - o It is important to maintain adequate hydration to prevent crystallization of the drug in the urine, this is important to help reduce the risk of acute renal failure
  - o GI upset is possible; Can be given with or without food

Albuterol (Proventil HFA, ProAir HFA, Ventolin HFA)
- Class: Beta-agonist
- Mechanism of Action: Stimulates beta-2 receptors leading to relaxation of smooth muscle and the opening of airways
- Common Uses: Acute relief of respiratory distress in asthma, COPD, and other respiratory disorders
- Memorable Side Effects: tachycardia, tremor, anxiousness, hypokalemia (rare), hyperglycemia (rare)
- Clinical Pearls:
  - o Rapid onset, meant to help with acute breathing issues
  - o It is often used with ipratropium (Duoneb/Combivent)
  - o Beta-blockers (i.e. propranolol) may blunt the effects of albuterol
  - o In patients who are taking multiple inhaled respiratory medications at the same time, albuterol should be done first to help open up the airways
  - o Patients who are frequently using their albuterol inhaler (or nebs) or presenting to the emergency room due to respiratory symptoms need to be assessed for adherence and possibly have controller medications adjusted
- Monitoring: Frequency of use, FEV1, peak-flow, pulse, blood pressure, and potassium (usually only necessary in high dosages), glucose (rarely clinically significant)
- Drug and Diet Considerations:
  - o Assess potassium intake and serum potassium if the patient is using a beta agonist frequently or has a history of hypokalemia
  - o Be aware of caffeine intake in combination with a beta-agonist as it can have an additive effect on blood pressure and heart rate

Albuterol and Ipratropium (Duoneb, Combivent)
- Class: Short acting beta-agonist and short acting anticholinergic
- See individual agents

Alendronate (Fosamax)
- Class: Bisphosphonate
- Mechanism of Action: Inhibits the action osteoclasts; osteoclasts break down bone and are responsible for bone resorption

- Common Uses: Treatment of osteoporosis
- Memorable Side Effects: Esophageal ulceration (administration procedure is important to decrease this risk), stomach upset, osteonecrosis of the jaw (rare)
- Clinical Pearls:
    - Have patient remain sitting or standing upright for 30 minutes following administration (this is to reduce the risk of esophageal irritation or ulceration)
    - After 5 years of bisphosphonate use, medication may be discontinued in some lower risk patients
    - Osteonecrosis of the jaw is extremely rare; patients at higher risk may include those with certain cancers, or who have had recent dental procedures
    - Be cautious with oral bisphosphonates in patients who already have esophageal or GI related concerns (GI bleed or ulcer history)
- Monitoring: Bone mineral density, calcium, vitamin D levels
- Drug and Diet Considerations:
    - Ensure the patient has adequate vitamin D and calcium intake – at least 1,200 mg per day of calcium and 1,000 units of vitamin D in females with osteoporosis
    - Esophagitis and GI upset is possible which could cause changes in appetite and weight loss – issues are more likely if alendronate is given on a daily basis versus weekly (weekly dosing is recommended)
    - The drug must be taken in the morning prior to breakfast with 6-8 ounces of plain water and nothing else
    - Wait at least 30 minutes prior to eating anything
    - If taken with food, juice, or other medications, the absorption (and effectiveness) of the drug will be reduced

Alfuzosin (Uroxatral)
- Class: Alpha blocker
- Mechanism of Action: Blocks alpha receptors causing smooth muscle relaxation and opening of the ureter
- Common Uses: Treatment of BPH symptoms and reduction of bladder obstruction
- Memorable Side Effects: Low blood pressure, increased fall risk, dizziness
- Clinical Pearls:
    - Usually dosed at night to try to avoid/minimize orthostasis risk
    - More selective for the prostate than other alpha blockers, (i.e. terazosin or doxazosin) so there is less risk of lowering blood pressure
    - Anticholinergics and pseudoephedrine can worsen BPH causing other alpha blockers, like tamsulosin, to be initiated or increased
    - May also be used to help patients pass a ureteral stone; relaxes the smooth muscle and opens up the ureter to ease flow
- Monitoring: Blood pressure, PSA as clinically indicated
- Drug and Diet Considerations:
    - Take after eating
    - Grapefruit juice may increase concentration

Alirocumab (Praluent)
- Class: Antilipemic, PCSK9 inhibitor

30

- Mechanism of Action: PCSK9 is a protein that destroys LDL receptors in the liver; by inhibiting this protein, it allows LDL receptors to do their job and to remove circulating LDL from the blood stream, thus lowering LDL
- Common Uses: LDL lowering, reduce the risk of cardiovascular events
- Memorable Side Effects: Injection site reactions, myopathy (minimal risk compared to statins), fatigue
- Clinical Pearls:
  - Additional agent to consider in high risk patients where statins have been insufficient at lowering cholesterol (LDL)
  - Injection only
  - Very expensive and access is often limited by insurance
- Monitoring: Lipids
- Drug and Diet Considerations:
  - Food does not affect the pharmacokinetics – can be administered anytime in relation to dietary intake
  - Encourage a lipid lowering diet for any patient taking a cholesterol medication

Allopurinol (Zyloprim)
- Class: Anti-gout, xanthine oxidase inhibitor
- Mechanism of Action: Xanthine oxidase is an enzyme necessary for uric acid production, allopurinol inhibits xanthine oxidase and thus decreases uric acid production
- Common Uses: Gout prophylaxis and reduction of high uric acid levels
- Memorable Side Effects: GI issues, rash
- Clinical Pearls:
  - Used for prophylaxis of gout, NOT treatment of an acute flare; NSAIDs, prednisone, or colchicine are generally used for an acute flare
  - Usually fairly well tolerated, but watch out for necessary dose adjustments in CKD as the drug is cleared by the kidneys
  - Keep an eye out for medications and supplements that can elevate uric acid; niacin, thiazide diuretics, some immunosuppressive drugs
- Monitoring: Uric acid, renal function
- Drug and Diet Considerations:
  - GI upset is possible, but likelihood is low when taken after meals
  - Adequate hydration is important to help flush uric acid out of the body – this can also be helpful in reducing the risk for uric acid based kidney stones
  - Alcohol, certain seafood (i.e. sardines, anchovies, shellfish, and tuna), liver, bacon, veal, and red meats have a higher purine content and may increase the risk for gout flares; assess diet and recommend a reduction in purines if a patient is having frequent gout attacks or elevated uric acid levels

Alprazolam (Xanax)
- Class: Antianxiety, benzodiazepine
- Mechanism of Action: Enhances activity of GABA (an inhibitory neurotransmitter that causes sedation and other CNS effects)
- Common Uses: Treatment of anxiety disorders, insomnia and alcohol withdrawal

- Memorable Side Effects: Sedation, confusion, fall risk, dizziness, slurred speech, ataxia
- Clinical Pearls:
  - Boxed warning when used in combination with opioids – increased risk for excessive sedation, respiratory depression, and death due to overdose
  - The best way to remember benzodiazepines is that they cause many similar effects to alcohol; "alcohol in a pill"
  - Benzodiazepines should not be abruptly discontinued
  - Flumazenil is antidote in overdose
  - The elderly are at higher risk for serious consequences from the adverse effects
  - Benzodiazepines are a controlled substance, meaning they may be abused or cause addiction
- Monitoring: Respiratory rate and cardiovascular parameters (usually only an issue with overdose or significant drug interactions)
- Drug and Diet Considerations:
  - If given with food, the peak concentration may be lower but the overall effect on total absorption is generally not clinically significant (can be given with or without food)
  - Grapefruit juice may increase concentrations and increase the risk of adverse effects and toxicity
  - The supplement St. John's wort may reduce concentrations of the drug

Alteplase (Activase, tPA)
- Class: Thrombolytic (clot buster)
- Mechanism of Action: Binds to fibrin and breaks up blood clots
- Common Uses: Improvement of patient survival after a stroke, pulmonary embolism or MI. Also used to open up central venous access (Cathflo)
- Memorable Side Effects: Bleeding
- Clinical Pearls:
  - Need to use this medication quickly at onset of stroke to have maximal benefit
  - Need to monitor for high blood pressure due to an increased risk of complications
- Monitoring: Blood pressure, PT/INR, CBC, bleed risk
- Drug and Diet Considerations:
  - Vitamin E, Omega-3 fatty acids, gingko, garlic, ginseng, turmeric, and fish oil supplements have been purported to have antiplatelet type activity which in theory could increase the risk of bleed – clinical significance is questionable; the most common resolution is to discontinue the supplements if they are not necessary
  - Alcohol may have an additive antiplatelet type effect and increase the risk of GI bleed

Aluminum Hydroxide (Maalox, Mylanta, Gaviscon)
- Class: Antacid, phosphate binder
- Mechanism of Action: Aluminum hydroxide neutralizes acid in the gut by binding hydrogen ions
- Common Uses: Treatment of GI upset and heartburn. Also used as a phosphate binder

- Memorable Side Effects: Constipation, hypomagnesemia, hypophosphatemia, aluminum accumulation
- Clinical Pearls:
  - Risk for aluminum accumulation in patients with poor kidney function (more likely with chronic use)
  - Generally avoided as a phosphate binder due to the risk of aluminum accumulation in CKD
  - May bind numerous medications and reduce absorption (i.e. levothyroxine, quinolone antibiotics, tetracycline antibiotics)
- Monitoring: Calcium and phosphorus levels (only in chronic use)
- Drug and Diet Considerations:
  - Take with food when used as a phosphate binder

Amantadine (Symmetrel)
- Class: Antiparkinson's agent, dopamine agonist, antiviral
- Mechanism of Action: A shortage of dopamine activity in the brain can lead to Parkinson's type symptoms; amantadine stimulates dopamine receptors thus enhancing overall dopamine activity
- Common Uses: Extrapyramidal symptoms and Parkinson's disorder
- Memorable Side Effects: Orthostasis, edema, hallucinations, purple spots on the skin, sedation, dry mouth, nausea, weight loss, OCD symptoms (rare)
- Clinical Pearls:
  - Has antiviral activity, but influenza resistance is high (use is avoided for this indication)
  - More dopamine activity can lead to an increase in GI adverse effects and psychiatric changes
- Monitoring: Blood pressure, renal function
- Drug and Diet Considerations:
  - Can be given with food if nausea occurs; weight loss and reduced appetite are possible
  - Rare associations with impulsive behaviors which could include, but is not limited to, binge eating
  - Alcohol may augment sedative adverse effect

Ambrisentan (Letairis)
- Class: Endothelin receptor antagonists:
- Mechanism of Action: Blocks endothelin receptors which helps relax the pulmonary blood vessels and ultimately lowers blood pressure
- Common Uses: Treatment of pulmonary arterial hypertension
- Memorable Side Effects: Headache, edema, flushing, increased bleeding risk
- Clinical Pearls:
  - REMS program due to fetal risks if females become pregnant
  - Can increase the risk of bleed especially in those on antiplatelet medications or anticoagulants
- Monitoring: Hemoglobin, pregnancy testing
- Drug and Diet Considerations:
  - May administer with or without food
  - Vitamin E, Omega-3 fatty acids, gingko, garlic, ginseng, turmeric, and fish oil supplements have been purported to have antiplatelet type activity which, in theory, could increase the risk of bleed –

clinical significance is questionable; the most common resolution is to discontinue the supplements if they are not necessary

Amiodarone (Cordarone)

- Class: Anti-arrhythmic
- Mechanism of Action: Multiple mechanisms including affecting sodium, potassium and calcium channels, as well as potentially having beta and alpha blocking activity
- Common Uses: Treatment of ventricular arrhythmia and atrial fibrillation
- Memorable Side Effects: Arrhythmias; low blood pressure, GI side effects (nausea, vomiting, anorexia, constipation), hypothyroid, elevated LFTs, pulmonary toxicity
- Clinical Pearls:
  - Unique in that it has a very long half-life – it takes about 40-55 days for half of the drug to be eliminated
  - Respiratory function should be monitored as amiodarone has a boxed warning for pulmonary fibrosis
  - Liver function needs to be monitored as it has a boxed warning for liver toxicity
- Monitoring: EKG, TSH, LFTs, blood pressure, lung function, potassium, magnesium, eye exams
- Drug and Diet Considerations:
  - With its potential to affect thyroid function, weight gain or weight loss is possible – check thyroid levels if the patient is experiencing symptoms of hypothyroidism or hyperthyroidism
  - If GI upset occurs, taking with meals is acceptable, consistency is recommended
  - Amiodarone contains iodine; be aware of this in relation to its effect on thyroid function
  - Grapefruit juice may increase concentrations of amiodarone; avoid use
  - The supplement St. John's wort may reduce concentrations of the drug
  - Out of range potassium or magnesium levels may increase the risk for arrhythmias

Amitriptyline (Elavil)

- Class: TCA (tri-cyclic antidepressant)
- Mechanism of Action: Inhibits reuptake of serotonin and norepinephrine
- Common Uses: Treatment of depression, neuropathy, pain syndromes, anxiety and PTSD
- Memorable Side Effects: Sedation, dry eyes, dry mouth, urinary retention, constipation, confusion, fall risk in elderly, QTc prolongation, weight gain, SIADH (rare)
- Clinical Pearls:
  - Generally not recommended in the elderly due to anticholinergic effects
  - Not a good first line choice for sleep or depression (other agents exist that are much safer)
  - May exacerbate BPH, dementia and constipation
  - Often dosed in the evening due to the adverse effect of sedation

- Monitoring: EKG and electrolytes in at risk patients (especially in high dosages or those on other QT prolonging medications), behavioral changes, weight, sodium (in patients with signs of hyponatremia),
- Drug and Diet Considerations:
    - Weight gain is possible and may be problematic
    - Slows the motility of the GI tract which could increase the risk for constipation – prevent by maintaining adequate fluids and non-constipating diet
    - If GI upset occurs, may give with food
    - Dry mouth may increase thirst and alter taste/pleasure of food
    - Poor dietary and fluid intake may place the patient at higher risk for complications from electrolyte abnormalities (i.e. hyponatremia, hypokalemia, or hypomagnesemia)

Amlodipine (Norvasc)

- Class: Antihypertensive, calcium channel blocker, dihydropyridine
- Mechanism of Action: Blocks calcium ions from entering voltage gated smooth muscle cells, resulting in relaxation (vasodilation)
- Common Uses: Treatment of hypertension, angina and Raynaud's syndrome
- Memorable Side Effects: Low blood pressure, edema and constipation
- Clinical Pearls:
    - Edema is more likely at higher dosages
    - Educate patients to get up slowly to minimize risk of orthostatic hypotension
    - Dihydropyridines typically do not affect the heart rate compared to non-dihydropyridines
- Monitoring: Blood pressure
- Drug and Diet Considerations:
    - Fluid retention (edema) is one of the most common adverse effects – altering fluid intake is usually not necessary as the drug is most often reduced or changed to another antihypertensive
    - Administer freely with or without food
    - St. John's wort may reduce effectiveness
    - Standard calcium supplementation typically will not impact the effectiveness of amlodipine; excessive doses of calcium may have a higher likelihood of blunting the effects of amlodipine

Amoxicillin (Amoxil)

- Class: Antibiotic, penicillin
- Mechanism of Action: Inhibits bacterial cell wall formation
- Common Uses: Treatment of bacterial infections such as ear infection, sinusitis, strep throat and skin infections
- Memorable Side Effects: Diarrhea, stomach upset, allergic reaction, rash
- Clinical Pearls:
    - Many patients have an allergy to penicillin; amoxicillin is from the same class and should not be used in patients with a severe allergy (if it is an intolerance like stomach upset, it may be prudent to try a "penicillin" type antibiotic again depending upon the patient's situation)

- o Diarrhea and GI upset are going to be the most common side effects; if symptoms are mild, hopefully the patient can manage to continue therapy
- Monitoring: Improvement of infection (i.e. fever and symptoms), lab work is typically not necessary with short term use
- Drug and Diet Considerations:
  - o Give with food to help reduce GI adverse effects
  - o Although food may lower the peak concentration of the drug, overall absorption is not changed
  - o Bland foods that reduce GI upset and diarrhea can be helpful
  - o Maintain adequate fluid intake to avoid dehydration especially if diarrhea is a significant problem

Amoxicillin/clavulanate (Augmentin)

- Class: Antibiotic, penicillin, beta-lactamase inhibitor
- Mechanism of Action: Inhibits bacterial cell wall formation; clavulanate inhibits bacterial beta-lactamase which can inactivate amoxicillin which ultimately preserves the drug and increases effectiveness
- Common Uses: Treatment of bacterial infections such as ear infection, sinusitis, strep throat, and skin infections
- Memorable Side Effects: Diarrhea, stomach upset, allergy, rash
- Clinical Pearls:
  - o Many patients have an allergy to penicillin; amoxicillin is from the same class and should not be used in patients with a severe allergy (if it is an intolerance like stomach upset, it may be prudent to try a "penicillin" type antibiotic again depending upon the patient's situation)
  - o Diarrhea and GI upset are going to be the major/common side effects with amoxicillin; with mild GI upset and/or diarrhea, hopefully the patient can tough it out and continue therapy
- Monitoring: Improvement of infection (i.e. fever and symptoms), lab work is typically not necessary with short term use
- Drug and Diet Considerations:
  - o Give with food to help reduce GI adverse effects
  - o Although food may lower the peak concentration of the drug, overall absorption is not changed
  - o Bland foods that reduce GI upset and diarrhea can be helpful
  - o Maintain adequate fluid intake to avoid dehydration especially if diarrhea is a significant problem
  - o Small amounts of potassium and/or phenylalanine may be present in some dosage forms

Amphetamine/Dextroamphetamine (Adderall)

- Class: CNS stimulant
- Mechanism of Action: Facilitates an increase in the release of norepinephrine and dopamine leading to CNS stimulation
- Common Uses: Management of ADHD
- Memorable Side Effects: Anxiety, insomnia, poor appetite, weight loss, twitching, shakiness, hypertension, tachycardia, emotional lability
- Clinical Pearls:

- o Remembering that this medication ramps you up (stimulant) will help you remember its side effects (anxiety, insomnia, weight loss, poor appetite, increased BP, increased pulse etc.)
  - o Be cautious in adult patients who may already be at cardiovascular risk (hypertension, congenital defects, etc.)
  - o Schedule 2 controlled substance, addictive and has high abuse potential
- Monitoring: Blood pressure, pulse, weight, cardiac monitoring (in patients with preexisting cardiac condition or at risk for cardiac complications) and growth in pediatric patients
- Drug and Diet Considerations:
  - o Food should have minimal impact on overall effectiveness, with or without food is acceptable
  - o Use caution with other foods/supplements that may have additive effects to heart rate, blood pressure, and insomnia (i.e. caffeine)
  - o Vitamin C may reduce the effectiveness by acidifying the urine which can enhance renal elimination of the drug (usually not clinically significant, but often we can discontinue the vitamin C supplement in patients who have a relatively normal diet)
  - o Assessing appetite and risk for anorexia is particularly important in pediatric patients

Amphotericin B (Ambisome, Fungizone)

- Class: Antifungal
- Mechanism of Action: Binds ergosterol which alters cell membranes and leads to fungal death
- Common Uses: Treatment of severe fungal infections
- Memorable Side Effects: Infusion reaction with flu-like symptoms (fever, GI upset, chills, headache), hypotension, tachypnea, renal failure, electrolyte imbalances
- Clinical Pearls:
  - o 4 different formulations available and they are not interchangeable; 2 major formulations include:
    - ▪ Ambisome is the lipid-based formulation
    - ▪ Fungizone is the conventional formulation
  - o Premedication may be necessary for infusion reactions (i.e. NSAIDs, acetaminophen, diphenhydramine, or corticosteroids)
- Monitoring: Renal function, electrolytes, CBC, EKG (as clinically indicated), LFTs
- Drug and Diet Considerations:
  - o Hypokalemia and hypomagnesemia are both possible, monitor electrolytes and replace as indicated
  - o Anorexia and diarrhea may be problematic if long term use is indicated
  - o Liposomal (lipids) amphotericin B contains 0.27 kcal per 5 mg; adjustments may be necessary in TPN patients

Ampicillin/Sulbactam (Unasyn)

- Class: Antibiotic, penicillin
- Mechanism of Action: Inhibits bacterial cell wall formation

- Common Uses: Treatment of a wide variety of bacterial infections including endocarditis, Group B strep prevention, sepsis and upper respiratory infections
- Memorable Side Effects: GI upset, diarrhea, allergy, rash, Clostridium difficile diarrhea
- Clinical Pearls:
  - Cross-reactivity with other penicillin antibiotics is common in severe allergic reaction
  - Available as injection only
- Monitoring: Signs of infection improvement (i.e. fever and symptoms), routine lab work is typically not necessary with short term use
- Drug and Diet Considerations:
  - GI upset and diarrhea is the most common adverse effect and could contribute to a short term reduction in caloric intake
  - Bland foods that reduce GI upset and diarrhea can be helpful
  - If diarrhea is problematic, maintain adequate hydration to avoid dehydration

Anastrozole (Arimidex)

- Class: Antineoplastic, aromatase inhibitor
- Mechanism of Action: Binds the aromatase enzyme and blocks conversion of androgens to estrogens which can starve a tumor of estrogen and block tumor growth
- Common Uses: Treatment of postmenopausal women diagnosed with breast cancer
- Memorable Side Effects: Menopausal symptoms (hot flashes), GI upset, flushing, osteoporosis risk, cholesterol elevations
- Clinical Pearls:
  - May increase the risk of cardiovascular events in patients who have a history of heart disease
- Monitoring: Bone mineral density and lipids
- Drug and Diet Considerations:
  - May be given with or without food
  - Ensure adequate calcium and vitamin D intake given osteoporosis risks
  - Implement lipid-lowering diet in patients at risk for hypercholesterolemia

Anidulafungin (Eraxis)

- Class: Antifungal, echinocandin
- Mechanism of Action: Inhibition of 1,3 beta-D glucan synthase (key enzyme involved in fungal cell wall synthesis)
- Common Uses: Alternative to fluconazole if the patient has a resistant fungal infection
- Memorable Side Effects: Low blood pressure, GI upset, diarrhea, edema, tachycardia, infusion reaction and electrolytes imbalances (rare)
- Clinical Pearls:
  - Typically better tolerated than other IV antifungals (i.e. azole antifungals and amphotericin B)
  - IV only
- Monitoring: Liver function, renal function (as clinically indicated), CBC (as clinically indicated)
- Drug and Diet Considerations:

o   No major dietary concerns

Apixaban (Eliquis)
- Class: Anticoagulant
- Mechanism of Action: Inhibits clotting factor 10A
- Common Uses: Prevention of stroke in patients with atrial fibrillation, DVT/PE prophylaxis or treatment
- Memorable Side Effects: Bleeding
- Clinical Pearls:
    o   Overall, less risk of drug interactions
    o   Patients do NOT need to do routine INRs
    o   Twice daily dosing is a downside compared to other anticoagulants
- Monitoring: CBC and renal function
- Drug and Diet Considerations:
    o   Administer with or without food
    o   Vitamin E, Omega-3 fatty acids, gingko, garlic, ginseng, turmeric, and fish oil supplements have been purported to have antiplatelet type activity which in theory could increase the risk of bleed – clinical significance is questionable; the most common resolution is to discontinue the supplements if they are not necessary
    o   Alcohol may have an additive antiplatelet type effect and increase the risk of GI bleed
    o   Grapefruit juice may increase concentrations

Aprepitant (Emend)
- Class: NK-1 receptor antagonist
- Mechanism of Action: Inhibition of neurokinin-1 receptor which can help stimulate antiemetic activity in the brain
- Common Uses: Helps prevent chemotherapy induced nausea and vomiting
- Memorable Side Effects: Sedation and blood pressure changes
- Clinical Pearls:
    o   Often used to augment the antiemetic action of ondansetron and corticosteroids in chemotherapy induced nausea and vomiting
    o   Hypersensitivity reaction possible, but rare
    o   Initially, aprepitant is typically dosed one hour before chemotherapy
- Monitoring: No routine lab work is necessary
- Drug and Diet Considerations:
    o   Grapefruit juice may increase drug concentrations
    o   May be administered with or without food

Arformoterol (Brovana)
- Class: Long acting beta-agonist
- Mechanism of Action: Stimulates beta-2 receptors leading to relaxation of smooth muscle and opening of airways
- Common Uses: Prevents bronchoconstriction in COPD
- Memorable Side Effects: tachycardia, tremor, anxiousness, hypokalemia (rare), hyperglycemia (rare)
- Clinical Pearls:
    o   Increased risk of asthma death in patients who take long acting beta agonists as monotherapy (given with corticosteroids)

- o Nebulized medication
- Monitoring: Frequency of use, FEV1, peak-flow, pulse, blood pressure, and potassium (usually only necessary in high dosages), glucose (rarely clinically significant)
- Drug and Diet Considerations:
  - o Assess potassium intake and blood levels of potassium if the patient is using a beta agonist frequently or has a history of hypokalemia
  - o Be aware of caffeine intake in combination with a beta-agonist as it can have an additive effect on blood pressure and heart rate
  - o Monitor diabetes patients for elevations in blood sugar
  - o Administration is unaffected by dietary intake

Aripiprazole (Abilify)
- Class: Antipsychotic (2nd generation)
- Mechanism of Action: Blocks dopamine receptors
- Common Uses: Treatment of mental/mood disorders such as schizophrenia, bipolar disorder, depression, dementia related behaviors like aggression, hallucinations and delusions (off-label)
- Memorable Side Effects: Sedation, fall risk, orthostatic BP changes, EPS and metabolic syndrome
- Clinical Pearls:
  - o May worsen Parkinson's disease symptoms
  - o NMS (neuroleptic malignant syndrome) is a very rare but very serious complication with antipsychotic medications; symptoms include fever, hyperreflexia, confusion, delirium and tremor
  - o May contribute to QTc prolongation
- Monitoring: Weight, lipids, HbA1c, blood sugars
- Drug and Diet Considerations:
  - o Increased appetite and risk for metabolic syndrome; this can occur, but is less common with aripiprazole compared to other antipsychotics like olanzapine
  - o Increased blood sugars can result in our diabetes patients, monitor blood sugars closely at initiation of therapy and during treatment
  - o Some dosage forms may contain lactose
  - o High-fat meal can slow down absorption rate – this is typically not clinically significant
  - o Can be administered with or without meals

Asenapine (Saphris)
- Class: Antipsychotic
- Mechanism of Action: Blocks dopamine receptors
- Common Uses: Treatment of mental/mood disorders such as schizophrenia, bipolar disorder, dementia related behaviors like aggression, hallucinations and delusions (off-label)
- Memorable Side Effects: Sedation, fall risk, orthostatic BP changes, EPS, metabolic syndrome
- Clinical Pearls:
  - o May worsen Parkinson's disease symptoms
  - o NMS (neuroleptic malignant syndrome) is a very rare but very serious complication with antipsychotic medications; symptoms include fever, hyperreflexia, confusion, delirium and tremor
  - o May contribute to QTc prolongation

- Monitoring: Weight, lipids, HbA1c, blood sugars
- Drug and Diet Considerations:
  - Increased appetite and risk for metabolic syndrome
  - Increased blood sugars can result in our diabetes patients, monitor blood sugars closely at initiation of therapy and during treatment
  - Sublingual tablet – avoid eating and drinking around the time of administration (at least 10 minutes)
  - Alcohol may exacerbate CNS depressant effects

Aspirin (Ecotrin)
- Class: Antiplatelet, NSAID
- Mechanism of Action: Low dose aspirin inhibits thromboxane (an important factor that causes platelet aggregation); Inhibits Cyclooxygenase-1 and 2 (COX-1 and COX-2); results in a reduction in prostaglandins which promote pain, fever, and inflammation
- Common Uses: Cardiovascular prophylaxis and treatment of pain, fever, and inflammation
- Memorable Side Effects: GI ulcer, bleeding, worsening kidney function, edema, hypertension, tinnitus
- Clinical Pearls:
  - Available over-the-counter
  - Generally avoided in pediatric patients due to the risk of Reye's syndrome
  - Due to effects on platelets, it is typically held for a period of time before/after surgery to reduce the risk of bleeding
  - May exacerbate heart failure (higher, analgesic dosages)
- Monitoring: CBC, platelets, bleed risk
- Drug and Diet Considerations:
  - Take with food to help reduce the risk of GI upset; GI upset is dose dependent (higher dose, more likely to have GI complaints)
  - Full glass of water or milk may also help reduce GI upset
  - Certain supplements and food like raisins, paprika, licorice, and curry powder may increase salicylate activity leading to an increase risk of GI upset – monitor the patient for increased GI symptoms
  - Vitamin C may increase renal elimination and cause lower concentrations – usually not clinically significant but may want to monitor patient for reduced benefit of aspirin
  - Vitamin E, Omega-3 fatty acids, gingko, garlic, ginseng, turmeric, and fish oil supplements have been purported to have antiplatelet type activity which, in theory, could increase the risk of bleed – clinical significance is questionable; the most common resolution is to discontinue the supplements if they are not necessary
  - Alcohol may have an additive antiplatelet type effect and increase the risk of GI bleed

Aspirin and Extended-Release Dipyridamole (Aggrenox)
- Class: Antiplatelet
- Mechanism of Action: Low dose aspirin inhibits thromboxane (an important factor that causes platelet aggregation); dipyridamole blocks adenosine which is necessary for platelet aggregation
- Common Uses: Reduces the risk for certain types of ischemic strokes

- Memorable Side Effects: Headache, GI ulcer, bleeding
- Clinical Pearls:
  - Rare cases of elevated LFTs have been reported with dipyridamole
- Monitoring: CBC, platelets, bleed risk
- Drug and Diet Considerations:
  - May be given with or without food
  - May contain lactose/sucrose
  - Certain supplements and food like raisins, paprika, licorice, and curry powder may increase salicylate activity leading to an increase risk of GI upset – monitor the patient for increased GI symptoms
  - Vitamin E, Omega-3 fatty acids, gingko, garlic, ginseng, turmeric, and fish oil supplements have been purported to have antiplatelet type activity which, in theory, could increase the risk of bleed – clinical significance is questionable; the most common resolution is to discontinue the supplements if they are not necessary
  - Alcohol may have an additive antiplatelet type effect and increase the risk of GI bleed

Atenolol (Tenormin)
- Class: Beta-blocker, antihypertensive
- Mechanism of Action: Selectively blocks beta-1 receptors which reduces cardiac action and ultimately lowers pulse and blood pressure
- Common Uses: Treatment of atrial fibrillation and hypertension
- Memorable Side Effects: Low blood pressure, bradycardia, lethargy
- Clinical Pearls:
  - Trick to remembering beta receptors: You have 1 heart and 2 lungs (beta-1 is primarily on the heart and beta-2 is primarily on the lungs)
  - Potential to blunt the effects of respiratory medications such as albuterol (greater risk at higher dosages)
- Monitoring: Blood pressure, pulse, respiratory status (if the patient has a history of breathing difficulties),
- Drug and Diet Considerations:
  - Relatively low incidence of GI upset
  - Absorption may be reduced with food, but usually the dose can be adjusted accordingly as long as it is taken in a consistent manner
  - May mask symptoms of hypoglycemia (except sweating) in diabetes patients

Atomoxetine (Strattera)
- Class: Norepinephrine reuptake inhibitor
- Mechanism of Action: Inhibits reuptake of norepinephrine
- Common Uses: Management of ADHD
- Memorable Side Effects: Sweating, dry mouth, GI upset, elevated BP, weight loss
- Clinical Pearls:
  - Non-controlled substance used for ADHD; many other agents for ADHD such as methylphenidate and amphetamine salts are controlled substances
  - Special warning regarding increased risk of suicidal thoughts and behaviors

42

- Monitoring: EKG evaluation for at risk patients, height, weight, appetite, sleep, blood pressure, pulse
- Drug and Diet Considerations:
    - Risk of weight loss is a concern in pediatrics, atomoxetine generally causes less weight loss than traditional stimulants like methylphenidate and amphetamines
    - If encountered, adverse effects of nausea, dry mouth, reduced appetite, and vomiting can impact nutrition
    - No specific concerns with absorption and food intake, administer with or without food

Atorvastatin (Lipitor)
- Class: Statin, antilipemic
- Mechanism of Action: HMG Co-A reductase inhibitor (causes a decrease in LDL)
- Common Uses: Reduction of cholesterol (particularly LDL)
- Memorable Side Effects: muscle aches, rhabdomyolysis (rare but serious)
- Clinical Pearls:
    - Statins like atorvastatin are one of the mainstays of therapy to reduce cholesterol, and more particularly LDL (bad cholesterol)
    - Usually muscle aches are all over which can help you differentiate from other pain conditions or pain/soreness from an injury or overuse
    - Contraindicated in pregnancy
- Monitoring: Lipids, LFTs, CPK if experiencing muscle pain (myopathy)
- Drug and Diet Considerations:
    - Liver toxicity risk from chronic alcohol use may be increased if used in combination with statins
    - Low risk of elevating blood sugars in patients with diabetes (often not clinically significant)
    - Grapefruit juice can significantly increase the concentrations of atorvastatin – generally avoid using grapefruit juice
    - Can be taken with or without food
    - Encourage a lipid lowering diet for any patient taking a cholesterol medication

Atovaquone (Mepron)
- Class: Antiprotozoal
- Mechanism of Action: Blocks electron transport in the organism's mitochondria which stops important metabolic enzymes
- Common Uses: Treatment and prevention of Pneumocystis jiroveci pneumonia
- Memorable Side Effects: GI side effects, rash, insomnia, headache, respiratory changes such as cough and rhinitis
- Clinical Pearls:
    - Rare risk for hypersensitivity reactions
- Monitoring: LFTs
- Drug and Diet Considerations:
    - Administer with food
    - Certain dosages may contain benzyl alcohol
    - Significant GI adverse effects may cause dehydration and reduced dietary intake

Atropine
- Class: Anticholinergic
- Mechanism of Action: Blocks acetylcholine in the parasympathetic system which decreases secretions and increases cardiac output
- Common Uses: Reduction of salivary secretions in pre-op and end of life situations; management of emergency bradycardia
- Memorable Side Effects: Constipation, urinary retention, dry eyes, dry mouth, tachycardia
- Clinical Pearls:
  - Oral drops used frequently in hospice to decrease excessive salivation
  - Psychotic type symptoms are possible with high enough doses ("mad as a hatter")
  - Monitoring: Pulse, blood pressure, EKG monitoring is critical if using for bradycardia
- Drug and Diet Considerations
  - Consider increasing fiber and fluid intake for patients at risk for constipation (chronic use)
  - Dry mouth could impact dietary intake, thirst, and appetite
  - Note that these issues may not be a top priority in a hospice patient when dietary intake is understandably low

Azathioprine (Imuran)
- Class: Immunosuppressive agent
- Mechanism of Action: Blocks purine metabolism which impacts production of DNA, RNA, and protein; ultimately causes immune system suppression
- Common Uses: Prevention of organ rejection after a transplant and treatment of inflammatory bowel diseases, refractory rheumatoid arthritis and psoriasis
- Memorable Side Effects: GI upset, immunosuppression, infection risk, thrombocytopenia, increased LFTs
- Clinical Pearls:
  - Boxed warning for an increased risk of malignancy
  - TPMT or NUDT15 genetic variations could lead to an increased risk for toxicity
  - Dosage adjustments recommended in patients with poor renal function
  - Really important interaction with allopurinol (increases myelosuppressive effects)
- Monitoring: CBC, LFTs, renal function
- Drug and Diet Considerations:
  - May be given with food to reduce the risk for GI upset

Azithromycin (Zithromax, Z-Pak)
- Class: Antibiotic, macrolide
- Mechanism of Action: Inhibits protein synthesis in bacteria by binding to the 50s subunit of ribosomes
- Common Uses: Treatment of bacterial upper respiratory infections (i.e. ear infection, pneumonia, bronchitis, sinusitis), MAC, chlamydia, and gonorrhea
- Memorable Side Effects: GI upset; QTc prolongation possible (very rare)
- Clinical Pearls:

- o Common alternative to penicillin antibiotics (i.e. history of penicillin allergy)
- o Use cautiously in patients who may be at risk for QTc prolongation
- o Much less likely to cause drug interactions compared to other macrolides like erythromycin and clarithromycin
- o Keep oral suspension (liquid formulation) at room temp; this is unique from many other liquid antibiotics which are normally refrigerated
- Monitoring: LFTs and CBC if using long term or if signs of complications
- Drug and Diet Considerations
  - o Immediate release tablets and suspension can be taken with or without food
  - o Absorption of suspension may be increased if administered with food (ideal but not required)
  - o Extended release (rarely used) should be taken 1 hour before or 2 hours after eating
  - o GI upset and diarrhea can happen, but generally less frequent than a drug like amoxicillin
  - o Bland foods that reduce GI upset and diarrhea can be helpful
  - o If diarrhea is problematic, maintain adequate hydration to avoid dehydration

Aztreonam (Azactam)

- Class: Antibiotic, monobactam
- Mechanism of Action: Works by binding penicillin-binding-proteins and inhibits bacterial cell wall synthesis (structurally different from penicillin antibiotics)
- Common Uses: Treatment of pneumonia, meningitis, and other susceptible infections
- Memorable Side Effects: Neutropenia, elevated LFTs
- Clinical Pearls:
  - o Injectable agent only
- Monitoring: LFTs and renal function
- Drug and Diet Considerations
  - o No major dietary concerns

Baclofen (Lioresal)

- Class: Muscle relaxant
- Mechanism of Action: Not well understood, but thought to cause hyperpolarization and block reflexes in the spinal cord which produces muscle relaxation
- Common Uses: Treatment of muscle spasms
- Memorable Side Effects: Dry mouth, constipation, GI upset, sedation, fall risk, confusion
- Clinical Pearls:
  - o May be used for spasms associated with multiple sclerosis
  - o Anticholinergic side effects can be problematic, especially in the elderly
  - o Can be given intrathecally via implantable pump
- Monitoring: No routine lab work
- Drug and Diet Considerations

- GI adverse effects such as nausea, vomiting, constipation and dry mouth are possible, occurring in less than 10% of patients, and may impact dietary intake,
- Additive central nervous system depression can occur when combined with alcohol (monitor for excessive sedation, confusion, and fall risk, especially in elderly)
- May be given with or without food

Baloxavir (Xofluza)
- Class: Anti-influenza agent; endonuclease inhibitor
- Mechanism of Action: Inhibits endonuclease which is necessary for influenza replication
- Common Uses: Treatment of influenza
- Memorable Side Effects: GI upset, skin and anaphylaxis reactions (rare)
- Clinical Pearls:
    - Activity against influenza type A and type B
- Monitoring: One time dose, lab monitoring is typically not necessary
- Drug and Diet Considerations:
    - Supplements like calcium carbonate, magnesium, zinc, selenium, and iron can block the absorption of baloxavir; avoid coadministration
    - Avoid dairy products or food with large amounts of calcium, iron, or magnesium
    - May be given with or without food

Beclomethasone (Qvar)
- Class: Inhaled corticosteroid
- Mechanism of Action: Inhaled steroid that helps to reduce inflammation
- Common Uses: Prevent and control symptoms in asthma and COPD
- Memorable Side Effects: Thrush, cough, rhinitis. Systemic corticosteroid effects are possible but not very likely as absorption is low (see prednisone for adverse effects of systemic corticosteroids)
- Clinical Pearls:
    - Educate patients that beclomethasone does not provide emergency relief of respiratory symptoms
    - Rinse mouth after administration to reduce the risk for thrush
- Monitoring: FEV1, peak-flow, growth in pediatric patients
- Drug and Diet Considerations:
    - As the dose of inhaled corticosteroid increases, there is a low possibility for systemic effects (see prednisone)
    - Administer without regard to food

Benazepril (Lotensin)
- Class: Antihypertensive, ACE inhibitor
- Mechanism of Action: Benazepril inhibits the angiotensin converting enzyme which reduces angiotensin 2 production; less angiotensin 2 equates to less vasoconstriction and lower blood pressure
- Common Uses: Treatment of hypertension, prevention of MI, management of heart failure and reduction of proteinuria
- Common Side Effects: Cough, kidney impairment, low blood pressure, angioedema, and hyperkalemia

46

- Clinical Pearls:
  - Angiotensin Receptor Blockers (ARBs) are the cousins to the ACE inhibitors, and are the first line substitute to a patient who has had a cough with an ACE inhibitor
  - ACE inhibitors are a classic cause of elevated potassium levels; if your patient has hyperkalemia, you must make sure the ACE inhibitor has been addressed
  - In some cases, patients of African descent may not respond to ACE inhibitors as well as other ethnicities
  - Contraindicated in pregnancy
  - ACE inhibitors are frequently used in patients with hypertension and a history of diabetes, stroke, CAD, CKD, or CHF
- Monitoring: Renal function, potassium, blood pressure
- Drug and Diet Considerations
  - Be cautious and monitor potassium closely in patients with high dietary intake of potassium as this could contribute to hyperkalemia in combination with this medication
  - Using an ACE inhibitor in a dehydrated patient may increase the risk for acute renal failure – ensure adequate hydration
  - May be given with or without food

Benzonatate (Tessalon)
- Class: Antitussive
- Mechanism of Action: Anesthetic effects on respiratory tract resulting in cough suppression
- Common Uses: Relief of cough
- Memorable Side Effects: Usually pretty well tolerated, GI upset, CNS effects (rare)
- Clinical Pearls:
  - It is very important to identify why patient is coughing (i.e. COPD, medication, GERD, infectious disease, etc.)
  - Be sure to reassess patient if cough has been chronic
  - ACE Inhibitors are classic cause of drug induced cough
- Monitoring: No lab work necessary
- Drug and Diet Considerations
  - Capsule should not be chewed
  - If chewed, it may cause numbness of the oral cavity and increase the risk of choking if food is ingested

Benztropine (Cogentin)
- Class: Anticholinergic, anti-Parkinson's agent
- Mechanism of Action: Blocks muscarinic (anticholinergic) receptors and also has antihistamine effects
- Common Uses: Treatment of EPS associated with antipsychotic medications and Parkinsonism
- Memorable Side Effects: Dry eyes, dry mouth, exacerbation of urinary retention (i.e. BPH), constipation, sedation, fall risk in the elderly, confusion
- Clinical Pearls:
  - Highly anticholinergic (can't spit, see, pee, or sh*t and increases confusion/fall risk) which can be especially problematic in geriatric patients – avoid if possible

- o Rarely used for Parkinson's because of the anticholinergic impacts in the elderly
- o Most common clinical use is for extrapyramidal disorders (movement side effects associated with antipsychotics)
- Monitoring: Pulse (rare risk for tachycardia at higher dosages)
- Drug and Diet Considerations:
  - o Slows the motility of the GI tract which could increase the risk for constipation – minimize problems by maintaining adequate fluids and non-constipating diet
  - o If GI upset occurs, may give with food
  - o Dry mouth may increase thirst and alter taste/pleasure of food
  - o Alcohol may exacerbate CNS depressant effects

Bethanechol (Urecholine)
- Class: Cholinergic agonist
- Mechanism of Action: Agonist activity at cholinergic receptors which improves urinary outflow
- Common Uses: Relief of urinary retention
- Memorable Side Effects: Nausea, diarrhea, sweating, flushing, dizziness, weakness, urinary frequency
- Clinical Pearls:
  - o May exacerbate breathing issues (opposes anticholinergic effects)
- Monitoring: Weight (if patient experiences nausea/vomiting)
- Drug and Diet Considerations:
  - o If sweating occurs, it may exacerbate the risk for dehydration – assess fluid status
  - o Assess for alteration in dietary intake if the patient experiences nausea/vomiting
  - o Give 1 hour before or 2 hours after meals

Bictegravir (Biktarvy – multiple drug combination)
- Class: Integrase inhibitor, antiretroviral
- Mechanism of Action: Inhibits the viral enzyme integrase by binding enzyme cations and preventing viral DNA integration into the host genome
- Common Uses: Treatment of HIV
- Memorable Side Effects: Usually pretty well tolerated, elevated LFTs, skin reaction risk/SJS (rare, but possible), CNS changes, GI adverse effects, CPK increase/myopathy
- Clinical Pearls:
  - o Integrase inhibitors are generally preferred now in place of protease inhibitors as they have less drug interactions and seem to be better tolerated
  - o Combined with emtricitabine and tenofovir alafenamide (Biktarvy)
- Monitoring: LFTs, HIV levels, CD4 count, Hepatitis B testing prior to initiation, CPK as clinically indicated, lipids as clinically indicated (must remember to monitor for all the medications in this combination)
- Drug and Diet Considerations:
  - o May be given without regard to food
  - o Monitor blood glucose in patients with diabetes and adjust diet accordingly (usually only a modest increase if there is one)

- o Supplements that are metal cations like magnesium, calcium, and iron may reduce absorption, give Biktarvy at least 2 hours before or 6 hours after these supplements

Bisacodyl (Dulcolax)
- Class: Stimulant laxative
- Mechanism of Action: Stimulates GI movement by irritating smooth muscle
- Common Uses: Constipation treatment
- Memorable Side Effects: Abdominal pain
- Clinical Pearls:
  - o Used to promote bowel movement
  - o Similar medication class as Sennosides
  - o Suppository formulation is an option for patients who may have difficulty swallowing/can't take oral tablets
  - o Can be used as needed
  - o May be used in the treatment/prevention of opioid induced constipation
- Monitoring: Bowel movements
- Drug and Diet Considerations:
  - o Review and assess diet contributing to constipation issues if this medication is necessary on a regular basis
  - o Ensure adequate fluid and fiber intake
  - o Avoid oral administration within an hour of milk, dairy, or antacids

Bismuth subsalicylate (Pepto-Bismol)
- Class: Dyspepsia agent, antidiarrheal agent
- Mechanism of Action: Possible antibacterial and antiviral activity may help with infectious diarrhea and stomach upset
- Common Uses: Treatment of diarrhea, dyspepsia and Helicobacter pylori
- Memorable Side Effects: Neurotoxicity and tinnitus at high dosages, increase in bleed risk, change in stool color, tongue discoloration
- Clinical Pearls:
  - o Neurotoxicity is rare, but possible with unsupervised, high doses
  - o Salicylate component can theoretically increase bleeding risk
- Monitoring: Bleeding risk, CBC with chronic use
- Drug and Diet Considerations:
  - o Monitor fluid and electrolyte status in a patient who may be experiencing diarrhea from an acute infection
  - o May be given with or without food

Bisoprolol (Zebeta)
- Class: Antihypertensive, beta-blocker
- Mechanism of Action: Blocks beta receptors leading to lower pulse/BP
- Common Uses: Treatment of hypertension and atrial fibrillation
- Memorable Side Effects: Low pulse, low BP, fatigue
- Clinical Pearls:
  - o Bisoprolol is relatively selective for beta-1 only
  - o Trick to remembering beta receptors: You have 1 heart and 2 lungs (beta-1 is primarily on the heart and beta-2 is primarily in the lungs)

- o Potential to blunt the effects of respiratory medications such as albuterol (greater risk at higher dosages)
- Monitoring: Blood pressure, pulse, respiratory status (if they have a history of breathing difficulties),
- Drug and Diet Considerations:
  - o Relatively low incidence of GI upset
  - o May mask symptoms of hypoglycemia in patients with diabetes (except sweating)
  - o May be taken with or without food

Bleomycin (Blenoxane)

- Class: Oncology agent, antibiotic
- Mechanism of Action: Binds to DNA which causes rupture of DNA and ultimately inhibits protein synthesis necessary for cell growth and replication
- Common Uses: Treatment of various types of cancers
- Memorable Side Effects: Hair loss, skin hyperpigmentation, hand-foot syndrome, anorexia, stomatitis, pain, lung toxicity, anaphylaxis, renal toxicity
- Clinical Pearls:
  - o Boxed warning for pulmonary toxicity and severe drug reaction of hypotension, CNS alterations, flu-like symptoms, and difficulty breathing
  - o Pulmonary toxicity risk increases with age and higher lifetime dosages
- Monitoring: Lung function (FEV1, FVC), renal function
- Drug and Diet Considerations:
  - o Monitor dietary intake as anorexia and weight loss are potential complications

Bosentan (Tracleer)

- Class: Endothelin receptor antagonists:
- Mechanism of Action: Blocks endothelin receptors which helps relax the pulmonary blood vessels, ultimately lowering blood pressure
- Common Uses: Treatment of pulmonary arterial hypertension
- Memorable Side Effects: Headache, edema, flushing, increased bleeding risk, elevation in LFTs
- Clinical Pearls:
  - o REMS program due to fetal risks if females become pregnant
  - o Boxed warning for hepatotoxicity
  - o Can increase risk of bleed especially in those on antiplatelet medications or anticoagulants
- Monitoring: Hemoglobin, LFTs, pregnancy testing
- Drug and Diet Considerations:
  - o Administer with or without food
  - o Vitamin E, Omega-3 fatty acids, gingko, garlic, ginseng, turmeric, and fish oil supplements have been purported to have antiplatelet type activity which, in theory, could increase the risk of bleed – clinical significance is questionable; the most common resolution is to discontinue the supplements if they are not necessary
  - o Possible increase in concentrations from the use of grapefruit juice

Brexpiprazole (Rexulti)

- Class: Antipsychotic (2nd generation)
- Mechanism of Action: Blocks dopamine receptors
- Common Uses: Adjunctive therapy for treatment of schizophrenia, bipolar disorder and depression. Off label use for dementia related behaviors like aggression, hallucinations and delusions
- Memorable Side Effects: Sedation, fall risk, orthostatic BP changes, EPS, metabolic syndrome
- Clinical Pearls:
  - May worsen Parkinson's disease symptoms
  - NMS (neuroleptic malignant syndrome) is a very rare but very serious complication with antipsychotic medications; symptoms include fever, hyperreflexia, confusion, delirium, tremor
  - May contribute to QTc prolongation
- Monitoring: Weight, lipids, HbA1c, blood sugars, blood pressure
- Drug and Diet Considerations:
  - Increased appetite and risk for metabolic syndrome; this can occur, but is less common with brexpiprazole compared to other antipsychotics like olanzapine
  - May exacerbate hyperglycemia in diabetes patients, monitor blood sugars closely with acute changes in the drug
  - Some dosage forms may contain lactose
  - High-fat meal can slow down absorption rate – this is typically not clinically significant
  - Can be administered with or without meals

Bromocriptine (Parlodel)

- Class: Dopamine agonist
- Mechanism of Action: Simulates dopamine-2 receptors which can help manage movement disorders and reduce prolactin production
- Common Uses: Treats elevated prolactin levels and symptoms of Parkinson's disease
- Memorable Side Effects: GI side effects (nausea/vomiting), hallucinations, psychiatric changes, dizziness, drop in blood pressure, can inhibit lactation (intentional or unintentional)
- Clinical Pearls:
  - Rare risk for fibrosis of cardiac valves
  - Syncope, drop in blood pressure may be exacerbated in the elderly
  - Worsening of or new onset impulse disorders such as gambling, eating, or sexual behaviors may occur
- Monitoring: Blood pressure, pulse, prolactin levels (as clinically indicated), renal and hepatic function
- Drug and Diet Considerations:
  - CNS depressant activity may be exacerbated by alcohol
  - To reduce GI adverse effects, give with food
  - Be aware of any excessive eating impulses as dopamine agonists can contribute to this concern

Brompheniramine (Respa-BR)

- Class: Antihistamine, anticholinergic

- Mechanism of Action: Blocks muscarinic (anticholinergic) receptors and also has antihistamine effects
- Common Uses: Treatment of insomnia, allergies, allergic reaction, itching and motion sickness
- Memorable Side Effects: Anticholinergic effects such as dry mouth, dry eyes, urinary retention, constipation, sedation, confusion
- Clinical Pearls:
  - Highly anticholinergic which can be very problematic in geriatric patients – avoid if possible
  - May have paradoxical insomnia reaction in pediatrics
- Monitoring: No routine lab work is typically necessary
- Drug and Diet Considerations
  - Slows the motility of the GI tract which could increase the risk for constipation – adequate fluids and non-constipating diet may be helpful
  - Alcohol may exacerbate CNS depressant effects
  - Dry mouth may increase thirst and alter taste/pleasure of food
  - May be given with or without food

Budesonide – oral (Entocort)

- Class: Corticosteroid
- Mechanism of Action: Suppresses leukocytes and ultimately reduces inflammation, suppresses adrenal function and the immune system
- Common Uses: Decrease the symptoms of dermatitis, arthritis flare, Crohn's disease, pneumonia, asthma exacerbation, etc. that stem from an acute inflammatory state
- Memorable Side Effects: GI side effects, insomnia and hyperglycemia; long term use may suppress the immune system, increase osteoporosis risk as well as cause adrenal insufficiency
- Clinical Pearls:
  - Oral budesonide is usually specifically reserved for ulcerative colitis or Crohn's disease because it has a high first pass effect and lower systemic absorption than other oral corticosteroids
  - Long term corticosteroid use can lead to increased risk of Cushing's syndrome (moon face), diabetes, and osteoporosis; make sure long term use is assessed frequently to minimize length and dose of steroids
  - Over time, the patient may develop tolerance to the insomnia adverse effect
  - Budesonide is also available as a nebulized inhaled corticosteroid (brand name – Pulmicort) for asthma/COPD/respiratory issues
- Monitoring: Blood sugar, bone mineral density, blood pressure, weight, risk for glaucoma, HPA suppression (usually only done with longer term use)
- Drug and Diet Considerations:
  - Grapefruit juice can increase the concentrations of budesonide
  - In patients on long term use, assess if vitamin D, calcium and bisphosphonates should be added to reduce osteoporosis risk
  - May cause an increase in blood sugars
  - Take with food to reduce GI upset
  - Capsule may be opened and sprinkled in 1 TBSP of applesauce (otherwise do not crush or chew)
  - May increase appetite and cause weight gain
  - Do not break or crush extended release tablet

Budesonide and Formoterol (Symbicort)

- Class: Inhaled corticosteroid and long acting beta-agonist
- Mechanism of Action: Provides anti-inflammatory effects through fluticasone and stimulates beta-2 receptors leading to relaxation of smooth muscle and opening of airways
- Common Uses: Prevention of bronchospasm associated with asthma or COPD
- Memorable Side Effects: Thrush, reduced bone mineral density (rare), HPS suppression (rare), tachycardia, tremor, anxiousness, hypokalemia (rare), hyperglycemia (rare)
- Clinical Pearls:
  - Inhaled corticosteroids have a very low rate of systemic absorption, so issues such as reduced bone mineral density, hyperglycemia, and HPA suppression are unlikely to be clinically significant
  - GINA guidelines indicate that this may be one of the only long acting agents used as needed for acute exacerbations of asthma
- Monitoring: Frequency of use, FEV1, peak-flow, pulse, blood pressure, and potassium (usually only necessary in high dosages), glucose (rarely clinically significant
- Drug and Diet Considerations:
  - Assess potassium intake and blood levels of potassium if the patient is using a beta agonist frequently or has a history of hypokalemia (rarely clinically significant)
  - Be aware of caffeine intake in combination with a beta-agonist, it can have an additive effect on blood pressure and heart rate
  - Monitor diabetes patients for elevations in blood sugar
  - As the dose of inhaled corticosteroid increases, there is a low potential for systemic effects (see prednisone)

Budesonide Oral Inhalation (Pulmicort, Pulmicort Flexhaler)

- Class: Inhaled corticosteroid
- Mechanism of Action: Inhaled steroid that helps to reduce inflammation
- Common Uses: Prevention of symptoms caused by asthma and COPD
- Memorable Side Effects: Thrush, cough and rhinitis; systemic corticosteroid effects are possible, but not likely, as absorption is low (see prednisone for adverse effects)
- Clinical Pearls:
  - Well tolerated
  - Educate patients that it is not meant to provide emergency relief of symptoms
  - Rinse mouth after administration
  - Comes with an option for a nebulized formulation
- Monitoring: FEV1, peak-flow, growth in pediatric patients
- Drug and Diet Considerations:
  - Monitor diabetes patients for elevations in blood sugar
  - As the dose of inhaled corticosteroid increases, there is a low potential for systemic effects (see prednisone)

Bumetanide (Bumex)

- Class: Loop diuretic

- Mechanism of Action: Inhibits sodium and chloride reabsorption in the ascending "Loop" of Henle in the kidney which results in an increase of fluid loss
- Common Use: Treatment of edema, hypertension, and heart failure
- Memorable Side Effects: Frequent urination, electrolyte depletion, low blood pressure, dehydration and renal impairment, tinnitus (rare, high dosages)
- Clinical Pearls:
  - Frequent urination can be significantly upsetting to patients and can greatly impact their wellbeing, including sleep interruptions; if possible, make sure loop diuretics are not given close to bedtime
  - Classic medication causes of edema include calcium channel blockers, pioglitazone, pregabalin, and NSAIDs
  - Loop diuretics deplete volume in the body, so patients run the risk of not having adequate perfusion through the kidney; assessing for elevations in creatinine from baseline can help us monitor for this risk
  - Urinary output and monitoring of weights can be very important patient factors to monitor and help assess the efficacy of how well the loop diuretic is working
- Monitoring: Renal function and electrolytes (all electrolytes may be depleted), weights, blood pressure, hearing (when used at high doses)
- Drug and Diet Considerations:
  - Potassium supplementation is usually required as bumetanide can cause significant hypokalemia, reinforce dietary potassium intake for those with a history of hypokalemia
  - Monitor for dehydration warning signs
  - Administration with or without food is acceptable

Buprenorphine/Naloxone (Suboxone)
- Class: Opioid use disorder agent, partial opioid agonist, opioid antagonist
- Mechanism of Action: Naloxone blocks full agonist opioids from providing euphoria and reduces the risk of overdose while buprenorphine partially binds opioid receptors and helps reduce withdrawal symptoms
- Common Uses: Management of opioid use disorder
- Memorable Side Effects: Opioid withdrawal symptoms when first initiated are possible (i.e. sweating, anxiety, GI upset, insomnia), liver function abnormalities (rare)
- Clinical Pearls:
  - Prevents euphoria from opioid agonists
  - Will precipitate opioid withdrawal, but partial opioid agonist of buprenorphine may help blunt the severity of withdrawal symptoms
- Monitoring: Liver function, blood pressure, withdrawal symptoms, pregnancy and HIV testing
- Drug and Diet Considerations:
  - Alcohol may exacerbate CNS depressant risks
  - Sublingual and buccal administration, avoid eating food and drinking fluid with this agent so it isn't inadvertently swallowed prior to oral absorption in the mouth

Bupropion (Wellbutrin, Zyban)
- Class: Antidepressant (non-SSRI)

- Mechanism of Action: Not well understood, thought to increase dopamine/norepinephrine (NOT serotonin)
- Common Uses: Treatment of depression, smoking cessation aid, and approved off-label for management of ADHD symptoms
- Memorable Side Effects: Insomnia, increases seizure risk, GI side effects
- Clinical Pearls:
  - Generally not used first line for depression unless a patient is also looking to stop smoking
  - Tends to be more activating versus sedating, which may lead to insomnia
  - Less risk of reduced libido compared to SSRIs
  - Avoid if the patient has a history of seizures
- Monitoring: Weight
- Drug and Diet Considerations:
  - One of the few antidepressants that is more likely to cause weight loss than weight gain which can benefit overweight patients (bupropion is a component of the weight loss drug, Contrave)
  - Take without regards to meals
  - Recommended to avoid cutting, chewing, or splitting of extended release tablets
  - Be aware of alcoholic patients who may be abruptly stopping alcohol use – they may be at increased risk for seizures if taking bupropion

Buspirone (Buspar)
- Class: Anti-anxiety
- Mechanism of Action: Not well known, possible effects on serotonin, dopamine
- Common Uses: Treatment of anxiety
- Memorable Side Effects: Sedation
- Clinical Pearls:
  - Usually a much safer choice, especially in the elderly, for treatment of anxiety versus benzodiazepines
  - Big disadvantage is the drug takes weeks to months to show an improvement of anxiety symptoms
  - Buspirone doesn't work on an as needed basis
  - Not a controlled substance in the U.S. (benzodiazepines are)
  - Usually dosed multiple times per day
- Monitoring: No routine lab work is necessary
- Drug and Diet Considerations:
  - Grapefruit juice can increase drug concentrations
  - Consistent administration with or without food is recommended as food can cause absorption to vary

Busulfan (Busulfex, Myleran)
- Class: Oncology agent, alkylating agent
- Mechanism of Action: Prevents DNA cross-linking which ultimately blocks proliferation and growth of cells
- Common Uses: Treatment of numerous types of cancers

- Memorable Side Effects: Nausea, vomiting, diarrhea, CNS effects such as insomnia and anxiety, edema, hypertension, skin reactions, low magnesium, potassium, calcium, hyperglycemia, myelosuppression, pulmonary toxicity, increased LFTs
- Clinical Pearls:
    o Boxed warning - risk of myelosuppression
    o Tablet and IV formulation; adverse effect profile and frequency may vary dependent upon the dosage form
- Monitoring: CBC, renal function, electrolytes, LFTs, lung function, blood pressure, pulse
- Drug and Diet Considerations:
    o Weight loss and poor nutrition may result on account of nausea and vomiting adverse effects
    o Assess the risk for electrolyte abnormalities and replace as appropriate
    o Weight gain may be indicative of edema adverse effect

Butalbital, Acetaminophen or Aspirin, Caffeine (Fioricet, Fiorinal)
- Class: Combination analgesic, barbiturate
- Mechanism of Action: Butalbital reduces motor activity and causes CNS depression; See other agents individually
- Common Uses: Management of headaches
- Memorable Side Effects: Sedation, dizziness, confusion, respiratory depression (butalbital)
- Clinical Pearls:
    o Controlled substance which carries a risk for dependence and addiction
    o Avoid use in geriatric patients
    o Fioricet contains acetaminophen and caffeine
    o Fiorinal contains aspirin and caffeine
- Monitoring: CBC, LFTs, renal function
- Drug and Diet Considerations:
    o Alcohol will exacerbate CNS depression risk
    o May be taken with or without food

Cabergoline (Dostinex)
- Class: Dopamine agonist, ergot derivative
- Mechanism of Action: Stimulates dopamine-2 receptors which can help manage movement disorders and reduce prolactin production
- Common Uses: Treatment of hyperprolactinemia, improvement of RLS symptoms and, inhibition of unwanted lactation
- Memorable Side Effects: GI side effects (nausea/vomiting), hallucinations/psychiatric changes, dizziness, drop in blood pressure, can inhibit lactation (intentional or unintentional)
- Clinical Pearls:
    o Rare risk for fibrosis of cardiac valves
    o Syncope, drop in blood pressure may be exacerbated in the elderly
    o Worsening or new onset of impulse disorders such as gambling, sexual behaviors, etc. may occur
- Monitoring: Blood pressure, pulse, prolactin levels (as clinically indicated)
- Drug and Diet Considerations:
    o CNS depressant activity may be exacerbated by alcohol

- o To reduce GI adverse effects, give with food
- o Be aware of any excessive eating impulses as dopamine agonists can contribute to this concern

Caffeine (No Doz, Stay Awake, Keep Alert)

- Class: PDE inhibitor, stimulant
- Mechanism of Action: Inhibits phosphodiesterase which increases cyclic AMP leading to CNS stimulation
- Common Uses: Improvement of mental alertness when fatigued
- Memorable Side Effects: GI upset, tachycardia, insomnia, anorexia, tremor/jitters, hypertension
- Clinical Pearls:
    - o Use cautiously in patients with a history of cardiovascular disease, seizures, insomnia, and anxiety
    - o May exacerbate GERD/GI bleed risk
- Monitoring: Heart rate, BP; may have effects on blood sugar in diabetes patients (especially at higher doses)
- Drug and Diet Considerations:
    - o May be given with or without food
    - o May exacerbate the effects of other stimulants (i.e. methylphenidate, amphetamine salts, modafinil, etc.)
    - o May increase concentrations of clozapine

Calcitonin (Miacalcin, Fortical)

- Class: Osteoporosis agent
- Mechanism of Action: Opposes the action of parathyroid hormone and inhibits the activity of osteoclasts which results in an increase in bone mineral density
- Common Uses: Treatment of osteoporosis
- Memorable Side Effects: Nasal irritation, rhinitis, flushing
- Clinical Pearls:
    - o Store upright and be sure it is primed before first use
    - o Refrigerate – 35 days max use once removed from fridge
    - o Can have benefit for compression fracture pain
- Monitoring: Bone mineral density, calcium, vitamin D levels
- Drug and Diet Considerations:
    - o Ensure the patient has adequate vitamin D and calcium intake – at least 1,200 mg per day of calcium and 1,000 units (25 mcg) of vitamin D in females with osteoporosis
    - o Give with or without food

Calcitriol (Rocaltrol)

- Class: Active vitamin D
- Mechanism of Action: Active vitamin D (1,25 hydroxyvitamin D3) binds vitamin D receptors which have numerous functions, some of which include lowering PTH, stimulating bone resorption of calcium and increasing calcium and phosphorus levels in the blood by stimulating gut absorption
- Common Uses: Prevention of hyperparathyroidism due to CKD and treatment of hypocalcemia
- Memorable Side Effects: Elevated calcium, otherwise pretty well tolerated
- Clinical Pearls:

57

- o Depending upon indication for calcitriol, calcium supplementation and levels should be assessed and evaluated with vitamin D
- Monitoring: Calcium, phosphate, PTH, renal function
- Drug and Diet Considerations:
  - o May take with or without food
  - o May need to adapt calcium and phosphorus intake depending upon levels and response to medication

Calcium acetate (PhosLo)

- Class: Phosphate binder
- Mechanism of Action: Binds with dietary phosphate in the gut and gets excreted in the feces
- Common Uses: Prevention of hyperphosphatemia associated with chronic kidney disease
- Memorable Side Effects: Hypercalcemia, GI (N/V/D)
- Clinical Pearls:
  - o Used as a phosphate binder usually in CKD as phosphate levels can build up in end stage renal disease
  - o Dosed with meals
  - o Need to monitor calcium as this medication can increase levels
- Monitoring: Phosphorus, calcium, parathyroid hormone (PTH)
- Drug and Diet Considerations:
  - o Be cautious of excessive calcium in the diet that could have additive effects to the drug
  - o Patients on this medication need to have adequate education about appropriate use and the need to lower their phosphorus levels
  - o Dietary maltitol (component of many "sugar-free" products) can increase the risk for diarrhea if the patient is taking the liquid formulation of calcium acetate
  - o The drug is ineffective if given without food

Calcium Carbonate (Os-Cal, Caltrate, Tums)

- Class: Supplement, antacid, phosphate binder
- Mechanism of Action: Neutralizes stomach acid leading to increased stomach pH; binds phosphorus in the gut to lower levels
- Common Uses: Calcium replacement for bone health, treatment for hyperphosphatemia and management of heartburn
- Memorable Side Effects: Hypercalcemia, constipation, hypophosphatemia
- Clinical Pearls:
  - o May cause rebound gastric acid secretion
  - o Vitamin D aids in calcium absorption
  - o RDA of calcium; 1,000 – 1,200 mg/day (upper end in elderly and patients at risk for osteoporosis)
  - o Give in divided doses; absorption is reduced as doses escalate above 600 mg
- Monitoring: Calcium, phosphorus, kidney function
- Drug and Diet Considerations:
  - o Giving with food helps aid absorption
  - o Common antibiotics such as quinolones, certain cephalosporins, and tetracycline derivatives may bind with calcium and reduce concentrations

- o Numerous other binding interactions such as bisphosphonates, baloxavir, and integrase inhibitors (HIV medications) may have concentrations reduced by calcium (not an all-inclusive list)

Canagliflozin (Invokana)
- Class: Anti-diabetes, SGLT-2 inhibitor
- Mechanism of Action: By inhibiting the Sodium–glucose co-transporter 2, this results in an increase in glucose excretion through the urine and lowering of blood sugar
- Common Uses: Control blood sugar in diabetes and adjunct therapy in heart failure
- Memorable Side Effects: Dehydration (high risk in patients taking diuretics or reduced fluid intake), increased risk for urinary tract infections and fungal infections like candidiasis, and potential drop in blood pressure
- Clinical Pearls:
  - o Caution in patients with a history of urinary tract infections; canagliflozin increases sugar in the urine which can act as a food source for organisms
  - o Monitor K+; hyperkalemia risk especially in patients on an ACE, ARB, potassium supplements, or those with a high potassium diet
  - o Rarely increases the risk for ketoacidosis
  - o Hypoglycemia risk is lower than with sulfonylureas
  - o Caution on an increased risk of bone fracture
  - o Volume depletion risk, leading to hypotension and dehydration
  - o Contraindicated in eGFR <30 (remember these drugs work in the kidney)
  - o Possible link to an increased risk for amputations
- Monitoring: Renal function, potassium, blood pressure, blood sugar, A1C
- Drug and Diet Considerations:
  - o Be cautious and monitor potassium closely in patients with high dietary intake of potassium; this could contribute to hyperkalemia in combination with this medication
  - o Monitor fluid intake as this medication can increase the risk for dehydration
  - o Patient should have an appropriate diabetes diet and education if taking this medication
  - o Administer with or without food

Candesartan (Atacand)
- Class: Antihypertensive, ARB
- Mechanism of Action: Blocks the angiotensin 2 (vasoconstrictor) receptor – ends up preventing vasoconstriction, aldosterone release, and lowers blood pressure
- Common Uses: Treatment of hypertension and heart failure
- Memorable Side Effects: Hyperkalemia, exacerbate/worsen kidney function, low blood pressure
- Clinical Pearls:
  - o When you think of ARBs and ACE inhibitors, you can lump the side effects together; overall, they are very similar

- One major exception to the above rule is the side effect of cough; patients who encounter this adverse effect from an ACE inhibitor may use an ARB as an alternative antihypertensive
- Kidney function changes and monitoring of potassium is critical when doses are changed or an ARB is initiated
- This worsening kidney function risk increases in patients who may be taking NSAIDs and/or diuretics
- As with any medication used to treat hypertension, we need to educate our patients to rise slowly when getting up to minimize the risk of orthostatic (postural) hypotension
- Monitoring: Renal function, potassium, blood pressure
- Drug and Diet Considerations
  - Be cautious and monitor potassium closely in patients with high dietary intake of potassium; this could contribute to hyperkalemia in combination with this medication
  - Administer with or without food

Captopril (Capoten)

- Class: Antihypertensive, ACE inhibitor
- Mechanism of Action: Inhibits angiotensin converting enzyme which prevents the production of angiotensin 2 and leads to lower BP; Angiotensin 2 is a potent vasoconstrictor
- Common Uses: Treatment of hypertension, heart failure and to improve survival after a heart attack
- Memorable Side Effects: Cough, kidney impairment, low blood pressure, hyperkalemia, angioedema, and agranulocytosis (specific to captopril, not necessarily all ACE inhibitors)
- Clinical Pearls:
  - ACE Inhibitors are notoriously known for causing a dry chronic cough
  - Angiotensin Receptor Blockers (ARBs) are the cousins to the ACE inhibitors and are the first line substitute to a patient who has had a cough with an ACE inhibitor
  - ACE inhibitors can exacerbate kidney impairment as well as contribute to acute renal failure especially in patients who are already on other potential renal toxic medications (i.e. diuretics, NSAIDs etc.) even though in conditions like heart failure, diuretics and ACE Inhibitors are often used together
  - ACE inhibitors can cause elevated potassium levels; if your patient has hyperkalemia, you must make sure the ACE inhibitor has been addressed
  - In some cases, patients of African descent may not respond to ACE inhibitors as well as other ethnicities
  - ACE inhibitors should not be used in combination with an ARB
  - ACE inhibitors (and ARBs) are frequently used in patients with hypertension and a history of diabetes, stroke, CAD, CKD, or CHF
  - Angioedema (swelling of the lips/airway) is classically caused by ACE inhibitors; it is an extremely rare, but very serious reaction requiring immediate discontinuation
- Monitoring: Renal function, potassium, blood pressure
- Drug and Diet Considerations:

- o Be cautious and monitor potassium closely in patients with high dietary intake of potassium as this could contribute to hyperkalemia in combination with this medication
- o Administer with or without food

Carbamazepine (Tegretol)
- Class: Antiepileptic
- Mechanism of Action: Multiple mechanisms, including altering sodium ion flow across cell membranes
- Common Uses: Prevention of seizures and pain relief associated with trigeminal neuralgia
- Memorable Side Effects: Sedation, dizziness, rash, hyponatremia (SIADH), N/V
- Clinical Pearls:
  - o Enzyme inducer that can cause numerous drug interactions; most often leads to a decrease in the concentration of other drugs
  - o Liver function, CBC, and sodium are important monitoring parameters
  - o Lots of wacky side effects such as rash, liver function, hyponatremia and CBC changes with this medication
  - o Levels likely not necessary for use in trigeminal neuralgia unless signs of toxicity
  - o Sedation, confusion, falls are possible with toxicity
  - o 4-12 mcg/mL is considered "normal" therapeutic concentration for seizures
- Monitoring: Sodium, renal function, CBC, LFTs, eye exams, carbamazepine level (depending upon clinical indication or signs of toxicity)
- Drug and Diet Considerations:
  - o Grapefruit juice can increase the concentration
  - o Carbamazepine can possibly contribute to folic acid, vitamin D, and various vitamin B deficiencies (cyanocobalamin, pyridoxine, riboflavin) – recommend supplementation especially if the patient is displaying any signs and symptoms of deficiency
  - o Most carbamazepine dosage forms should be given with food; nausea is a common adverse effect

Carbidopa/levodopa (Sinemet)
- Class: Anti-Parkinson's
- Mechanism of Action: Levodopa crosses the blood brain barrier and gets converted to dopamine; carbidopa prevents the peripheral breakdown of levodopa
- Common Uses: Treatment of Parkinson's disease symptoms and restless leg syndrome
- Memorable Side Effects: Nausea/vomiting, hallucinations, orthostasis
- Clinical Pearls:
  - o Levodopa replaces the body's dopamine supply (shortage of dopamine in Parkinson's)
  - o Can cause psychotic type symptoms (remember that antipsychotics block dopamine)
  - o GI upset/nausea is common

- o Frequent dosing (up to 6-8 times per day) may be necessary depending upon patient's symptoms
- o May see used at night for RLS
- Monitoring: LFTs, blood pressure, CBC, renal function, mental health (hallucinations), fluctuations in motor symptoms
- Drug and Diet Considerations:
  - o Significant protein intake could reduce the concentration of carbidopa/levodopa leading to an increase in Parkinson's symptoms (i.e. tremor, rigidity, postural changes)
  - o Large meals could delay absorption which could be problematic in patients who are very sensitive to changes in drug concentration
  - o May administer with food to reduce the risk of nausea and vomiting – consistency in the timing of administration is very important
  - o Iron supplements may decrease the absorption of carbidopa/levodopa – avoid administration within 2 hours of each other (if patients are stable and doing well with Parkinson's symptoms, it might make sense to not make adjustments if they are taking these together)

Carboplatin (Paraplatin)
- Class: Oncology agent, platinum compound
- Mechanism of Action: Blocks DNA synthesis and alters the natural double helix of DNA to inhibit cell growth
- Common Uses: Treatment of numerous types of cancer
- Memorable Side Effects: Deficiencies in calcium, magnesium, sodium, or potassium, neuropathy, vomiting, nausea, increased LFTs, myelosuppression, hair loss, renal toxicity, ototoxicity, hypersensitivity reactions
- Clinical Pearls:
  - o Boxed warnings for myelosuppression, nausea/vomiting, and anaphylaxis
- Monitoring: CBC, renal function, electrolytes, LFTs, hearing
- Drug and Diet Considerations:
  - o Weight loss and poor nutrition may result on account of nausea and vomiting adverse effects
  - o Assess for the need of fluid and electrolyte replacement in patients with vomiting

Cariprazine (Vraylar)
- Class: Antipsychotic
- Mechanism of Action: Blocks dopamine receptors
- Common Uses: Treatment of mental/mood disorders such as schizophrenia and bipolar disorder; off label for dementia-related behaviors like aggression, hallucinations, and delusions
- Memorable Side Effects: Sedation, fall risk, orthostatic BP changes, EPS, metabolic syndrome
- Clinical Pearls:
  - o Usually higher doses are required for younger patients with schizophrenia and/or bipolar disorder while lower doses can and should be used in the elderly
  - o Remember with antipsychotic medications that they block dopamine and can exacerbate conditions where there is a shortage of dopamine like Parkinson's disorder (remember that we use

dopamine to treat Parkinson's – i.e. carbidopa/levodopa or pramipexole)
- o Sedation, orthostatic hypotension, movement disorder side effects can all increase the risk of falls especially in our elderly patients
- o NMS (neuroleptic malignant syndrome) is a very rare but very serious complication with antipsychotic medications; a few symptoms of NMS include: fever, hyperreflexia, confusion, delirium and tremor
- o Antipsychotics increase risk of metabolic syndrome (diabetes, elevated lipids, weight gain, etc.) – it is important to periodically monitor for this, especially in younger patients with schizophrenia and/or bipolar who may be likely to require long term use of higher doses
- o Anticholinergic effects are possible as well with antipsychotics; dry eyes, dry mouth, exacerbation of urinary retention (i.e. BPH), constipation (SLUD – can't salivate, lacrimate, urinate or defecate)
- o Antipsychotics can contribute to QTC prolongation, which can be especially problematic in patients who are already at risk (i.e. on antiarrhythmic medications)
- Monitoring: Weight, lipids, HbA1c, blood sugars
- Drug and Diet Considerations:
  - o Increased appetite and risk for metabolic syndrome
  - o Increased blood sugars can happen in our diabetes patients, monitor blood sugars closely with acute changes in the drug
  - o May give with or without food
  - o Alcohol may exacerbate CNS depressant effect

Carisoprodol (Soma)
- Class: Skeletal muscle relaxant
- Mechanism of Action: Not well understood, acts in the CNS and produces muscle relaxation
- Common Uses: Musculoskeletal pain management
- Memorable Side Effects: Sedation, dizziness
- Clinical Pearls:
  - o Controlled substance, so there is a risk of it being habit forming
  - o Can cause cognitive changes like confusion and sedation especially in the elderly; caution patients about driving
  - o Limit to short term use if possible
  - o Rare, but possible increased risk of lowering seizure threshold in patients with seizure disorder
  - o Anticholinergic and sedative effects make skeletal muscle relaxants not well tolerated in the elderly
- Monitoring: Excessive sedation
- Drug and Diet Considerations:
  - o Given with or without food
  - o Be wary of alcohol use causing excessive sedation in combination with carisoprodol

Carmustine (BiCNU)
- Class: Oncology agent, alkylating agent

- Mechanism of Action: Prevents DNA cross-linking which ultimately prevents proliferation and growth of cells
- Common Uses: Treatment of numerous types of cancers
- Memorable Side Effects:
  - Implant formulation - Seizure risk, nausea, vomiting, constipation and fatigue
  - IV formulation – Renal failure, nausea, vomiting, diarrhea, rash, hair loss, gynecomastia, elevated LFTs, hypersensitivity reaction, pulmonary fibrosis, ophthalmic complications, seizure, and myelosuppression
- Clinical Pearls:
  - Boxed warnings for the risk of myelosuppression and lung toxicity
- Monitoring: CBC, renal function, electrolytes, LFTs, lung function, blood pressure and pulse during IV administration
- Drug and Diet Considerations:
  - Weight loss and poor nutrition may be a result of nausea and vomiting adverse effects

Carvedilol (Coreg)
- Class: Antihypertensive, beta-blocker
- Mechanism of Action: Blocks beta receptors leading to lower pulse/BP; also has some alpha blocking activity which is different from most beta-blockers
- Common Uses: Treatment of hypertension and atrial fibrillation
- Memorable Side Effects: Low pulse, low BP, fatigue
- Clinical Pearls:
  - Trick to remembering beta receptors: You have 1 heart and 2 lungs (beta-1 is primarily on the heart and beta-2 primarily in the lungs)
  - Carvedilol has the additive effect of blocking alpha receptors compared to other beta-blockers
  - Often in practice, providers will place a hold order on beta-blockers if the pulse is too low; this is done to reduce the risk of significant bradycardia
  - Clinically it may depend upon the situation, but in an ambulatory setting, you may see the order set to hold the beta blocker when pulse is less than 55 or 60
- Monitoring: Blood pressure, pulse, respiratory status (if they have a history of breathing difficulties),
- Drug and Diet Considerations:
  - Giving with food can help reduce the risk of orthostatic blood pressure
  - Has the potential to mask symptoms of hypoglycemia in diabetes patients

Caspofungin (Cancidas)
- Class: Antifungal, echinocandin
- Mechanism of Action: Inhibition of 1,3 beta-D glucan synthase (key enzyme involved in fungal cell wall synthesis)
- Common Uses: Alternative to fluconazole if the patient has a resistant infection
- Memorable Side Effects: Low blood pressure, GI upset, diarrhea, edema, tachycardia, infusion reaction, electrolytes imbalances possible, but rare
- Clinical Pearls:

- o Typically better tolerated and lower risk than other IV antifungals (i.e. azole antifungals and amphotericin B)
- Monitoring: Liver function
- Drug and Diet Considerations:
  - o No major diet concerns
  - o Monitor fluid and electrolyte status and alter dietary intake accordingly

Cefaclor (Ceclor)
- Class: 2nd generation cephalosporin antibiotic
- Mechanism of Action: Inhibits bacterial cell wall formation
- Common Uses: Treatment of bacterial skin infections, sinusitis, strep throat and bronchitis
- Memorable Side Effects: GI side effects most common, diarrhea, allergic reaction, rash
- Clinical Pearls:
  - o Common use is upper respiratory bacterial infection (sinusitis, bronchitis)
  - o Alternative to penicillin antibiotics; very low risk of cross reactivity, but possible
  - o Patients should begin improving within a couple days if drug is working/being taken appropriately
  - o If suspension is used, you must adequately shake to disperse the medication
- Monitoring: Renal function
- Drug and Diet Considerations:
  - o Generally given with food to reduce GI upset

Cefadroxil (Duracef)
- Class: 1st generation cephalosporin antibiotic
- Mechanism of Action: Inhibits bacterial cell wall formation
- Common Uses: Treatment of bacterial skin infections, strep throat and susceptible UTIs
- Memorable Side Effects: GI side effects most common, diarrhea, allergic reaction, rash
- Clinical Pearls:
  - o Common use is upper respiratory bacterial infection (sinusitis, bronchitis)
  - o Alternative to penicillin antibiotics; very low risk of cross reactivity, but possible
  - o Patients should begin improving within a couple days if drug is working/being taken appropriately
  - o If suspension is used, you must adequately shake to disperse the medication
- Monitoring: Renal function
- Drug and Diet Considerations:
  - o Generally given with food to reduce GI upset, but can be given without food

Cefazolin (Ancef)
- Class: 1ˢᵗ generation cephalosporin antibiotic
- Mechanism of Action: Inhibits bacterial cell wall formation
- Common Uses: Surgical prophylaxis and treatment of bacterial endocarditis and skin infections
- Memorable Side Effects: GI side effects most common, allergy, rash, seizure (rare)
- Clinical Pearls:
    - Often used in surgery prophylaxis to prevent infections
    - Alternative to penicillin antibiotics; very low risk of cross reactivity, but possible
    - If using for treatment of an active infection, patients should begin improving within a couple days if drug is working
- Monitoring: Signs of infection improvement (i.e. fever and symptoms), rash, lab work is typically not necessary with short term use but renal function and LFTs may be considered if there is a clinical reason
- Drug and Diet Considerations:
    - GI upset and diarrhea is the most common adverse effect and could contribute to a short term reduction in caloric intake
    - Bland foods that reduce GI upset and diarrhea can be helpful
    - Maintain adequate hydration to avoid dehydration if diarrhea is a significant problem
    - Consult prescriber/pharmacist if adverse effects are severe

Cefdinir (Omnicef)
- Class: 3ʳᵈ generation cephalosporin antibiotic
- Mechanism of Action: Inhibits bacterial cell wall formation
- Common Uses: Treatment of bacterial skin infections, ear infections, sinusitis and strep throat
- Memorable Side Effects: GI side effects most common, allergy, rash
- Clinical Pearls:
    - It is often used as an alternative to amoxicillin, however with its chemical structure, it is somewhat related to the penicillin's (cross reactivity risk is low)
    - As with most antibiotics, usual adverse effects are GI upset/diarrhea related
    - Usually dosed multiple times per day which can be an issue for patient adherence
- Monitoring: Signs of infection improvement (i.e. fever and symptoms), rash, lab work is typically not necessary with short term use but renal function and LFTs may be considered if there is a clinical reason
- Drug and Diet Considerations:
    - Typically given with food to reduce GI upset
    - Maintain adequate hydration to avoid dehydration if diarrhea is a significant problem
    - Consult prescriber/pharmacist if adverse effects are severe for an alternative antibiotic
    - Vitamins and supplements with iron may block absorption; separate by 2 hours or possibly hold the iron product until the course is completed

66

Cefepime (Maxipime)
- Class: 4th generation cephalosporin antibiotic
- Mechanism of Action: Inhibits bacterial cell wall formation
- Common Uses: IV agent for treatment of gram negative pathogens in bacteremia, intra-abdominal infections, osteomyelitis, pneumonia, and other infections
- Memorable Side Effects: Diarrhea, nausea, rash; rare, but possible changes in platelets and WBCs
- Clinical Pearls:
  - Has Pseudomonas activity
  - Can be given IM as well as IV
  - Not contraindicated with penicillin allergy, cross reactivity low, but need to at least be aware
  - With most antibiotics, symptoms should start to get better within 2-4 days
- Monitoring: Renal function
- Drug and Diet Considerations:
  - Diarrhea is possible, but is usually less than orally administered cephalosporins
  - Low phosphorus levels (rare)

Cefprozil (Cefzil)
- Class: 2nd generation cephalosporin antibiotic
- Mechanism of Action: Inhibits bacterial cell wall formation
- Common Uses: Treatment of bacterial skin infections, ear infections, strep throat and bronchitis
- Memorable Side Effects: GI side effects most common, diarrhea, allergic reaction, rash
- Clinical Pearls:
  - Common use is upper respiratory bacterial infection (sinusitis, bronchitis)
  - Alternative to penicillin antibiotics; very low risk of cross reactivity, but possible
  - Patients should begin improving within a couple days if drug is working/being taken appropriately
  - If suspension is used, you must adequately shake to disperse the medication
- Monitoring: Renal function
- Drug and Diet Considerations:
  - Generally given with food to reduce GI upset, but can be given without food

Ceftaroline (Teflaro)
- Class: 5th generation cephalosporin antibiotic
- Mechanism of Action: Inhibits bacterial cell wall formation
- Common Uses: IV agent for treatment of gram negative pathogens in pneumonia and skin and soft-tissue infections
- Memorable Side Effects: GI side effects, rash and rare changes in platelets and WBCs
- Clinical Pearls:

- o   Known for its activity against MRSA
- o   Not contraindicated with penicillin allergy, cross reactivity low, but need to at least be aware
- o   With most antibiotics, symptoms should start to get better within 2-4 days
- Monitoring: Renal function
- Drug and Diet Considerations:
  - o   Diarrhea is possible, but is usually less than orally administered cephalosporins; monitor fluids and electrolytes
  - o   Alterations in glucose levels and potassium are rare, but may consider monitoring in at risk patients

Ceftazidime (Fortaz)

- Class: 3rd generation cephalosporin antibiotic
- Mechanism of Action: Inhibits bacterial cell wall formation
- Common Uses: IV agent for treatment of gram negative pathogens in bacteremia, meningitis and other infections
- Memorable Side Effects: GI side effects, rash and rare changes in platelets and WBCs
- Clinical Pearls:
  - o   Has Pseudomonas activity
  - o   Can be given IM as well as IV
  - o   Not contraindicated with penicillin allergy, cross reactivity low, but need to at least be aware
  - o   With most antibiotics, symptoms should start to get better within 2-4 days
- Monitoring: Renal function
- Drug and Diet Considerations:
  - o   Diarrhea is possible, but is usually less than orally administered cephalosporins

Ceftriaxone (Rocephin)

- Class: 3rd generation cephalosporin antibiotic
- Mechanism of Action: Inhibits bacterial cell wall formation
- Common Uses: Treatment of bacterial pneumonia, gonorrhea and skin infections
- Memorable Side Effects: GI side effects, rash and rare changes in platelet and WBCs
- Clinical Pearls:
  - o   Very commonly used in pneumonia
  - o   Can be given IM as well as IV
  - o   Not contraindicated with penicillin allergy, cross reactivity low, but need to at least be aware
  - o   Be more cautious if patient has allergy to another cephalosporin
  - o   With most antibiotics, symptoms should start to get better within 2-4 days
- Monitoring: No routine lab work is usually done in short term cases
- Drug and Diet Considerations:
  - o   IV calcium or Lactated Ringers can form a precipitate with ceftriaxone if given together
  - o   GI upset and diarrhea is possible, but is usually less than orally administered cephalosporins

Cefuroxime (Ceftin, Zinacef)

- Class: 2nd generation cephalosporin antibiotic
- Mechanism of Action: Inhibits bacterial cell wall formation
- Common Uses: Treatment of bacterial skin infections, ear infection, sinusitis and strep throat
- Memorable Side Effects: GI side effects most common, allergy, rash
- Clinical Pearls:
  - Common use is upper respiratory bacterial infection (sinusitis or ear infection)
  - Alternative to penicillin antibiotics; very low risk of cross reactivity, but possible
  - Oral or IV formulation available
  - Patients should begin improving within a couple days if drug is working/being taken appropriately
  - If suspension is used, you must adequately shake to disperse the medication
- Monitoring: CBC, LFTs, and renal monitoring is typically done only if the patient is taking a prolonged course or doing chronic prophylaxis for an infection
- Drug and Diet Considerations:
  - Can take oral formulation with meals to ease GI upset and diarrhea risk
  - Taste disturbances can happen but are infrequent

Celecoxib (Celebrex)

- Class: COX-2 inhibitor, analgesic
- Mechanism of Action: Inhibits cyclooxygenase-2 preferentially (COX-2); results in a reduction in prostaglandins which cause pain, fever and inflammation
- Common Uses: Management of pain and inflammation
- Memorable Side Effects: GI ulcer (less than traditional NSAIDs), worsening kidney function, edema, hypertension, inhibits platelets (which can exacerbate bleed risk)
- Clinical Pearls:
  - COX-2 inhibitors can cause GI bleed, but the risk is much less than traditional NSAID; risk increases in the elderly and those on medications that increase risk of bleeding (anticoagulants and antiplatelet medications)
  - COX-2 inhibitors can contribute to edema and exacerbate CHF (congestive heart failure); be on the lookout and have celecoxib reassessed if you see a patient with a CHF exacerbation or a patient requiring an increase of diuretics, like furosemide
  - Celecoxib can cause worsening kidney function (creatinine should be monitored); this risk can be greatly increased in patients on ACE inhibitors or ARBs and/or diuretics
  - When you think of celecoxib, think NSAID side effects with less GI risk
  - Boxed warning for increased risk of heart attack (MI) and stroke
- Monitoring: Renal function, hemoglobin, platelets (contained within CBC), blood pressure, signs of bruising or bleeding

- Drug and Diet Considerations:
  - Stomach issues are less common with celecoxib compared to traditional NSAIDs, like ibuprofen; ok to give with food
  - Dehydration coupled with celecoxib may increase the risk for acute renal failure

Cephalexin (Keflex)

- Class: 1st generation cephalosporin antibiotic
- Mechanism of Action: Inhibits bacterial cell wall formation
- Common Uses: Treatment of bacterial skin infections, ear infection, sinusitis and strep throat
- Memorable Side Effects: GI upset, diarrhea, allergic reaction, rash
- Clinical Pearls:
  - Very common antibiotic used for skin infections, upper respiratory problems like strep throat, bronchitis and ear infection
  - It is often used as an alternative to amoxicillin, however with its chemical structure, it is somewhat related to the penicillin's (cross reactivity risk is low)
  - As with most antibiotics, usual adverse effects are GI upset/diarrhea related
  - Usually dosed multiple times per day which can be an issue for patient adherence
  - With or without food is ok
- Monitoring: Lab work is not typically necessary with short term use; consider renal labs, LFTs, and CBC if being used chronically
- Drug and Diet Considerations:
  - Zinc can reduce the absorption; take zinc at least 3 hours after cephalexin
  - Can be given with or without food but is often given with food to reduce the risk for GI upset

Cetirizine (Zyrtec)

- Class: Antihistamine
- Mechanism of Action: Blocks histamine-1 receptors
- Common Uses: Relief of allergy symptoms
- Memorable Side Effects: Sedation (much less than 1st generation antihistamines like diphenhydramine or hydroxyzine), mildly anticholinergic
- Clinical Pearls:
  - Generally used first line for seasonal allergies as they are more tolerable than first generation antihistamines
  - Less sedating and less anticholinergic effects than first generation
  - Remember that histamine 1 receptor blockers are generally called antihistamines, while histamine 2 receptor blockers are acid blockers used for GI issues (ranitidine, famotidine, etc.)
  - Often with antihistamines, if one doesn't work, patients may try another one from the same class (loratadine, fexofenadine, etc.)
  - Over-the-counter availability
- Monitoring: No routine lab work is necessary
- Drug and Diet Considerations:
  - Absorption may be slightly reduced with food, but it is likely not clinically significant so can give with or without food

70

- o   It has mild anticholinergic side effects so dry mouth could potentially alter taste and desire to eat
- o   Alcohol may exacerbate mild sedative effects

Chlorambucil (Leukeran)

- Class: Oncology agent, nitrogen mustard
- Mechanism of Action: Prevents DNA cross-linking which ultimately prevents proliferation and growth of cells
- Common Uses: Treatment of certain lymphomas and leukemias
- Memorable Side Effects: Myelosuppression, anemia, skin reactions, liver toxicity, thrombocytopenia, neuropathy, infertility, pulmonary fibrosis, GI adverse effects
- Clinical Pearls:
  - o   Boxed warning for the risk of myelosuppression and has carcinogenic and infertility activity
  - o   Oral agent
- Monitoring: CBC, LFTs
- Drug and Diet Considerations:
  - o   Give on an empty stomach as food can lower absorption

Chlordiazepoxide (Librium)

- Class: Antianxiety, benzodiazepine
- Mechanism of Action: Enhances activity of GABA (an inhibitory neurotransmitter that causes sedation)
- Common Uses: Treatment of anxiety, seizure and, insomnia
- Memorable Side Effects: Sedation, confusion, fall risk, dizziness
- Clinical Pearls:
  - o   The best way I remember benzodiazepines is that they are very close to "alcohol in a pill"
  - o   Sedation, slurred speech, trouble walking (ataxia), etc. are all common with benzos/alcohol; they are also used in alcohol withdrawal
  - o   Be cautious with patients on higher doses of benzodiazepines to make sure they aren't abruptly stopped
  - o   Educate patients on possible impairment when driving/operating machinery or motor vehicles
  - o   Unlike SSRIs for anxiety, a great advantage of benzos is that they work quickly and can be used as needed
  - o   Fall risk in the elderly is a big downside to using these medications
  - o   Benzos are a controlled substance; they can cause addiction and dependence
  - o   May be used for acute behavioral issues as well as seizure
  - o   Flumazenil is antidote in overdose
- Monitoring: Routine lab monitoring typically isn't necessary unless clinically indicated; respiratory rate in overdose
  - o   Alcohol intake can have additive side effects of sedation, confusion, slurred speech, and other CNS depressant effects
  - o   May give with or without food

Chlorpheniramine (Chlor-Trimeton)
- Class: Antihistamine, anticholinergic
- Mechanism of Action: Blocks muscarinic (anticholinergic) receptors and also has antihistamine effects
- Common Uses: Relief of allergy symptoms and prevention of motion sickness
- Memorable Side Effects: Anticholinergic effects such as dry mouth, dry eyes, urinary retention, constipation, sedation and confusion
- Clinical Pearls:
    - Highly anticholinergic (can't spit, see, pee, or sh*t and increases confusion/fall risk) which can be especially problematic in geriatric patients – avoid if possible
    - May have paradoxical insomnia reaction in pediatrics
- Monitoring: No routine lab work is typically necessary
- Drug and Diet Considerations:
    - Slows the motility of the GI tract which could increase the risk for constipation; maintain adequate fluids and non-constipating diet
    - Alcohol may exacerbate CNS depressant effects
    - Dry mouth may increase thirst and alter taste/pleasure of food
    - May be given with or without food

Chlorpromazine (Thorazine)
- Class: Antiemetic, dopamine blocker, 1st generation antipsychotic
- Mechanism of Action: Blocks dopamine receptors in the brain which can help manage psychosis and mania episodes
- Common Uses: Treatment of psychotic disorders, hiccups and nausea/vomiting
- Memorable Side Effects: Sedation, fall risk, orthostatic BP changes, EPS, metabolic syndrome (typically not an issue with short term use)
- Clinical Pearls:
    - If chlorpromazine is used on a regular basis, monitor for development of tardive dyskinesia
    - Elderly may be more susceptible to adverse effects
- Monitoring: EKG, and possibly electrolytes in at risk patients (especially in overdose), lipids, blood glucose (metabolic syndrome risk)
- Drug and Diet Considerations:
    - May give with food to decrease GI upset
    - CNS depressant activity which could be exacerbated by alcohol

Chlorthalidone (Hygroton, Thalitone, Chlorthalid)
- Class: Antihypertensive, thiazide diuretic
- Mechanism of Action: Inhibits sodium/chloride transporter in the distal tubules
- Common Use: Treatment of hypertension and heart failure symptoms caused by fluid retention
- Memorable Side Effects: frequent urination, electrolyte depletion, low blood pressure, and increased risk of kidney failure, photosensitivity
- Clinical Pearls:
    - One of the major differences between loops and thiazides are that thiazides can INCREASE serum calcium while loops will reduce it
    - While loop diuretics can cause hyperuricemia (elevated uric acid possibly contributing to or exacerbating gout), thiazides are classically known to do this; be on the lookout for chlorthalidone when gout medications are being added or patients are reporting gout flares

- o Kidney function and electrolytes are going to be the primary labs to monitor – potassium supplementation is common in patients taking diuretics
- o Watch the timing of diuretics like chlorthalidone; evening dosing can cause frequent nighttime urination
- Monitoring: Renal function, electrolytes, blood pressure, uric acid (in patients with gout)
- Drug and Diet Considerations:
  - o A low potassium or low magnesium diet could increase the risk for deficiency in combination with the drug
  - o Hypercalcemia is possible; monitor calcium and vitamin D intake
  - o This drug is dehydrating so be aware of acute renal failure risk in patients who have reduced fluid intake (i.e. acutely ill, geriatric patients, etc.)
  - o Alcohol may exacerbate low blood pressure and urinary frequency
  - o Modest increases in glucose may happen in our diabetes patients (typically not clinically significant)
  - o Possible cause of weight loss

Cholestyramine (Questran)

- Class: Antilipemic, bile acid sequestrant, antidiarrheal
- Mechanism of Action: Binds bile acids in the intestine which inhibits reuptake into systemic circulation; this will promote the loss of LDL which is bound to bile salts
- Common Uses: Reduction of cholesterol and treatment of diarrhea and pruritus with cholestasis
- Memorable Side Effects: Constipation, GI upset and pain, myalgia
- Clinical Pearls:
  - o Can help bulk up stools and manage diarrhea symptoms in patients
  - o Lots of binding interactions with other medications that can reduce absorption
  - o Use cautiously in patients with high triglycerides
  - o Rare risk for acidosis
- Monitoring: Lipids
- Drug and Diet Considerations:
  - o May increase the risk of fat soluble vitamin deficiencies (A, D, E, and K) as well as folic acid and iron deficiency
  - o Take vitamins and drugs that interact one hour before cholestyramine or 4 hours after
  - o Give with meals

Cilostazol (Pletal)

- Class: Vasodilator and antiplatelet agent
- Mechanism of Action: Inhibits phosphodiesterase 3 which ultimately increases cyclic AMP; an increase in cyclic AMP can lead to inhibition of platelet activity, relaxation of vascular smooth muscle and vasodilation
- Common Uses: Improvement of intermittent claudication
- Memorable Side Effects: GI upset, headache, edema, low BP, dizziness
- Clinical Pearls:
  - o Possible CYP2C19 and CYP3A4 interactions

- o Can increase risk of bleed especially in those on antiplatelet medications/anticoagulants
- o Contraindicated in patients with heart failure
- Monitoring: Blood pressure, CBC
- Drug and Diet Considerations:
  - o Administer on empty stomach
  - o Vitamin E, Omega-3 fatty acids, gingko, garlic, ginseng, turmeric, and fish oil supplements have been purported to have antiplatelet type activity which, in theory, could increase the risk of bleed – clinical significance is questionable; the most common resolution is to discontinue the supplements if they are not necessary
  - o Alcohol may have an additive antiplatelet type effect and increase the risk of GI bleed
  - o Grapefruit juice can significantly increase drug levels

Cimetidine (Tagamet)
- Class: H2 blocker
- Mechanism of Action: Blocks histamine 2 receptors (H2 blocker) which results in reduced gastric acid secretion and a higher pH in the stomach
- Common Uses: Treatment of GERD, heartburn and GI bleed prophylaxis
- Memorable Side Effects: Pretty well tolerated overall, drowsiness, dry mouth
- Clinical Pearls:
  - o H2 blockers are cleared by the kidney; they can accumulate in CKD and require dose adjustments
  - o Generally less effective at suppressing stomach acid than PPIs
  - o Available over the counter
  - o CNS effects likely more common in elderly, at higher doses, and in patients with kidney disease
  - o Generally used before PPIs if something more than Tums (calcium carbonate) is needed in pregnancy
  - o Cimetidine is generally avoided of all the H2 blockers due to the risk of drug interactions
- Monitoring: No routine lab work is typically necessary; LFTs, hemoglobin when clinically indicated
- Drug and Diet Considerations:
  - o Reduced stomach acid (high pH) may impair the absorption of iron supplements
  - o Associations with B12 deficiency in chronic users
  - o Given with meals

Cinacalcet (Sensipar)
- Class: Anti-hyperparathyroid agent, calcimimetic
- Mechanism of Action: Acts by altering the calcium-sensing receptor on the parathyroid gland which lowers PTH calcium, and phosphorus (essentially mimics the action of calcium without increasing calcium levels)
- Common Uses: Treatment of hyperparathyroidism
- Memorable Side Effects: Low calcium, GI upset, low blood pressure
- Clinical Pearls:
  - o May exacerbate QTc prolongation risk if calcium gets too low
  - o Avoid use if calcium is already low
  - o Low calcium may increase seizure risk
- Monitoring: Calcium, phosphorus, parathyroid hormone (PTH), renal function

74

- Drug and Diet Considerations:
  - Administer with meals
  - Pay attention to calcium and phosphorus intake and may need to adjust diet accordingly

Ciprofloxacin (Cipro)

- Class: Quinolone, antibiotic
- Mechanism of Action: Inhibits bacterial DNA synthesis
- Common Uses: Treatment of UTIs
- Memorable Side Effects: GI side effects, QTc prolongation (rare), and there is a boxed warning for the risk of tendon rupture, neuropathy, and CNS changes
- Clinical Pearls:
  - Commonly used for the treatment of UTI's; great coverage against many gram negative bacteria
  - Dose adjustments might be necessary in patients with poor kidney function
  - Should not be co-administered with iron or calcium products as this can significant reduce absorption and possibly lead to treatment failure
  - Generally NOT used for pneumonia (Other quinolones like levofloxacin and moxifloxacin can be) due to its poor activity against Strep. pneumoniae
  - Usually dosed multiple times per day (at least twice)
- Monitoring: In the short term, lab monitoring is typically not necessary; in longer term therapy, renal function, LFTs, CBC, and risk for hypoglycemia in diabetes may be assessed
- Drug and Diet Considerations:
  - Antacids, iron, calcium, zinc, magnesium, aluminum, and dairy products can interfere with the absorption of this drug; administer oral ciprofloxacin 2 hours before or up to 6 hours after any of the above listed products
  - Caffeine can interact with ciprofloxacin and its effects may be exacerbated due to an interaction; monitor for signs of caffeine toxicity (tachycardia, insomnia, anxiety, etc.) and suggest a reduction in caffeine intake for heavy users

Cisplatin (Platinol)

- Class: Oncology agent, platinum compound
- Mechanism of Action: Blocks DNA synthesis and alters the natural double helix of DNA to inhibit cell growth
- Common Uses: Treatment of numerous types of cancers
- Memorable Side Effects: Neuropathy, CNS toxicity, nausea, vomiting, diarrhea, myelosuppression, hair loss, renal toxicity, ototoxicity, hypersensitivity reactions
- Clinical Pearls:
  - Boxed warnings for myelosuppression, nausea/vomiting, nephrotoxicity, and neuropathy
- Monitoring: CBC, renal function, electrolytes, LFTs, hearing
- Drug and Diet Considerations:

- o Weight loss and poor nutrition may be a result of nausea and vomiting adverse effects
- o Assess for need for fluid and electrolyte replacement in patients with vomiting

Citalopram (Celexa)
- Class: SSRI, antidepressant
- Mechanism of Action: SSRI – selective serotonin reuptake inhibitor; increases serotonin in the brain
- Common Uses: Treatment of depression, anxiety and PTSD
- Memorable Side Effects: GI side effects (N/V/D), can cause sedation or activation depending upon the patient, changes in mental status, hyponatremia (rare)
- Clinical Pearls:
  - o The dose of citalopram should be limited/monitored closely in the elderly as well as patients on omeprazole
  - o SSRIs are generally considered the first line medication to treat depression, they are generally well tolerated and less risky than other antidepressants in regards to suicidal ideations
  - o Stomach/GI complaints/diarrhea are the most common side effects
  - o There may be an increased risk of suicidal thinking when first starting these medications (there is a BOXED warning for this risk)
  - o Although not terribly common, hyponatremia (low sodium) is a possible unique side effect with SSRIs and much more likely in patients already prone to hyponatremia – classic example would be patients who are taking diuretics, which can also lower sodium
  - o Remember that these drugs are not an immediate fix! In most cases, SSRIs take weeks, sometimes months, before a patient will start improving; however, side effects will be apparent from the start of the medication, making it difficult to coach our patients to continue the medication in the first few weeks after starting
  - o SSRIs are used in pregnancy, but the risk versus the benefit needs to be assessed on a case by case basis
  - o SSRIs can decrease libido
- Monitoring: EKG, potassium and magnesium if the patient is at risk for QTc prolongation; sodium level if the patient is displaying symptoms of hyponatremia
- Drug and Diet Considerations:
  - o Weight gain or weight loss can happen with SSRIs; monitor for changes over time once started, increased, reduced, or discontinued
  - o Diarrhea can happen, but isn't incredibly common; assess fluid status, notify provider if the patient is reporting this side effect
  - o If the patient has a prolonged QT interval, out of range electrolytes like potassium and magnesium could increase the risk for Torsades de Pointes
  - o Low sodium can be a rare adverse effect
  - o Can be taken with or without food
  - o Alcohol has additive, unpredictable effects when used with SSRIs
  - o St John's wort has additive effects on any drug that has serotonergic type activity

Clarithromycin (Biaxin)
- Class: Macrolide, antibiotic

- Mechanism of Action: Inhibits protein synthesis in bacteria (macrolide class of antibiotics)
- Common Uses: Treatment of upper respiratory infections (i.e. ear infection, pneumonia, bronchitis, sinusitis) and Helicobacter pylori
- Memorable Side Effects: GI upset and QTc prolongation possible (very rare)
- Clinical Pearls:
  - Numerous drug interactions, compared to azithromycin, rarely used as an antibiotic due to this reason
  - Dosed multiple times per day; azithromycin much simpler dosing
- Monitoring: LFTs and CBC if using long term or if signs of complications
- Drug and Diet Considerations:
  - GI upset and diarrhea can happen, but generally less frequent than an antibiotic like amoxicillin
  - Maintain adequate hydration to avoid dehydration if diarrhea is a significant problem
  - Can be administered without regard to meals (ER formulation should be given with food)

Clemastine (Tavist)
- Class: First generation antihistamine
- Mechanism of Action: Blocks histamine receptors
- Common Uses: Treatment of insomnia, management of allergies, allergic reactions and itching
- Memorable Side Effects: Anticholinergic effects such as dry mouth, dry eyes, urinary retention, constipation, sedation, confusion
- Clinical Pearls:
  - Highly anticholinergic (can't spit, see, pee, or sh*t and increases confusion/fall risk) which can be especially problematic in geriatric patients – avoid if possible
  - May have paradoxical insomnia reaction in pediatrics
- Monitoring: No routine lab work is typically necessary
- Drug and Diet Considerations:
  - Slows the motility of the GI tract which could increase the risk for constipation; maintain adequate fluids and non-constipating diet
  - Alcohol may exacerbate CNS depressant effects
  - Dry mouth may increase thirst and alter taste/pleasure of food
  - May be given with or without food

Clindamycin (Cleocin)
- Class: Antibiotic, lincosamide
- Mechanism of Action: Inhibits bacterial protein synthesis
- Common Uses: Treatment of skin, bone, and joint infections
- Memorable Side Effects: GI side effects, colitis (C. diff risk), metallic taste
- Clinical Pearls:
  - Has some activity against MRSA (methicillin resistant Staphylococcus aureus) where penicillin antibiotics would not be effective
  - Possible alternative for patients who need antibiotic prophylaxis undergoing dental procedures who can't tolerate or have an allergy to penicillin antibiotics

- One of the common antibiotics that may contribute to C. diff development (quinolones, cephalosporins, and penicillins may contribute as well)
- Frequent administration is kind of a nuisance; usually 3-4 times per day
- Monitoring: Risk for diarrhea; short term lab work is typically not necessary
- Drug and Diet Considerations:
  - Give with a full glass of water to reduce the risk of GI ulceration; oral administration only
  - If the patient is reporting severe diarrhea continuing after the drug has been stopped, be aware of the risk for Clostridium difficile-associated diarrhea and be sure to notify provider
  - Alteration of taste (metallic taste) can happen and may contribute to changes in eating patterns; typically this is short term
  - Can be given with or without meals

Clomipramine (Anafranil)

- Class: TCA (tri-cyclic antidepressant)
- Mechanism of Action: Inhibits reuptake of serotonin and possibly norepinephrine
- Common Uses: Treatment of depression, neuropathy, pain syndromes, anxiety and PTSD
- Memorable Side Effects: Anticholinergic, confusion; fall risk in elderly
- Clinical Pearls:
  - Old TCA generally not recommended in the elderly due to anticholinergic effects
  - Highly anticholinergic (can't spit, see, pee, or sh*t and increases confusion/fall risk) which can be especially problematic in geriatric patients – avoid if possible
  - In addition, cognitive impairment is not a good thing in the elderly due to possibility of preexisting dementia
  - TCAs may have some benefit in neuropathy, generally much cheaper than SNRIs, like duloxetine, which can be also beneficial in neuropathy
  - Not a good first line choice for sleep or depression; other agents exist that are much safer
  - Look out for TCAs causing the prescribing cascade! Artificial tears for dry eyes, constipation medications, BPH medications, like tamsulosin, dementia medications, or artificial saliva
  - Often dosed in the evening due to the adverse effect of sedation
- Monitoring: EKG, and possibly electrolytes, in at risk patients (especially in overdose), behavioral changes, weight, sodium (in patients with signs of hyponatremia),
- Drug and Diet Considerations:
  - Weight gain is possible and may be problematic
  - Slows the motility of the GI tract which could increase the risk for constipation; maintain adequate fluids and non-constipating diet
  - If GI upset occurs, no issues in giving the drug with food
  - Dry mouth may increase thirst and alter taste/pleasure of food
  - Poor intake may place the patient at higher risk for complications from electrolyte abnormalities (i.e. hyponatremia, hypokalemia, or hypomagnesemia)
  - Alcohol may exacerbate sedative adverse effect

Clonazepam (Klonopin)

- Class: Antianxiety, benzodiazepine
- Mechanism of Action: Enhances activity of GABA; an inhibitory neurotransmitter that causes sedation
- Common Uses: Management of anxiety and insomnia
- Memorable Side Effects: Sedation, confusion, fall risk, dizziness
- Clinical Pearls:
  - The best way I remember benzodiazepines is that they are very close to "alcohol in a pill"
  - Sedation, slurred speech, trouble walking (ataxia), etc. are all common with benzos/alcohol; they are also commonly used in alcohol withdrawal
  - Be cautious with patients on higher doses of benzodiazepines to make sure they aren't abruptly stopped
  - Educate patients on driving/operating machinery
  - Unlike SSRIs for anxiety, a great advantage of benzos are that they work quickly and can be used as needed
  - Falls in the elderly is a big downside to using these medications
  - Benzos are a controlled substance; they can cause addiction and dependence
  - Flumazenil is antidote in overdose
- Monitoring: Routine lab monitoring typically isn't necessary unless clinically indicated
- Drug and Diet Considerations:
  - Alcohol intake can have additive side effects of sedation, confusion, slurred speech, and other CNS depressant effects
  - Grapefruit juice may increase the concentrations of clonazepam

Clonidine (Catapres)

- Class: Antihypertensive, alpha-2 agonist
- Mechanism of Action: Centrally acting alpha-2 agonist which results in decreased sympathetic activity and drop in blood pressure
- Common Uses: Treatment of hypertension and management of ADHD symptoms
- Memorable Side Effects: Drowsiness, dizziness, dry mouth
- Clinical Pearls:
  - Not the best in the elderly (on Beer's list)
  - Mainly used in hypertension, but occasionally will see it used off label for various psych issues
  - Comes in a patch formulation (and oral tabs) which may be advantageous for patients who can't swallow or take pills
  - Low blood pressure and pulse is possible
  - Sedating which can be a significant problem especially in the elderly
  - Can be used in relief of opioid withdrawal management
  - Rebound hypertension is a risk if abruptly discontinued
- Monitoring: Blood pressure, pulse
- Drug and Diet Considerations:
  - Alcohol can exacerbate the CNS depressant effect from clonidine
  - Can be given with or without food

Clopidogrel (Plavix)

- Class: Antiplatelet, thienopyridine
- Mechanism of Action: Blocks ADP receptors (leads to inhibition of platelets)
- Common Uses: Prevention of heart attacks and strokes
- Memorable Side Effects: Bleeding (GI, nose bleeds etc.)
- Clinical Pearls:
  - Clopidogrel is often used after a heart attack (MI) with aspirin to prevent further heart attacks; how long a patient should remain on this medication can vary depending upon cardiac and/or stroke risk; length of therapy should be addressed by the primary provider and in many situations may be 12 months, but can be longer or indefinite depending upon risk factors
  - Clopidogrel is a substitute if a patient cannot take or tolerate aspirin to help prevent stroke or heart attack
  - Due to its ability to inhibit platelets, the major complication is bleeding; assess patients for bruising, blood in the stool, any abnormal sign of bleeding
- Monitoring: CBC with platelets
- Drug and Diet Considerations:
  - Grapefruit juice may reduce effectiveness of clopidogrel
  - Generally avoid supplements that may be associated with antiplatelet activity such as ginseng, garlic, glucosamine, vitamin E, etc. or at a minimum, monitor for bruising and bleed risk
  - Can be administered with or without food

Clorazepate (Tranxene)

- Class: Antianxiety, benzodiazepine
- Mechanism of Action: Enhances activity of GABA (an inhibitory neurotransmitter that causes sedation)
- Common Uses: Treatment of anxiety, seizure and insomnia
- Memorable Side Effects: Sedation, confusion, fall risk, dizziness
- Clinical Pearls:
  - The best way I remember benzodiazepines is that they are very close to "alcohol in a pill"
  - Sedation, slurred speech, trouble walking (ataxia), etc. are all common with benzos/alcohol; they are also commonly used in alcohol withdrawal
  - Be cautious with patients on higher doses of benzodiazepines to make sure they aren't abruptly stopped
  - Educate patients on driving/operating machinery (remember that benzodiazepines are often used for sleep as well as anxiety)
  - Unlike SSRIs for anxiety, a great advantage of benzos is that they work quickly and can be used as needed
  - Fall risk in the elderly is a big downside to using these medications
  - Benzos are a controlled substance; they can cause addiction and dependence
  - Can be used for acute behavioral issues as well as seizure
  - Flumazenil is antidote in overdose
- Monitoring: Routine lab monitoring typically isn't necessary unless clinically indicated; respiratory rate in overdose risk, CBC, LFTs as clinically indicated
- Drug and Diet Considerations:

- o Alcohol intake can have additive side effects of sedation, confusion, slurred speech, and other CNS depressant effects
- o May give with or without food

Clotrimazole troche (Mycelex)
- Class: Antifungal
- Mechanism of Action: Ultimately inhibits formation in fungal cell membrane
- Common Uses: Treatment of thrush
- Memorable Side Effects: Elevated LFTs, upper GI/mouth irritation
- Clinical Pearls:
  - o Acts topically in the mouth/throat area and has very low systemic absorption
- Monitoring: LFTs if clinically indicated or if using prolonged therapy
- Drug and Diet Considerations:
  - o The drug should dissolve in the mouth so administration with food or fluid is not appropriate as it will prevent this action

Clozapine (Clozaril, Fazaclo)
- Class: Antipsychotic
- Mechanism of Action: Blocks dopamine receptors
- Common Uses: Treatment of severe schizophrenia, bipolar disorder and off label for dementia-related behaviors like aggression, hallucinations and delusions
- Memorable Side Effects: Sedation, fall risk, orthostatic BP changes, EPS, metabolic syndrome, low white blood cell count, lowers seizure threshold, cardiomyopathy
- Clinical Pearls:
  - o Multiple boxed warnings: Risk for agranulocytosis, hypotension, seizures, cardiomyopathy
  - o Usually higher doses are required for younger patients with schizophrenia and/or bipolar disorder while lower doses can and should be used in the elderly
  - o Remember with antipsychotic medications that they block dopamine and can exacerbate conditions where there is a shortage of dopamine like Parkinson's disorder (remember that we use dopamine to treat Parkinson's – i.e. carbidopa/levodopa or pramipexole)
  - o Sedation, orthostatic hypotension, movement disorder side effects can all increase the risk of falls, especially in our elderly patients
  - o NMS (neuroleptic malignant syndrome) is a very rare but very serious complication with antipsychotic medications; a few symptoms of NMS include: fever, hyperreflexia, confusion, delirium and tremor
  - o Antipsychotics increase the risk of metabolic syndrome (diabetes, elevated lipids, weight gain, etc.) – it is important to periodically monitor for this, especially in younger patients with schizophrenia and/or bipolar who may be likely to require long term use of higher doses; olanzapine is one of the worst antipsychotics as far as this side effect goes

- May have some anticholinergic activity (can't spit, see, pee, or sh*t and increases confusion/fall risk) which can be especially problematic in geriatric patients
- Antipsychotics can contribute to QTc prolongation, which can be especially problematic in patients who are already at risk (i.e. on antiarrhythmic medications)
- Usually reserved for patients who have failed other antipsychotics
- Monitoring: CBC, ANC, weight, BMI, lipids, HbA1c, blood sugars, EKG as clinically appropriate, electrolytes (potassium and magnesium important if the patient is at risk for QTc prolongation)
- Drug and Diet Considerations:
  - Increased appetite and risk for metabolic syndrome; clozapine is one of the higher risk antipsychotics
  - Increased blood sugars can result in our diabetes patients, monitor blood sugars closely with acute changes in the drug
  - Alcohol may exacerbate the CNS depressant effect
  - Oral medication can be administered with or without meals
  - Caffeine may increase concentrations

Cobicistat (Tybost)
- Class: Pharmacokinetic booster, cytochrome p450 inhibitor
- Mechanism of Action: Boosts the concentration of protease inhibitors like atazanavir or darunavir which ultimately helps to bind to the site where protein cleavage occurs and prevents protease from releasing essential proteins
- Common Uses: Combined with other agents for the treatment of HIV infection
- Memorable Side Effects: Hepatic impairment, elevated bilirubin, hyperglycemia, elevated lipase and amylase, GI upset, increases in LDL and triglycerides
- Clinical Pearls:
  - Tremendous amount of potential drug interactions
- Monitoring: Lipids, glucose, HIV parameters (i.e. viral load and CD4 count), CBC, renal function
- Drug and Diet Considerations:
  - Take with food
  - Monitor hyperglycemia risk and may need to adjust diet accordingly
  - Lipid-lowering diet could help reduce the adverse effect of hypercholesterolemia

Codeine / APAP (Tylenol #3)
- Class: Analgesic, opioid, (see acetaminophen)
- Mechanism of Action: Binds opioid receptors inhibiting CNS pain pathways to provide pain relief; acetaminophen is believed to inhibit prostaglandin production, but does not have anti-inflammatory effects like NSAIDs
- Common Uses: Management of pain disorders, both chronic and acute
- Memorable Side Effects: Constipation, sedation, respiratory depression, CNS effects like confusion, delirium, etc., liver toxicity (acetaminophen in large doses >4 grams/day)
- Clinical Pearls:
  - Codeine is a prodrug of morphine; when it enters the body, it gets metabolized to morphine which has opioid activity and is primarily responsible for pain relief

- o With opioids we need to remember that prevention of constipation is important
- o Another combination product with acetaminophen, need to educate/monitor patients for use of other medications that contain acetaminophen
- o Sedation and CNS effects are often problematic with opioids
- o Driving/working machinery is certainly risky when using opioids as they can cause significant sedation; tolerance occurs with chronic use
- o Codeine with acetaminophen is a schedule 3 controlled substance
- Monitoring: Bowel movements, pain management, risk for addiction
- Drug and Diet Considerations:
  - o Alcohol can exacerbate the CNS depressant effect from codeine
  - o Giving with food and water can reduce the risk of GI upset
  - o Encourage a constipation friendly diet consisting of fiber, fluids and exercise as codeine can be very constipating
  - o Possible increase in activity of codeine when administered with grapefruit juice
  - o See acetaminophen for information on that medication

Colchicine (Colcrys)
- Class: Anti-gout agent
- Mechanism of Action: Inhibits beta-tubulin ultimately inhibiting action of neutrophils that may contribute to gout symptoms
- Common Uses: Gout prophylaxis and treatment
- Memorable Side Effects: Diarrhea, nausea
- Clinical Pearls:
  - o Diarrhea is a very prominent side effect
  - o Cleared by the kidney, so may need to use lower doses in CKD
  - o Can be used for acute gout flare or prophylaxis (unique from allopurinol which is only used for prophylaxis of gout)
- Monitoring: Renal function, CBC, LFTs, uric acid (due to gout diagnosis, not necessarily because of the drug)
- Drug and Diet Considerations:
  - o Very high incidence of diarrhea with the medication; be sure to assess fluid status and ask about this adverse effect
  - o Avoid grapefruit juice as it can significantly raise concentrations of colchicine
  - o Colchicine may cause certain vitamin deficiencies (i.e. B12) particularly if diarrhea is a problem
  - o Can be given with or without food
  - o Niacin may increase uric acid and increase the risk of gout flares

Colestipol (Colestid)
- Class: Antilipemic, bile acid sequestrant, antidiarrheal
- Mechanism of Action: Binds bile acids in the intestine which inhibits reuptake back into systemic circulation; this will promote the loss of LDL which is bound to bile salts
- Common Uses: Reduction of cholesterol, diarrhea and pruritus with cholestasis
- Memorable Side Effects: Constipation, GI upset and pain, myalgia
- Clinical Pearls:

- o Can help bulk up stools and manage diarrhea symptoms in patients
- o Lots of binding interactions with other medications that can reduce absorption
- o Use cautiously in patients with high triglycerides
- o Rare risk for acidosis
- Monitoring: Lipids
- Drug and Diet Considerations:
  - o May increase the risk of fat soluble vitamin deficiencies (A, D, E and K) as well as folic acid and iron deficiency
  - o Take vitamins and drugs that interact one hour before colestipol or 4 hours after
  - o Give with meals

Conjugated Estrogen (Premarin)
- Class: Estrogen derivative
- Mechanism of Action: Mimics body's natural estrogen
- Common Uses: Treatment of menopausal symptoms, osteoporosis, uterine bleeding and vaginal atrophy due to menopause
- Memorable Side Effects: GI side effects, clot formation (DVT/PE), increased risk of endometrial and breast cancer
- Clinical Pearls:
  - o Most often used for estrogen replacement in postmenopausal women
  - o Alleviates troublesome hot flashes
  - o Big risk is increase in certain types of cancer as well as clot formation (DVT); long term use is not recommended if possible
  - o Positive bone effects which is beneficial for patients with osteoporosis
- Monitoring: Risk for blood clots, lipids, TSH in patients receiving a supplement, blood pressure
- Drug and Diet Considerations:
  - o Reduced folic acid absorption; need to assess for deficiency risk
  - o Can be given with or without food
  - o Monitor for an increase in blood sugar (usually not clinically significant)
  - o Grapefruit juice may increase concentration

Cromolyn (NasalCrom, Gastrocrom)
- Class: Mast cell stabilizer
- Mechanism of Action: Mast cells release histamine and leukotrienes which can cause allergic reaction-type symptoms; cromolyn prevents the release from mast cells
- Common Uses: Management of symptoms in allergic rhinitis and asthma
- Memorable Side Effects: Nasal irritation, cough, sneezing (nasal administration)
- Clinical Pearls:
  - o Nasal is the most commonly used method of administration in practice
  - o OTC availability
- Monitoring: No routine lab work is necessary for nasal administration
- Drug and Diet Considerations:
  - o No concerns with nasal administration

Cyclobenzaprine (Flexeril)

- Class: Skeletal muscle relaxant
- Mechanism of Action: Acts in the CNS and produces muscle relaxation
- Common Uses: Reduction of muscle spasms
- Memorable Side Effects: Anticholinergic activity, sedation, fall risk, confusion
- Clinical Pearls:
    - Normally used to relax the muscles in the case of muscle spasms, hopefully this medication only needs to be used for a short period of time
    - Elderly may have an increased risk for side effects like anticholinergic effects, sedation, dizziness; thus increasing fall risk
    - Onset of action is pretty quick, approximately one hour, so this medication can be used on an as needed basis
    - With the sedation side effect, we always need to caution our patients about driving, using machinery, etc.
    - Dry mouth is common especially with frequent use
- Monitoring: No routine lab work is recommended
- Drug and Diet Considerations:
    - Alcohol can exacerbate the CNS depressant effect from cyclobenzaprine
    - Dry mouth may alter eating habits
    - Monitor for constipation and encourage a constipation friendly diet including fiber, fluids and exercise, if necessary
    - Administering with a meal may increase the percentage of the drug that is absorbed; pay attention to increased effects of cyclobenzaprine if it is given with food

Cyclophosphamide (Cytoxan, Procytox)

- Class: Oncology agent, nitrogen mustard, alkylating agent
- Mechanism of Action: Prevents DNA cross-linking which ultimately prevents proliferation and growth of cells
- Common Uses: Treatment of numerous types of cancers
- Memorable Side Effects: Hemorrhagic cystitis, bladder toxicity, diarrhea, nausea and vomiting, hyponatremia, myelosuppression, hair loss
- Clinical Pearls:
    - Mesna may be used in combination with cyclophosphamide to reduce the risk for bladder toxicity
- Monitoring: CBC, LFTs, renal function, electrolytes, EKG (as clinically indicated),
- Drug and Diet Considerations:
    - Monitor for adequate hydration to reduce the risk for bladder complications
    - Monitor sodium due to risk of SIADH and hyponatremia, may need to replace as clinically indicated
    - Weight loss and poor nutrition may be a result of nausea and vomiting adverse effects

Cyclosporine (Sandimmune, Gengraf, Neoral)

- Class: Immunosuppressant, calcineurin inhibitor

- Mechanism of Action: Blocks T-cell activation by binding the FKBP-12 protein as part of the process to inhibit calcineurin activity
- Common Uses: Organ rejection prevention
- Memorable Side Effects: Hypertension, immunosuppression, elevated lipids, hyperglycemia, hyperkalemia, GI upset
- Clinical Pearls:
    - Numerous drug interactions through CYP3A4 that can alter concentrations
    - Dosage forms have varying bioavailability, any changes should prompt close monitoring of levels
    - Boxed warning that it should be used by an experienced clinician who specializes in areas where this medication might be used
    - Additional boxed warnings for nephrotoxicity, hypertension, immunosuppression, and bioavailability risks with different dosage forms
    - When you may want to reassess levels
        - Monitor adherence
        - Changes in drug therapy and monitoring of drug interactions
        - Adjusting of dose
        - Signs of toxicity or rejection
- Monitoring: Drug levels, blood sugars in diabetes patients, electrolytes, renal function, CBC, blood pressure, LFTs
- Drug and Diet Considerations:
    - Consistency of administration is critical, but can be given with or without meals
    - Avoid the use of grapefruit juice as it may increase drug concentrations
    - Be aware of blood glucose, lipid effects, and elevations of potassium in relation to diet and the use of this medication

Cyproheptadine (Periactin)

- Class: 1st generation antihistamine, anticholinergic
- Mechanism of Action: Blocks muscarinic (anticholinergic) receptors and also has antihistamine effects by blocking H1 receptors; in addition, has antiserotonergic properties
- Common Uses: Relief of allergy symptoms, treatment of serotonin syndrome and appetite stimulation
- Memorable Side Effects: Anticholinergic effects such as dry mouth, dry eyes, urinary retention, constipation, sedation, confusion
- Clinical Pearls:
    - Highly anticholinergic (can't spit, see, pee, or sh*t and increases confusion/fall risk) which can be especially problematic in geriatric patients – avoid if possible
    - May have paradoxical insomnia reaction in pediatrics
- Monitoring: Weight
- Drug and Diet Considerations:
    - Slows the motility of the GI tract which could increase the risk for constipation – adequate fluids and non-constipating diet may be helpful in prevention
    - May be helpful in stimulating appetite
    - Alcohol may exacerbate CNS depressant effects
    - Dry mouth may increase thirst and alter taste/pleasure of food

- o   May be given with or without food

Cytarabine (Cytosar-U, Ara-C)
- Class: Oncology agent, pyrimidine analog
- Mechanism of Action: Becomes activated when converted to aracytidine triphosphate which ultimately helps stop DNA polymerase
- Common Uses: Treatment of numerous types of cancers
- Memorable Side Effects: Vomiting, nausea, increased LFTs, myelosuppression, ophthalmic toxicity, CNS changes, anemia, GI ulceration
- Clinical Pearls:
  - o   May exacerbate gout
  - o   As doses escalate, the risk for neurotoxicity, GI ulceration, hepatic, and cardiovascular complications increases
- Monitoring: CBC, renal function, electrolytes, LFTs, uric acid
- Drug and Diet Considerations:
  - o   Weight loss and poor nutrition may be a result of nausea and vomiting adverse effects
  - o   Assess for diet implications on hyperuricemia risk

Dabigatran (Pradaxa)
- Class: Anticoagulant, thrombin inhibitor
- Mechanism of Action: Direct thrombin inhibitor which leads to prevention of blood clots
- Common Uses: Reduces risk of DVT, anticoagulation in atrial fibrillation
- Memorable Side Effects: Bleeding
- Clinical Pearls:
  - o   Bleed risk! Monitor for bruising, low hemoglobin, blood in stools, nose bleeds, etc.
  - o   GI bleed risk is especially problematic when used with NSAIDs (ibuprofen, naproxen, etc.)
  - o   Reversal agent is idarucizumab
  - o   Twice daily dosing makes it a little inconvenient
  - o   Have provider assess for dose adjustment in patients with CKD
  - o   Alternative to warfarin and routine INR is not necessary
- Monitoring: CBC, renal function, bleeding risk, LFTs
  - o   Note: Routine INRs are not required
- Drug and Diet Considerations:
  - o   May give with or without food
  - o   Increased concentrations and risk of toxicity and bleeding is possible if the patient chews or breaks open the capsules
  - o   Vitamin E, Omega-3 fatty acids, gingko, garlic, ginseng, turmeric, and fish oil supplements have been purported to have antiplatelet type activity which in theory could increase the risk of bleed – clinical significance is questionable; the most common resolution is to discontinue the supplements if they are not necessary
  - o   Alcohol may have an additive antiplatelet type effect and increase the risk of GI bleed

Dacarbazine (DTIC, DIC)
- Class: Oncology agent, alkylating agent

- Mechanism of Action: Prevents DNA cross-linking which ultimately prevents proliferation and growth of cells
- Common Uses: Treatment of metastatic cancers
- Memorable Side Effects: Hair loss, nausea, vomiting, weight loss, myelosuppression, thrombocytopenia, hepatotoxicity, infertility
- Clinical Pearls:
  - Boxed warning for the risk of myelosuppression, liver toxicity and its carcinogenic and infertility activity
- Monitoring: CBC, LFTs
- Drug and Diet Considerations:
  - High incidence of nausea and vomiting may increase the risk for weight loss and nutritional deficiencies
  - Avoid large meals with emetogenic foods prior to infusion

Danazol (Danocrine)

- Class: Androgen
- Mechanism of Action: As an androgen, it blocks pituitary release of FSH and LH
- Common Uses: Treatment of endometriosis and prophylaxis of hereditary angioedema
- Memorable Side Effects: Acne, amenorrhea, cardiovascular risks, hypertension, elevated lipids, weight gain, decreased libido, hepatitis
- Clinical Pearls:
  - Fetal risks: boxed warning in pregnancy
  - Boxed warning for hepatotoxicity, intracranial hypertension, and blood clot risk
- Monitoring: LFTs, CBC, lipids, blood pressure
- Drug and Diet Considerations:
  - Monitor weight changes
  - Assess need for lipid-friendly diet due to the risk for hypercholesterolemia
  - Foods with high fat content may increase absorption

Dapagliflozin (Farxiga)

- Class: Antidiabetic, SGLT-2 inhibitor
- Mechanism of Action: By inhibiting the sodium–glucose co-transporter 2, this results in an increase in glucose excretion through the urine and lowering of blood sugar
- Common Uses: Diabetes management and an adjunct medication in heart failure
- Memorable Side Effects: Dehydration (high risk in patients taking diuretics or reduced fluid intake), increased risk for urinary tract infections and fungal infections, like candidiasis, and potential drop in blood pressure
- Clinical Pearls:
  - Caution in patients with a urinary infection history (drug increases sugar to the urine which can feed the organism)
  - Monitor K+; hyperkalemia risk especially in patients on ACE, ARB, potassium supplements, or those with a high potassium diet
  - Rarely can increase the risk for ketoacidosis
  - Hypoglycemia risk not as bad as with sulfonylureas
  - Caution on an increase in bone fracture risk
  - Hypotension, volume depletion risk, dehydration

- o Contraindicated in eGFR <30 (remember these drugs work in the kidney)
- Monitoring: Renal function, potassium, blood pressure, blood sugar, HbA1c
- Drug and Diet Considerations:
  - o Be cautious and monitor potassium closely in patients with high dietary intake of potassium as this could contribute to hyperkalemia in combination with this medication
  - o Monitor fluid intake; this medication can increase the risk for dehydration
  - o Patient should have an appropriate diabetes education if taking this medication
  - o Administer with or without food

Dapsone
- Class: Antibiotic
- Mechanism of Action: Blocks para-aminobenzoid acid which is necessary for bacterial production of folic acid
- Common Uses: Treatment of leprosy, dermatitis herpetiformis, idiopathic thrombocytopenic purpura, and PCP prophylaxis
- Memorable Side Effects: Hemoglobin reduction, hemolysis, agranulocytosis, skin reactions, GI upset, neuropathy
- Clinical Pearls:
  - o Patients with a sulfa allergy may have cross reactivity to this medication
- Monitoring: CBC, LFTs, blood sugar in diabetic patients, G6PD deficiency risk
- Drug and Diet Considerations:
  - o May give with food if stomach upset occurs

Daptomycin (Cubicin)
- Class: Antibiotic, cyclic lipopeptide
- Mechanism of Action: Inhibits synthesis of DNA, RNA, and protein by causing bacterial cell depolarization
- Common Uses: Provides gram positive coverage and MRSA coverage to treat bacterial infections
- Memorable Side Effects: Myalgia, rhabdomyolysis, CPK elevation, neuropathy, eosinophilic pneumonia
- Clinical Pearls:
  - o Higher risk of myopathy/muscle pain if previously on statin, if possible avoid using together
  - o Do not use in pneumonia as drug is inactivated by lung surfactants
- Monitoring: CPK, renal function
- Drug and Diet Considerations:
  - o No major concerns

Darafenacin (Enablex)
- Class: Bladder anticholinergic
- Mechanism of Action: Blocks muscarinic receptors (anticholinergic medication) in the bladder which increases urine volume in the bladder and potentially decreases frequency/urge

- Common Uses: Treatment of overactive bladder and bladder spasms
- Memorable Side Effects: Anticholinergic effects possible: dry mouth, dry eyes, urinary retention and constipation
- Clinical Pearls:
  - Anticholinergic effects
  - Solifenacin is less likely to cause anticholinergic effects than older bladder agents like oxybutynin as it is more selective for the bladder
  - Long acting product available, nice for once daily dosing
  - Be sure to assess if the medication is working for incontinence/frequency
  - Keep an eye out for patients on diuretics; if frequency is the major issue, make sure that diuretics are at the minimum effective dose (not always possible to reduce diuretics with CHF history)
  - Frequency can be especially problematic in patients who have an active social life as well as night when trying to sleep
- Monitoring: LFTs as clinically indicated
- Drug and Diet Considerations:
  - Slows the motility of the GI tract which could increase the risk for constipation; maintain adequate fluids and non-constipating diet
  - If GI upset occurs, there are no issues in giving the drug with food
  - Dry mouth may increase thirst and alter taste/pleasure of food
  - Grapefruit juice may increase concentrations

Darbepoetin alfa (Aranesp)
- Class: Erythropoiesis stimulating agent (ESA)
- Mechanism of Action: Stimulates the production of red blood cells; mimics the body's natural erythropoietin which is produced by the kidney
- Common Uses: Treatment of anemia from CKD and from chemotherapy/cancer
- Memorable Side Effects: Hypertension, GI, injection site reaction, increase clot risk (boxed warning)
- Clinical Pearls:
  - Injection only
  - Lack of iron stores may inhibit response
  - Monitor hemoglobin/hematocrit for response (should increase)
  - Risk of hypertension
  - There should be hold parameters in place if hemoglobin gets too high
  - Longer acting form of erythropoietin; advantage of less frequent dosing
  - Important boxed warning on increased risk of MI, stroke, blood clots
- Monitoring: Hemoglobin typically needs to be monitored frequently to assess response, iron stores, blood pressure
- Drug and Diet Considerations:
  - Iron has to be assessed and monitored as iron deficiency is one of the most common causes of treatment failure/non-response

Darunavir (Prezista)
- Class: Protease inhibitor, antiretroviral
- Mechanism of Action: Binds to site where protein cleavage occurs and prevents protease from releasing essential proteins

90

- Common Uses: HIV treatment
- Memorable Side Effects: Buffalo hump, fat redistribution, metabolic effects like increased cholesterol and hyperglycemia, hepatotoxicity, skin reaction, nausea, vomiting, diarrhea
- Clinical Pearls:
  - Metabolic risks are a significant downside to long term use in younger populations
  - Numerous drug interactions through CYP3A4
  - Typically dose with a booster (ritonavir)
- Monitoring: Lipids, glucose, HIV parameters (i.e. viral load and CD4 count), LFTs
- Drug and Diet Considerations:
  - Monitor hyperglycemia risk and may need to adjust diet accordingly
  - Lipid-lowering diet could help reduce the adverse effect of hypercholesterolemia
  - Take with food to maximize absorption

Daunorubicin (Cerubidine)
- Class: Oncology agent, anthracycline
- Mechanism of Action: Inhibits DNA/RNA synthesis by inhibiting topoisomerase 2; leads to blockade of intercalation of DNA base pairs
- Common Uses: Treatment of numerous types of cancers
- Memorable Side Effects: Cardiotoxicity, nausea and vomiting, hair loss, anemia, stomatitis, neutropenia, thrombocytopenia diarrhea, elevated uric acid, change in urine color
- Clinical Pearls:
  - Dexrazoxane and/or beta-blockers may help with cardiotoxicity complication
  - IV agent only
  - Extravasation risk
- Monitoring: CBC, LFTs, renal function, electrolytes, uric acid (as clinically indicated) blood sugar in diabetic patients, EKG
- Drug and Diet Considerations:
  - Monitor for adequate hydration particularly if the patient has diarrhea and vomiting or excessive fluid loss
  - Weight loss and poor nutrition may be a result of nausea, vomiting or stomatitis adverse effects
  - Blood sugar fluctuations may happen in diabetes patients

Denosumab (Prolia)
- Class: Anti-osteoporosis agent, bone-modifying agent
- Mechanism of Action: Monoclonal antibody that targets RANKL and prevents activation of RANK which is important in activating the action of osteoclasts; thus reducing bone resorption and increasing bone strength
- Common Uses: Osteoporosis treatment
- Memorable Side Effects: Low calcium, muscle pain, injection pain, weakness
- Clinical Pearls:
  - Alternative to bisphosphonates particularly in the situation where oral bisphosphonates and not tolerated due to GI issues
  - Twice yearly injection

- o More expensive than oral bisphosphonates
- Monitoring: Bone mineral density, calcium, vitamin D levels, magnesium, phosphorus, renal function
- Drug and Diet Considerations:
  - o Ensure the patient has adequate vitamin D and calcium intake – at least 1,200 mg per day of calcium and 1,000 units (25 mcg) of vitamin D in females with osteoporosis

Desipramine (Norpramin)

- Class: Tri-cyclic antidepressant (TCA)
- Mechanism of Action: – Inhibits reuptake of serotonin and possibly norepinephrine
- Common Uses: Depression, neuropathy, pain syndromes, anxiety, PTSD and bulimia
- Memorable Side Effects: Constipation, dry eyes, dry mouth, urinary retention, sedation, confusion, fall risk in elderly, hypotension
- Clinical Pearls:
  - o Old TCA generally not recommended in the elderly due to anticholinergic effects
  - o Highly anticholinergic (can't spit, see, pee, or sh*t and increases confusion/fall risk) which can be especially problematic in geriatric patients – avoid if possible
  - o In addition, cognitive impairment is not a good thing in the elderly due to possibility of preexisting dementia
  - o TCAs may have some benefit in neuropathy, generally much cheaper than SNRIs, like duloxetine, which can be also beneficial in neuropathy
  - o Not a good first line choice for sleep or depression (other agents exist that are much safer)
  - o Look out for TCAs causing the prescribing cascade! Artificial tears for dry eyes, constipation medications, BPH medications like tamsulosin, dementia medications, or artificial saliva
  - o Often dosed in the evening due to the adverse effect of sedation
- Monitoring: EKG, and possibly electrolytes, in at risk patients (especially in overdose), behavioral changes, weight, sodium (in patients with signs of hyponatremia),
- Drug and Diet Considerations:
  - o Slows the motility of the GI tract which could increase the risk for constipation, maintain adequate fluids and non-constipating diet
  - o If GI upset occurs, no issues in giving the drug with food
  - o Dry mouth may increase thirst and alter taste/pleasure of food
  - o Poor intake may place the patient at higher risk for QTc complications from electrolyte abnormalities (i.e. hyponatremia, hypokalemia, or hypomagnesemia)
  - o Alcohol may exacerbate sedative adverse effect

Desmopressin (DDAVP, Nocdurna)

- Class: Vasopressin analog
- Mechanism of Action: Acts as antidiuretic hormone which ultimately leads to reabsorption of water and reduced urine volume; it can also increase von Willebrand factor which can help reduce bleeding time

- Common Uses: Treatment of nocturia, diabetes insipidus and Von Willebrand disease
- Memorable Side Effects: Hyponatremia, dry mouth, weight gain, edema, hypotension (IV)
- Clinical Pearls:
    o Boxed warning for life-threatening hyponatremia
    o Multiple different dosages forms; oral, nasal, sublingual, injectable
- Monitoring: Sodium and other electrolytes, renal function, blood pressure (IV)
- Drug and Diet Considerations:
    o Fluid/water intoxication is possible and fluid intake may need to be reduced
    o Assess sodium intake and levels to ensure avoidance of hyponatremia

Dexlansoprazole (Dexilant)
- Class: Proton pump inhibitor (PPI)
- Mechanism of Action: Inhibits proton pumps in the stomach leading to a less acidic environment
- Common Uses: Treatment of GERD, ulcers and Barrett's esophagus
- Memorable Side Effects: Usually pretty well tolerated; Long term use: increased fracture risk, decrease B12 levels, C. diff risk, low magnesium
- Clinical Pearls:
    o PPIs are the most potent acid blocker on the market
    o For some patients PPIs may not work very quickly; it might take a few days for maximal effect
    o For the above reason, as needed (PRN) PPIs can possibly be effective, but are generally not used
    o Use short term if possible due to increased risk of osteoporosis, C. Diff, low magnesium, and B12 deficiency if used long term
    o Barrett's esophagus, high risk GI medications (i.e. NSAIDs, prednisone), or chronic GI bleed are examples where patients may require indefinite therapy
    o If GI bleed is problematic, monitoring hemoglobin and/or hemoccult (blood in the stool) might be appropriate to assess possible blood loss
- Monitoring: Magnesium (chronic use), B12
- Drug and Diet Considerations:
    o When it is used chronically, it is a possible cause or contributing factor to B12 and magnesium deficiency
    o PPIs are typically best given about 30 minutes before a meal
    o Reduced stomach acid (high pH) may impair the absorption of iron supplements

Dexmethylphenidate (Focalin)
- Class: CNS stimulant
- Mechanism of Action: Blocks reuptake of norepinephrine and dopamine leading to CNS stimulation; by blocking reuptake, you end up with more norepinephrine and dopamine in the synapse leading to more activity
- Common Uses: Management of ADHD symptoms and off label use for depression/fatigue

- Memorable Side Effects: Anxiety, insomnia, poor appetite, weight loss, hypertension, tachycardia, emotional lability
- Clinical Pearls:
  - Remembering that this medication ramps you up will help you remember its side effects: anxiety, insomnia, weight loss, poor appetite, increased BP, and increased pulse
  - When used in pediatrics, poor appetite can be a significant problem and should be assessed
  - Elevated BP and pulse monitoring important
  - Be cautious in adult patients who may have cardiovascular risks
  - Schedule 2 controlled substance, highly addictive
- Monitoring: Blood pressure, pulse, weight, cardiac monitoring (in patients with preexisting cardiac condition or at risk for cardiac complications) and growth in pediatric patients
- Drug and Diet Considerations:
  - Food should have minimal impact on overall effectiveness, with or without food is ok
  - Use caution with other foods/supplements that may have additive effects to heart rate, blood pressure, and insomnia (i.e. caffeine)
  - Vitamin C may reduce the effectiveness by acidifying the urine which can enhance renal elimination of the drug; usually not clinically significant, but often we can discontinue the vitamin C supplement in patients who have adequate intake through food sources
  - Assessing appetite and the risk for anorexia is important
  - Caffeine may increase stimulant effects

Dextromethorphan (Delsym, Robitussin DM, Triaminic, and Numerous Other OTC Names)

- Class: Antitussive
- Mechanism of Action: Reduces coughing by suppressing the medullary cough reflex
- Common Uses: Cough suppressant
- Memorable Side Effects: Usually pretty well tolerated, GI effects are possible, CNS effects (rare)
- Clinical Pearls:
  - It is very important to identify why patient is coughing (especially if the symptoms are chronic)
  - If coughing has been going on a long time be sure patients get assessed
  - ACE inhibitors are classic cause of drug induced cough
  - An atypical cause of cough that won't resolve is heartburn or GERD, especially in elderly or young
  - Asthma is another potential cause of chronic cough
  - Has been associated with drug misuse/abuse
- Monitoring: No lab work necessary
- Drug and Diet Considerations
  - Some formulations may contain sugar, alcohol, and/or sodium

Diazepam (Valium)

- Class: Antianxiety, antiepileptic

- Mechanism of Action: Enhances activity of GABA, an inhibitory neurotransmitter that causes sedation
- Common Uses: Treatment of anxiety, muscle spasms, seizures and insomnia
- Memorable Side Effects: Sedation, confusion, fall risk, dizziness
- Clinical Pearls:
  - The best way I remember benzodiazepines is that they are very close to "alcohol in a pill"
  - Diazepam specifically has a long half-life in the elderly, so significant potential for accumulation of the drug exists when used in the elderly
  - Sedation, slurred speech, trouble walking (ataxia), etc. are all common with benzos/alcohol; they are also commonly used in alcohol withdrawal
  - Be cautious with patients on higher doses of benzodiazepines to make sure they aren't abruptly stopped
  - Educate patients on driving/operating machinery (remember that benzodiazepines are often used for sleep as well as anxiety)
  - Unlike SSRIs for anxiety, a great advantage of benzos are that they work quickly and can be used as needed
  - Falls in the elderly is a big downside to using these medications
  - Benzos are a controlled substance, they can cause addiction and dependence
  - Rectal/injectable formulation can be used in acute treatment of seizures
  - Flumazenil is antidote in overdose
- Monitoring: Routine lab monitoring typically isn't necessary unless clinically indicated
- Drug and Diet Considerations:
  - Alcohol intake can have additive side effects of sedation, confusion, slurred speech, and other CNS depressant effects
  - Grapefruit juice may increase drug levels and the risk for adverse effects

Diclofenac (Voltaren)
- Class: NSAID, analgesic
- Mechanism of Action: Inhibits Cyclooxygenase-1 and 2 (COX-1 and COX-2); results in a reduction in prostaglandins which cause pain, fever, inflammation
- Common Uses: Management of pain, fever and inflammation
- Memorable Side Effects: GI ulcer, worsening kidney function, edema, hypertension, inhibits platelets (can exacerbate bleed risk)
- Clinical Pearls:
  - NSAIDs are one of the most common causes of GI bleeding; this risk increases in the elderly and those on medications that increase risk of bleeding (anticoagulants and antiplatelet medications)
  - Due to effects on platelets, NSAIDs are typically held before/after surgery to reduce the risk of bleeding
  - NSAIDs can contribute to edema and exacerbate CHF (congestive heart failure); be on the lookout and have NSAIDs reassessed if you see a patient with a CHF exacerbation or a patient requiring increasing diuretics, like furosemide

- o NSAIDs can cause worsening kidney function (creatinine should be monitored); this risk can be greatly increased in patients on ACE inhibitors or ARBs and/or diuretic type medications
- o Due to above reasons of kidney function, GI bleed risk, and CHF, NSAIDs are not the safest medication in the elderly
- o Although generally considered riskier in the elderly, a big advantage of NSAIDs over acetaminophen is that they can reduce inflammation
- o Pregnancy category C/D when >30 weeks gestation; NSAIDs are generally avoided in pregnancy and especially after 30 weeks gestation
- Monitoring: Renal function, hemoglobin, platelets (contained within CBC), blood pressure, signs of bruising or bleeding, weight (risk for edema)
- Drug and Diet Considerations:
  - o Because of significant incidence of GI upset, it is recommended to give with food or milk
  - o Dehydration may exacerbate the risk for acute renal failure
  - o Excessive alcohol may increase GI bleed risk
  - o Vitamin E, Omega-3 fatty acids, gingko, garlic, ginseng, turmeric, and fish oil supplements have been purported to have antiplatelet type activity which in theory could increase the risk of bleed – clinical significance is questionable; the most common resolution is to discontinue the supplements if they are not necessary

Dicloxacillin

- Class: Antibiotic, penicillin
- Mechanism of Action: Inhibits bacterial cell wall formation
- Common Uses: Treatment of susceptible Staphylococcus and Streptococcus skin infections
- Memorable Side Effects: GI side effects most common, allergy, rash
- Clinical Pearls:
  - o Many patients have an allergy to penicillin; dicloxacillin is from the same class and should not be used in patients with a severe allergy (if it is an intolerance like stomach upset, it may be prudent to try a "penicillin" type antibiotic again depending upon the patient's situation)
  - o Diarrhea and GI upset are going to be the major/common side effects with penicillin antibiotics; with mild GI upset and/or diarrhea, hopefully the patient can continue therapy
  - o We are going to want to monitor the response of the patient, hopefully they will begin feeling better by day 2 or 3 of treatment
  - o Temperature would be an important thing to monitor for patients who were significantly febrile
- Monitoring: Signs of infection improvement (i.e. fever and symptoms), rash, lab work is typically not necessary with short term use; CBC, renal function, and ALT might be considered for longer term therapy
- Drug and Diet Considerations:
  - o Should be given 1 hour before or 2 hours after meals which makes it less desirable to use compared to amoxicillin

Dicyclomine (Bentyl)

- Class: GI antispasmodic, anticholinergic

- Mechanism of Action: Blocks acetylcholine receptors
- Common Uses: Treatment of irritable bowel syndrome
- Memorable Side Effects: Anticholinergic effects (can't spit, see, pee or poop)
- Clinical Pearls:
  - Primary use is to help relieve GI spasms/pain due to irritable bowel syndrome
  - Anticholinergic (slows the GI tract and decreases spasms) side effects can be prominent especially in the elderly population
  - Usually dosed multiple times throughout the day
  - If diarrhea is an issue associated with a patient's IBS, the anticholinergic effect of constipation can contribute to the patient's benefit
- Monitoring: No routine lab work is recommended
- Drug and Diet Considerations:
  - Alcohol can exacerbate the CNS depressant effect
  - The side effect of dry mouth could affect eating habits
  - Administering with a meal may increase the percentage of the drug that is absorbed; pay attention to increased effects of cyclobenzaprine if it is given with food

Diflunisal (Dolobid)

- Class: NSAID, antipyretic, analgesic
- Mechanism of Action: Inhibits cyclooxygenase-1 and 2 (COX-1 and COX-2); results in a reduction in prostaglandins which cause pain, fever, inflammation
- Common Uses: Reduction of pain, fever and inflammation
- Memorable Side Effects: GI ulcer, worsening kidney function, edema, hypertension, inhibits platelets (can exacerbate bleed risk)
- Clinical Pearls:
  - NSAIDs are one of the most common causes of GI bleeding; this risk increases in the elderly and those on medications that increase risk of bleeding (anticoagulants and antiplatelet medications)
  - Because of the side effects of GI upset/bleeding, NSAIDs should be taken with food
  - Ibuprofen does have a relatively shorter half-life compared to other NSAIDs and usually needs to be dosed more frequently
  - Due to effects on platelets, NSAIDs are typically held before/after surgery to reduce the risk of bleeding
  - NSAIDs can contribute to edema and exacerbate CHF (congestive heart failure); be on the lookout and have NSAIDs reassessed if you see a patient with a CHF exacerbation or a patient requiring increasing diuretics, like furosemide
  - NSAIDs can cause worsening kidney function (creatinine should be monitored); this risk can be greatly increased in patients on ACE inhibitors or ARBs and/or diuretic type medications
  - Due to above reasons on kidney function, GI bleed risk, and CHF, NSAIDs are not the safest medication in the elderly (acetaminophen is generally preferred for generalized pain with a few exceptions)
  - Although generally considered riskier in the elderly, a big advantage of NSAIDs over acetaminophen is that they can reduce inflammation

- o Pregnancy category C/D when >30 weeks gestation; NSAIDs are generally avoided in pregnancy and especially after 30 weeks gestation
- Monitoring: Renal function, hemoglobin, platelets (contained within CBC), blood pressure, signs of bruising or bleeding, weight (risk for edema)
- Drug and Diet Considerations:
  - o Because of significant incidence of GI upset, it is recommended to give with food or milk
  - o Dehydration coupled with NSAIDs may increase the risk for acute renal failure
  - o Excessive alcohol may increase GI bleed risk
  - o Vitamin E, Omega-3 fatty acids, gingko, garlic, ginseng, turmeric, and fish oil supplements have been purported to have antiplatelet type activity which in theory could increase the risk of bleed – clinical significance is questionable; the most common resolution is to discontinue the supplements if they are not necessary

Digoxin (Digitek, Lanoxin)

- Class: Antiarrhythmic, cardiac glycoside
- Mechanism of Action: Inhibition of sodium/potassium ATPase
- Common Uses: Treatment of atrial fibrillation and heart failure
- Memorable Side Effects: Nausea, vomiting, bradycardia, cognitive changes, weight loss, visual changes (usually at very high levels)
- Clinical Pearls:
  - o Classic symptoms of digoxin toxicity involve GI side effects, bradycardia, cognitive changes and weight loss
  - o Often providers will use hold parameters in healthcare settings to prevent pulse from going to low (i.e. hold digoxin if pulse is less than 60)
  - o Digoxin is cleared by the kidney; it can accumulate and be much more likely to cause toxicity in the elderly as patients tend to have worse kidney function as they age
  - o Higher doses are usually used in atrial fibrillation as compared to heart failure
  - o Upper limit of normal for a digoxin level is considered 2 ng/mL
  - o Patients with low levels of potassium are at greater risk of toxicity, it is really important to assess potassium as many patients on digoxin may also be on diuretics (usually for heart failure) that can deplete potassium
- Monitoring: Electrolytes (potassium, magnesium, and calcium are the most critical), renal function, pulse, EKG
- Drug and Diet Considerations:
  - o Consistency is key with administration so the dose can be adjusted accordingly; take the same time and the same way every day
  - o Fiber, pectin, and large meals would be more likely to reduce the absorption of the drug and lower concentrations
  - o Low potassium and/or magnesium levels could increase the risk for toxicity – note substantial diet changes, monitor levels, and notify prescriber as appropriate
  - o Elevated calcium levels may increase the risk of digoxin toxicity; most likely caused by unusually high intake of vitamin D and/or calcium supplements

Dihydroergotamine (DHE, Migranal, "ergotamine")

- Class: Anti-migraine, ergot derivative
- Mechanism of Action: Serotonin 5HT agonist – which causes vasoconstriction and also reduces pro-inflammatory neuropeptide activity
- Common Uses: Acute relief of migraine
- Memorable Side Effects: Dizziness, GI upset, runny nose (nasal administration), hypertension
- Clinical Pearls:
    - Cardiovascular complications limit its use compared to triptans
    - Nasal and IV administration routes
    - Significant risk for CYP3A4 drug interactions
    - Avoid in pregnancy
- Monitoring: Blood pressure
- Drug and Diet Considerations:
    - Given as needed for migraine, so administration at any point is fine with regards to food

Diltiazem (Cardizem CD, Cartia XT)

- Class: Calcium channel blocker (non-dihydropyridine), antiarrhythmic
- Mechanism of Action: Blocks calcium channels resulting in vasodilation and cardiac relaxation
- Common Uses: Treatment of atrial fibrillation and hypertension
- Memorable Side Effects: Low pulse, low BP, constipation, edema
- Clinical Pearls:
    - Very important distinction: verapamil and diltiazem (non-dihydropyridines) are the calcium channel blockers that act on the heart AND blood vessels; you will not see amlodipine and nifedipine used in atrial fibrillation, because their activity is primarily on the vessels. This also means that pulse monitoring will not be necessary with nifedipine and amlodipine
    - The higher you push the dose on these medications, the more likely you will see the side effect of edema; keep an eye out for new diuretic prescriptions to treat the edema caused by the calcium channel blockers
    - Simvastatin is a common medication that interacts with diltiazem
    - Diltiazem comes in several different formulations (long acting, short acting, etc.), make sure you have the right one
- Monitoring: Blood pressure, pulse, EKG
- Drug and Diet Considerations:
    - Grapefruit juice can increase concentrations of the drug
    - St. John's wort can lower concentrations of diltiazem
    - Standard calcium supplementation typically will not impact the effectiveness of diltiazem; excessive doses of calcium may have a higher likelihood of blunting the effects of the drug

Dimenhydrinate (Dramamine)

- Class: Antihistamine, anticholinergic
- Mechanism of Action: Blocks muscarinic (anticholinergic) receptors and also has antihistamine effects
- Common Uses: Prevention of motion sickness

- Memorable Side Effects: Anticholinergic effects such as dry mouth, dry eyes, urinary retention, constipation, sedation, confusion
- Clinical Pearls:
    - Avoid, minimize use in geriatric patients
    - May have paradoxical insomnia reaction in pediatrics
- Monitoring: No routine lab work is typically necessary
- Drug and Diet Considerations:
    - Slows the motility of the GI tract which could increase the risk for constipation; maintain adequate fluids and non-constipating diet
    - Alcohol may exacerbate CNS depressant effects
    - Dry mouth may increase thirst and alter taste/pleasure of food
    - May be given with or without food

Diphenhydramine (Benadryl)

- Class: Antihistamine, anticholinergic
- Mechanism of Action: Blocks muscarinic (anticholinergic) receptors and also has antihistamine effects
- Common Uses: Management of symptoms associated with insomnia, allergies, allergic reaction, itching and motion sickness
- Memorable Side Effects: Anticholinergic effects such as dry mouth, dry eyes, urinary retention, constipation, sedation, confusion
- Clinical Pearls:
    - Highly anticholinergic (can't spit, see, pee, or sh*t and increases confusion/fall risk) which can be especially problematic in geriatric patients – avoid if possible
    - May have paradoxical insomnia reaction in pediatrics
- Monitoring: No routine lab work is typically necessary
- Drug and Diet Considerations:
    - Slows the motility of the GI tract which could increase the risk for constipation; maintain adequate fluids and non-constipating diet
    - Alcohol may exacerbate CNS depressant effects
    - Dry mouth may increase thirst and alter taste/pleasure of food
    - May be given with or without food

Diphenoxylate/atropine (Lomotil)

- Class: Antidiarrheal
- Mechanism of Action: Diphenoxylate inhibits GI motility, atropine is highly anticholinergic
- Common Uses: Treatment of diarrhea
- Memorable Side Effects: Well tolerated - abdominal distress, possible anticholinergic effects, but not likely as atropine dose is very low
- Clinical Pearls:
    - Controlled substance
    - Can be used as needed
    - Be sure patients who are on this chronically have been assessed for medical and possible medication concerns for chronic diarrhea
- Monitoring: Bowel movement frequency
- Drug and Diet Considerations:
    - Assess benefit of medication and if the patient continues to have diarrhea concerns, monitor fluid and electrolytes

- o Diphenoxylate can have mild CNS depressant effects that could be synergistic with alcohol (typically not at standard, approved dosages)

Disulfiram (Antabuse)
- Class: Aldehyde dehydrogenase inhibitor
- Mechanism of Action: By inhibiting aldehyde dehydrogenase, this drug prevents oxidation and ultimately causes a buildup of acetaldehyde; acetaldehyde can cause flushing, headache, and GI upset
- Common Uses: Alcohol use disorder
- Memorable Side Effects: Disulfiram reaction as noted above if used with alcohol, sedation, taste disturbances (bitter), hepatic impairment (rare)
- Clinical Pearls:
    - o Even relatively small amounts of alcohol which may be found in some liquid formulations of medications can cause this reaction
    - o Patients may stop taking this medication if they know they are going to drink
- Monitoring: LFTs, CBC
- Drug and Diet Considerations:
    - o Avoid if the patient has recently used alcohol; wait at least 12 hours from last intake
    - o Educate patient they must avoid any products that may have even small quantities of alcohol (vinegars, ciders, extracts, etc.)

Divalproex (Valproic Acid, Depakote)
- Class: Antiepileptic, mood stabilizer
- Mechanism of Action: Increases GABA (inhibitory neurotransmitter)
- Common Uses: Treatment of seizures, bipolar disorder and migraine prophylaxis
- Memorable Side Effects: Sedation, dizziness, N/V/stomach pain, hair loss – lots of rare side effects: possible effects on platelets, ammonia levels, LFTs, CBC alterations
- Clinical Pearls:
    - o Checking drug levels usually not as important when using for mood or headaches (compared to seizures), unless trying to rule out toxicity
    - o Frequent dosing - 2 or 3 times per day
    - o Critical to ensure patient adherence; especially for seizures
    - o If using for seizures, be sure to have the patient assessed for meds that lower seizure threshold (bupropion and tramadol are classic examples)
    - o Does have some drug interactions (i.e. lamotrigine)
    - o Pregnancy category X
- Monitoring: Ammonia (if they have signs of confusion or CNS changes), LFTs, CBC (platelets included), drug levels if signs of toxicity (or depending upon indication), weight
- Drug and Diet Considerations:
    - o GI upset can occur with significant frequency in some patients – ok to administer with food
    - o Depakote sprinkle capsule may be opened and given with applesauce or pudding in patients who cannot swallow pills

101

- o Alcohol could contribute to CNS depressant effect as well as have synergistic negative effects on the liver
- o Weight gain has been reported with valproic acid

Docetaxel (Taxotere, Docefrez)
- Class: Oncology agent, Taxane
- Mechanism of Action: Stimulates tubulin dimers, interferes with the M phase and ultimately blocks necessary DNA, RNA, and protein synthesis
- Common Uses: Treatment of numerous types of cancers
- Memorable Side Effects: Edema, neuropathy, CNS toxicity, muscle soreness, stomatitis, nausea, vomiting, diarrhea, myelosuppression, hair loss, hypersensitivity reactions
- Clinical Pearls:
  - o Fluid retention is one of the most common complications with this medication
  - o Pre-medicate with dexamethasone to reduce the risk of hypersensitivity reactions
- Monitoring: Weight due to risk of fluid retention, CBC, LFTs, renal function, vital signs with infusion
- Drug and Diet Considerations:
  - o Weight loss and poor nutrition may result on account of nausea, vomiting, and stomatitis adverse effects
  - o Weight gain may occur on account of fluid retention
  - o Certain IV formulations may contain alcohol

Dolutegravir (Isentress)
- Class: Integrase inhibitor, antiretroviral
- Mechanism of Action: Inhibits the viral enzyme integrase by binding enzyme cations and preventing viral DNA integration into the host genome
- Common Uses: HIV treatment
- Memorable Side Effects: Usually well tolerated, elevated LFTs, skin reaction risk/SJS (rare, but possible), CNS changes, GI adverse effects, CPK increase/myopathy
- Clinical Pearls:
  - o Generally preferred now in place of protease inhibitors as they have less drug interactions and seem to be better tolerated
  - o Typically included in healthcare associated post-exposure prophylaxis (PEP) regimens
- Monitoring: LFTs, HIV levels, CD4 count, Hepatitis B testing prior to initiation, CPK and lipids as clinically indicated
- Drug and Diet Considerations:
  - o May be given without regard to food
  - o Monitor blood glucose in patients with diabetes and adjust diet accordingly (usually only a modest increase if there is one)
  - o Some of the ingredients in multivitamins, supplements, or antacids, (calcium, magnesium, or iron) may block absorption, take dolutegravir 2 hours before and or 6 hours after

Donepezil (Aricept)
- Class: Dementia agent, acetylcholinesterase inhibitor

- Mechanism of Action: Inhibits acetylcholinesterase which increases acetylcholine in the CNS
- Common Uses: Treatment of Alzheimer's dementia
- Memorable Side Effects: GI (N/V/D), weight loss, insomnia, bradycardia
- Clinical Pearls:
  - One of the more common drug causes of weight loss in the elderly
  - Will NOT reverse dementia, but may help with some symptom improvement
  - Dementia medications in general can contribute to behavioral changes (good or bad)
- Monitoring: Weight, GI adverse effects, pulse
- Drug and Diet Considerations:
  - Significant cause of weight loss and poor appetite
  - Assess for GI upset and loose stools
  - Typically dosed at night with or without food (to minimize GI risk) even though there is a small possibility for insomnia

Dopamine

- Class: Adrenergic agonist
- Mechanism of Action: Stimulates adrenergic and dopamine receptors
- Common Uses: Treatment of shock caused by heart failure
- Memorable Side Effects: BP, pulse changes, N/V, arrhythmia
- Clinical Pearls:
  - At low doses may actually cause renal vasodilation
  - At higher doses more likely to act like epinephrine (stimulates heart and vasoconstriction to increase pulse and BP)
- Monitoring: Blood pressure, heart rate, cardiac status, renal function, EKG, blood glucose
- Drug and Diet Considerations:
  - Volume replacement and norepinephrine may be appropriate before this agent is used depending upon clinical circumstances
  - Likely to be used as a short term IV agent, typically no concerns with diet/nutrition

Doripenem (Doribax)

- Class: Carbapenem, antibiotic
- Mechanism of Action: Binds penicillin-binding proteins and inhibits production of the bacterial cell wall; cilastatin blocks elimination of the drug by inhibiting dehydropeptidase in the renal tubules
- Common Uses: Broad spectrum antibiotic used in many resistant, severe infections (i.e. complicated UTIs involving resistant organisms)
- Memorable Side Effects: Infusion reaction, diarrhea, GI upset, lowers seizure threshold
- Clinical Pearls:
  - Usually reserved for very severe, resistant infections
  - Good coverage for gram negatives
    - Generally they do not cover MRSA or VRE
- Monitoring: Renal function, CBC, LFTs (as clinically indicated)
- Drug and Diet Considerations:
  - Minimal concerns with short term use

103

- o Monitor fluid and electrolyte status if diarrhea is problematic

Doxazosin (Cardura)
- Class: Alpha blocker, antihypertensive
- Mechanism of Action: Blocks alpha receptors causing smooth muscle relaxation, vasodilation and opening of the ureter
- Common Uses: Treatment of BPH, urinary obstruction and hypertension
- Memorable Side Effects: Low BP, dizziness
- Clinical Pearls:
  - o Non-selective alpha blocker, so can be used for both hypertension and BPH
  - o Risk of orthostasis is higher with a non-selective alpha blocker
  - o In the case of worsening urinary retention due to BPH and initiation of these agents, be sure to assess if your patient is on anticholinergic medications (diphenhydramine, TCAs, etc.)
  - o Usually dosed at night to minimize the risk of orthostasis
  - o Risk of floppy iris syndrome for those undergoing eye surgery
- Monitoring: Blood pressure
- Drug and Diet Considerations:
  - o Administer with or without food
  - o Grapefruit juice may increase concentrations

Doxepin (Sinequan, Silenor)
- Class: TCA, antidepressant
- Mechanism of Action: Inhibits reuptake of serotonin and possibly norepinephrine
- Common Uses: Treatment of depression, anxiety, insomnia and used topically to relieve itching
- Memorable Side Effects: Anticholinergic effects such as dry mouth, dry eyes, urinary retention, constipation, sedation, confusion
- Clinical Pearls:
  - o Generally avoid in the elderly due to the risk for anticholinergic adverse effects
  - o Not a good first line choice for sleep or depression; other agents exist that are much safer
- Monitoring: EKG, and possibly electrolytes in at risk patients (especially in overdose or patients who may be at risk for QTc prolongation), weight, sodium (in patients with signs of hyponatremia)
- Drug and Diet Considerations:
  - o Weight gain is possible and may be problematic
  - o Slows the motility of the GI tract which could increase the risk for constipation; maintain adequate fluids and non-constipating diet
  - o Food (particularly fatty foods) can increase bioavailability
  - o Dry mouth may increase thirst and alter taste/pleasure of food
  - o Poor dietary intake may place the patient at higher risk for complications from electrolyte abnormalities (i.e. hyponatremia, hypokalemia, or hypomagnesemia)

Doxorubicin (Adriamycin)
- Class: Oncology agent, anthracycline

- Mechanism of Action: Inhibits DNA/RNA synthesis by inhibiting topoisomerase 2; leads to blockade of intercalation of DNA base pairs
- Common Uses: Treatment of numerous types of cancers
- Memorable Side Effects: Cardiotoxicity, nausea and vomiting (very high risk when combined with cyclophosphamide), hair loss, anemia, stomatitis, neutropenia, thrombocytopenia diarrhea, elevated uric acid, change in urine color
- Clinical Pearls:
  - Dexrazoxane and/or beta-blockers may help with cardiotoxicity complication
  - IV agent only
  - Liposomal formulation of doxorubicin may have improved tolerability (less cardiac effects, myelosuppression, and hair loss toxicity), but may have a higher risk of hand-foot syndrome
  - Extravasation risk
- Monitoring: CBC, LFTs, renal function, electrolytes, uric acid (as clinically indicated) blood sugar in diabetic patients, EKG
- Drug and Diet Considerations:
  - Monitor for adequate hydration particularly if the patient has diarrhea and vomiting or excessive fluid loss
  - Weight loss and poor nutrition may result on account of nausea and vomiting or stomatitis adverse effect
  - Blood sugar fluctuations may happen in diabetes patients

Doxycycline (Vibramycin)

- Class: Tetracycline, antibiotic
- Mechanism of Action: Inhibits bacterial protein synthesis
- Common Uses: Often an alternative to penicillin antibiotics to treat skin infections, pneumonia, etc.
- Memorable Side Effects: GI side effects, photosensitivity (increased risk of sunburn), rash
- Clinical Pearls:
  - Can cause birth defects (category D)
  - It is from the tetracycline class, so if patients have a tetracycline allergy, it shouldn't be used
  - Can make patients more susceptible to sunburn
  - Possibility to cause tooth discoloration; usually long term use or multiple courses
- Monitoring: LFTs, renal function, and CBC (only in cases with clinical concerns or in long term therapy)
- Drug and Diet Considerations:
  - Avoid taking calcium, iron, magnesium, zinc, and antacids at the same time as doxycycline; take calcium 2 hours before or 4 hours after doxycycline to ensure adequate absorption
  - May give with meals if GI upset is a problem
  - Long term, chronic alcohol use may decrease drug concentrations
  - Meals with large amounts of dairy or high-fat may cause small reductions in concentrations

Doxylamine (OTC Sleep-Aid)

- Class: Antihistamine, anticholinergic

- Mechanism of Action: Blocks muscarinic (anticholinergic) receptors and also has antihistamine effects
- Common Uses: Treatment of insomnia, and prevention of motion sickness
- Memorable Side Effects: Anticholinergic effects such as dry mouth, dry eyes, urinary retention, constipation, sedation, confusion
- Clinical Pearls:
  - Avoid, minimize use in geriatric patients
  - Occasionally used for morning sickness in pregnancy
  - May have paradoxical insomnia reaction in pediatrics
- Monitoring: No routine lab work is typically necessary
- Drug and Diet Considerations:
  - Slows the motility of the GI tract which could increase the risk for constipation; maintain adequate fluids and non-constipating diet
  - Alcohol may exacerbate CNS depressant effects
  - Dry mouth may increase thirst and alter taste/pleasure of food
  - May be given with or without food

Dronabinol (Marinol)
- Class: Appetite stimulant, marijuana derivative
- Mechanism of Action: Stimulates cannabinoid (primarily CB1) receptors which can help improve appetite
- Common Uses: Improvement of poor appetite
- Memorable Side Effects: Sedation, confusion, euphoria, dizziness, may have modest effects on heart rate and blood pressure
- Clinical Pearls:
  - In addition to stimulating appetite, it can have antiemetic-type effects
  - Controlled substance that carries a risk of addiction and dependence
- Monitoring: Weight, blood pressure, heart rate
- Drug and Diet Considerations:
  - Typically dosed 30-60 minutes before meals
  - Large meals with a higher fat component may increase bioavailability but delay the peak

Dulaglutide (Trulicity)
- Class: Antidiabetic, GLP-1 agonist
- Mechanism of Action: Enhances glucose dependent insulin secretion, slows gastric emptying, and reduces post prandial glucagon to reduce blood sugars
- Common Uses: Management of type 2 diabetes
- Memorable Side Effects: Nausea, vomiting, hypoglycemia if taken in combination with insulin or sulfonylurea, pancreatitis concerns exist, but are rare
- Clinical Pearls:
  - Dosed once weekly
  - Boxed warning to avoid medication in certain types of thyroid tumors
  - Promotes fullness, weight loss can be a beneficial effect
  - Typically better in HbA1c reduction than most oral diabetes medications
- Monitoring: Blood sugar, HbA1c, renal function as clinically indicated
- Drug and Diet Considerations:
  - Can be administered without regard to meals

- o Reduces appetite which can be helpful in obese type 2 diabetes patients
- o Implementation of a diabetic diet

Duloxetine (Cymbalta)
- Class: SNRI, antidepressant
- Mechanism of Action: Selective serotonin and norepinephrine reuptake inhibitor (SNRI)
- Common Uses: Treatment of depression and relief of nerve pain due to diabetes, fibromyalgia
- Memorable Side Effects: GI side effects, can exacerbate hypertension (usually only at higher doses), CNS changes
- Clinical Pearls:
  - o Has effects on both serotonin and norepinephrine
  - o Duloxetine is indicated to help with pain syndromes as well depression; neuropathic pain in particular is where you will likely see it used most frequently
  - o GI and central nervous system side effects (CNS) are most common
  - o Decreased libido can be an issue for patients taking duloxetine
  - o Be careful with the risk of serotonin syndrome especially in patients on other serotonergic medications
- Monitoring: No routine lab work, but may check sodium, LFTs, blood pressure, or renal function if clinical concerns arise
- Drug and Diet Considerations:
  - o Can be given with or without food
  - o Adverse effects of nausea and dry mouth could impact nutrition, monitor if new concerns arise with initiation or dose escalation
  - o Capsule can be open and sprinkled in apple sauce

Dutasteride (Avodart)
- Class: 5-apha reductase inhibitor
- Mechanism of Action: Inhibits 5-alpha reductase which results in less dihydrotestosterone
- Common Uses: Treatment of BPH
- Memorable Side Effects: Impotence, weakness
- Clinical Pearls:
  - o Not for immediate relief of acute urinary retention due to BPH
  - o Takes weeks to months for clinical benefit
  - o Well tolerated, impotence is the most common side effect
  - o Keep an eye out for drugs, like anticholinergics, that exacerbate BPH
- Monitoring: Prostate specific antigen (PSA)
- Drug and Diet Considerations:
  - o Can be given with or without food
  - o Small increase in concentration is possible with grapefruit juice, but unlikely to be clinically significant

Edoxaban (Savaysa)
- Class: Anticoagulant

107

- Mechanism of Action: Inhibits clotting factor 10A
- Common Uses: Prevention of stroke in patients with atrial fibrillation, DVT/PE prophylaxis or treatment
- Memorable Side Effects: Bleeding
- Clinical Pearls:
  - Less risk of drug interaction versus warfarin
  - Patients do NOT need to do routine INRs compared to warfarin
  - With bleed risk being the major side effect, hemoglobin (CBC) is important to monitor
  - Should not be used in a patient with CrCl >95m/min
- Monitoring: CBC, renal function
- Drug and Diet Considerations:
  - Administer with or without food
  - Vitamin E, Omega-3 fatty acids, gingko, garlic, ginseng, turmeric, and fish oil supplements have been purported to have antiplatelet type activity which in theory could increase the risk of bleed – clinical significance is questionable; the most common resolution is to discontinue the supplements if they are not necessary
  - Alcohol may have an additive antiplatelet type effect and increase the risk of GI bleed

Efavirenz (Sustiva)
- Class: Antiretroviral, non-nucleoside reverse transcriptase inhibitor
- Mechanism of Action: They bind to a hydrophobic site of the HIV Reverse Transcriptase and inactivate it; active conversion to triphosphate forms is not required, like in NRTIs
- Common Uses: HIV treatment
- Memorable Side Effects: Hallucinations, psychiatric changes, abnormal dreams, hepatotoxicity, rash, lowers seizure threshold
- Clinical Pearls:
  - Rash will usually occur with the first few days/weeks of starting the medication
  - May contribute to QTc prolongation risks
  - Resistance risk may be high especially if this medication is used alone
- Monitoring: LFTs, lipid panel, HIV parameters
- Drug and Diet Considerations:
  - Given on an empty stomach at bedtime to minimize CNS adverse effects
  - Cushing's-type appearance may happen as a result of this medication; this can include obesity and buffalo hump complications
  - Recognize the risk for hypercholesterolemia and consider a lipid friendly diet and/or removing the agent
  - Alcohol may exacerbate CNS side effects; avoid use if possible
  - High fat meal may increase concentrations

Elbasvir/grazoprevir (Zepatier)
- Class: Hepatitis C antiviral, polymerase inhibitor
- Mechanism of Action: Elbasvir inhibition of NS5A which is a viral phosphoprotein necessary for replication, assembly, and viral secretion; grazoprevir inhibits HCV NS3/4A protease

108

- Common Uses: Treatment of hepatitis C
- Memorable Side Effects: Fatigue, headache, increase in LFTs
- Clinical Pearls:
    - Potential association with new onset diabetes
    - Boxed warning for risk of hepatitis B reactivation
    - Very high cure rates (~95%)
    - Duration of treatment ranges from 8 to 24 weeks, but typically 12 weeks
- Monitoring: CBC, liver function, renal function, INR
- Drug and Diet Considerations:
    - May be given with or without food
    - May alter blood sugars, monitor in patients with diabetes

Eletriptan (Relpax)
- Class: Anti-migraine, triptan
- Mechanism of Action: Serotonin 5HT agonist; which causes vasoconstriction and reduction in inflammation associated with migraine
- Common Uses: Acute relief of migraine
- Memorable Side Effects: Dizziness, changes in CNS
- Clinical Pearls:
    - Meant for acute relief of migraine, not prophylaxis
    - Be sure to assess frequent use; if using frequently, need to have control of migraines assessed and add controller medication if necessary (valproic acid, propranolol, topiramate, etc.)
    - Often used with NSAIDs (i.e. naproxen) in migraine treatment
    - Does have serotonin activity so could potentially contribute to serotonin syndrome (higher risk in patients already on SSRIs, tramadol, etc.)
- Monitoring: Blood pressure, EKG when clinically indicated to assess risk for QTc prolongation
- Drug and Diet Considerations:
    - Given as needed for migraine, so administration at any point is fine with regards to food
    - If administered near the time of fatty foods, bioavailability may be increased

Elvitegravir (Vitekta)
- Class: Integrase inhibitor, antiretroviral
- Mechanism of Action: Inhibits the viral enzyme, integrase, by binding enzyme cations and preventing viral DNA integration into the host genome
- Common Uses: HIV treatment
- Memorable Side Effects: Elevated LFTs, skin reaction risk/SJS (rare, but possible), CNS changes, GI adverse effects, CPK increase/myopathy
- Clinical Pearls:
    - Generally preferred now in place of protease inhibitors as they have less drug interactions and seem to be better tolerated
- Monitoring: CBC, LFTs, HIV levels, CD4 count, hepatitis B testing prior to initiation
- Drug and Diet Considerations:
    - Administered with food

- o Supplements that have antacid activity like calcium carbonate and magnesium products may block absorption; separate by a minimum of 2 hours
- o St. John's wort decreases serum concentrations and should be avoided

Empagliflozin (Jardiance)

- Class: Antidiabetic, SGLT-2 inhibitor
- Mechanism of Action: Inhibition of the sodium–glucose co-transporter 2, this results in an increase in glucose excretion through the urine and lowering of blood sugar
- Common Uses: Treatment of diabetes and adjunct therapy in heart failure
- Memorable Side Effects: Dehydration (high risk in patients taking diuretics or reduced fluid intake), increased risk for urinary tract infections and fungal infections, like candidiasis, and potential drop in blood pressure
- Clinical Pearls:
  - o Caution in patients with a urinary infection history; drug increases sugar to the urine which can facilitate the grow of organisms
  - o Monitor K+; hyperkalemia risk, especially in patients on ACE, ARB, potassium supplements, or those with a high potassium diet, etc.
  - o Rarely can increase the risk for ketoacidosis
  - o Hypoglycemia risk not as bad as sulfonylureas
  - o Caution on an increase in bone fracture risk
  - o Contraindicated in eGFR <30 (remember these drugs work in the kidney)
- Monitoring: Renal function, potassium, blood pressure, blood sugar, HbA1c
- Drug and Diet Considerations:
  - o Be cautious and monitor potassium closely in patients with high dietary intake of potassium as this could contribute to hyperkalemia in combination with this medication
  - o Monitor fluid intake; this medication can increase the risk for dehydration
  - o Patient should have an appropriate diabetes diet and education if taking this medication
  - o Administer with or without food

Emtricitabine (Emtriva)

- Class: Antiretroviral, nucleoside reverse transcriptase inhibitor (NRTI)
- Mechanism of Action: Converted to active triphosphate forms which competes with natural substrates to inhibit reverse transcriptase; the HIV virus uses the enzyme reverse transcriptase to convert RNA into DNA
- Common Uses: HIV treatment
- Memorable Side Effects: Lactic acidosis/fatty liver warning, GI adverse effects, elevation in cholesterol, fatigue, neuropathy, darkening of skin
- Clinical Pearls:
  - o In combination products such as Sustiva, Atripla
  - o Boxed warning on risk of hepatitis B exacerbations
- Monitoring: Liver function, HIV viral load, CD4 count, renal function, hepatitis B testing prior to initiation
- Drug and Diet Considerations:

110

- o Monitor cholesterol and implement cholesterol lowering diet in patients who may have elevated levels due to the adverse effects of the drug
- o May be given with or without meals

Enalapril (Vasotec)
- Class: Antihypertensive, ACE inhibitor
- Mechanism of Action: Inhibition of the angiotensin converting enzyme which prevents the production of angiotensin 2. Angiotensin 2 is a potent vasoconstrictor; blocking angiotensin 2 equates to less vasoconstriction, and lower blood pressure
- Common Uses: Hypertension, acute MI, heart failure
- Common Side Effects: Cough, kidney impairment, low blood pressure, and hyperkalemia
- Clinical Pearls:
  - o ACE inhibitors are notoriously known for causing a dry chronic cough
  - o If you ever have a patient with a chronic cough, you must assess if they are on an ACE inhibitor.
  - o Angiotensin Receptor Blockers (ARBs) are the cousins to the ACE inhibitors, and are the first line substitute to a patient who has had a cough with an ACE inhibitor
  - o ACE inhibitors can exacerbate kidney impairment as well as contribute to acute renal failure especially in patients who are already on other potential renal toxic medications (i.e. diuretics, NSAIDs, etc.) even though in conditions like heart failure, diuretics and ACE inhibitors are often used together
  - o ACE inhibitors are a classic cause of elevated potassium levels; if your patient has hyperkalemia, you must make sure the ACE inhibitor has been addressed
  - o In some cases, patients of African descent may not respond to ACE inhibitors as well as other ethnicities
  - o A mistake I've seen clinicians make is using an ACE inhibitor with an ARB; this is generally not recommended
  - o ACE inhibitors (and ARBs) are frequently used in patients with hypertension and a history of diabetes, stroke, CAD, CKD, and CHF
  - o Angioedema (swelling of the lips/airway) is classically caused by ACE inhibition; it is an extremely rare, but very serious adverse reaction that requires immediate discontinuation
- Monitoring: Renal function, potassium, blood pressure
- Drug and Diet Considerations:
  - o Be cautious and monitor potassium closely in patients with high dietary intake of potassium as this could contribute to hyperkalemia in combination with this medication
  - o Administer with or without food

Enoxaparin (Lovenox)
- Class: Anticoagulant, low molecular weight heparin
- Mechanism of Action: Primarily inhibits factor 10A clotting factor (anticoagulant)

111

- Common Uses: Treatment and prevention of blood clots to reduce the risk of heart attacks and DVT
- Memorable Side Effects: Bleed risk
- Clinical Pearls:
    - Bleeding risk is the major adverse effect that needs to be monitored with any medication that inhibits clotting factors
    - It is a heparin based product (low molecular weight heparin) so risk of heparin induced thrombocytopenia is there, but much lower than heparin
    - Checking INRs with enoxaparin is not necessary; weight based dosing
    - Platelets and hemoglobin are two important monitoring parameters (part of a CBC)
    - Often patients are bridged to warfarin with orders to start warfarin, and follow INR; when INR is 2 or greater, discontinue enoxaparin
    - Significantly higher dose of enoxaparin recommended for treatment of blood clot (DVT) versus prevention
    - Injection only is a downside and why patients are often transitioned to an oral anticoagulant
- Monitoring: CBC, platelets, bleed risk, renal function, potassium (not likely to be done in short term use unless clinical circumstances dictate)
- Drug and Diet Considerations:
    - Vitamin E, Omega-3 fatty acids, gingko, garlic, ginseng, turmeric, and fish oil supplements have been purported to have antiplatelet type activity which in theory could increase the risk of bleed – clinical significance is questionable; the most common resolution is to discontinue the supplements if they are not necessary
    - Alcohol may have an additive antiplatelet-type effect and increase the risk of GI bleed
    - Very rare risk for hyperkalemia, be aware of any diet contributions as well as other medications if the patient's potassium is elevated

Entacapone (Comtan)

- Class: Anti-Parkinson's, COMT inhibitor
- Mechanism of Action: Inhibition of catechol-O-methyltransferase prevents further breakdown of levodopa which ultimately increases dopamine levels
- Common Uses: Management of Parkinson's symptoms
- Memorable Side Effects: Nausea/vomiting, hallucinations, orthostasis, dyskinesia, sedation (adverse effect profile will look similar to carbidopa/levodopa)
- Clinical Pearls:
    - Utilized with carbidopa/levodopa
- Monitoring: LFTs, blood pressure
- Drug and Diet Considerations:
    - May be given with or without meals
    - Only used when the patient is taking carbidopa/levodopa
    - Alcohol may exacerbate depressive effects from the medication
    - May bind iron and reduce levels (typically not clinically significant)
    - Monitor for potential weight loss which could be associated with entacapone, carbidopa/levodopa, Parkinson's disorder, or a combination

Epinephrine (EpiPen, Adrenalin)
- Class: Alpha and beta agonist
- Mechanism of Action: Stimulates alpha and beta receptors
- Common Uses: Treatment of anaphylactic reactions, hypotension/shock
- Memorable Side Effects: Tachycardia, hypertension, anxiety, insomnia, dry mouth, urinary retention
- Clinical Pearls:
    o Ramps you up; increase in BP, pulse, anxiety, irritability, etc.
    o Drug found in "Epi-pen" for severe allergic reactions
    o Epinephrine is used in the ACLS algorithm as well
- Monitoring: Heart rate, blood pressure, EKG, blood glucose
- Drug and Diet Considerations:
    o Unlikely to have any issues with diet considerations given the medication is virtually never used long term
    o Could potentially contribute to alterations in blood sugar, insulin resistance, and hypokalemia (unlikely to be of significant concern in an emergency situation with short term use)

Eplerenone (Inspra)
- Class: Antihypertensive, potassium sparing diuretic, aldosterone antagonist
- Mechanism of Action: Increases water and sodium excretion (diuretic) but spares potassium (can increase potassium levels)
- Common Uses: Treatment of heart failure and cirrhosis with ascites
- Memorable Side Effects: Hyperkalemia, low BP, hyponatremia, dehydration
- Clinical Pearls:
    o Much like all diuretics, in relation to the effects on the kidney, the risk of overdiuresis (promoting too much fluid loss) can worsen kidney function by inadequate flow through the kidney
    o The development of gynecomastia is less likely with eplerenone versus spironolactone
    o We can often reduce the potassium supplementation (especially patients on high doses of KCL supplements) burden by using potassium sparing diuretics
- Monitoring: Renal function, potassium, blood pressure
- Drug and Diet Considerations:
    o Be cautious and monitor potassium closely in patients with high dietary intake of potassium as this could contribute to hyperkalemia in combination with this medication
    o Can be given with or without food
    o Grapefruit juice can increase concentrations

Ertapenem (Invanz)
- Class: Carbapenem, antibiotic
- Mechanism of Action: Binds penicillin-binding proteins and inhibits production of the bacterial cell wall
- Common Uses: Broad spectrum antibiotic used to treat many resistant, severe infections (i.e. complicated UTIs or intra-abdominal infections involving resistant organisms)
- Memorable Side Effects: Diarrhea, GI upset, lowers seizure threshold
- Clinical Pearls:

113

- o Usually reserved for very severe, resistant infections
- o Known for its coverage of ESBL+ bacteria such as E. coli, Klebsiella, etc.
- o Does not cover Pseudomonas
- Monitoring: Renal function
- Drug and Diet Considerations:
  - o Minimal concerns with shorter term use
  - o Monitor fluid and electrolyte status if diarrhea is problematic

Erythromycin (Ery-tab)
- Class: Macrolide, antibiotic
- Mechanism of Action: Inhibits protein synthesis in bacteria
- Common Uses: Treatment of upper respiratory infections (ear infection, pneumonia, bronchitis, sinusitis); also used chronically for gastroparesis
- Memorable Side Effects: GI most common, QTc prolongation rare, but possible
- Clinical Pearls:
  - o Numerous drug interactions (compared to azithromycin), rarely used as an antibiotic due to this reason
  - o Dosed multiple times per day (azithromycin much simpler dosing)
  - o Used chronically at low doses to improve gastroparesis; slow GI motility common with diabetes
- Monitoring: LFTs and CBC if using long term or if signs of complications
- Drug and Diet Considerations:
  - o GI upset and diarrhea can happen, but generally less frequent than a drug like amoxicillin
  - o Maintain adequate hydration to avoid dehydration if diarrhea is a significant problem
  - o Timing of administration depends upon the dosage form used; Ery-Tab can be administered without regard to meals

Erythropoietin (Procrit, Epogen)
- Class: Erythropoiesis stimulating agent (ESA)
- Mechanism of Action: Stimulates the production of red blood cells
- Common Uses: Treatment of anemia from CKD and chemotherapy/cancer
- Memorable Side Effects: Hypertension, GI, Injection site reaction, increase clot risk (boxed warning)
- Clinical Pearls:
  - o Lack of iron may inhibit response
  - o Monitor hemoglobin/hematocrit; an increase indicates response to treatment
  - o Risk of hypertension
  - o There should be hold parameters in place (i.e. hold if hemoglobin is greater than 11)
  - o Important boxed warning on increased risk of MI, stroke, blood clots
- Monitoring: Hemoglobin typically needs to be monitored frequently to assess response, iron stores, blood pressure
- Drug and Diet Considerations:
  - o Iron has to be assessed and monitored as iron deficiency is one of the most common causes of treatment failure/non-response

Escitalopram (Lexapro)

- Class: Antidepressant, SSRI
- Mechanism of Action: selective serotonin reuptake inhibitor; increases serotonin in the brain
- Common Uses: Treatment of depression, anxiety and PTSD
- Memorable Side Effects: GI side effects (N/V/D), sedation or activation depending upon the patient, changes in mental status, hyponatremia (rare)
- Clinical Pearls:
  - SSRIs are generally considered the first line medication to treat depression, they are generally well tolerated, and less risky than other antidepressants in the situation of suicide attempt through overdosing on pills
  - Stomach/GI complaints like stomach upset and/or diarrhea are the most common complications
  - Boxed warning for an increased risk of suicidal thinking when first starting these medications
  - Although not terribly common, hyponatremia (low sodium) is a possible unique side effect with SSRIs and much more likely in patients already prone to hyponatremia; classic example would be patients who are taking diuretics, which can also lower sodium
  - Remember that these drugs are not an immediate fix! In most cases, SSRIs take weeks sometimes months before a patient will start improving; however side effects will be apparent from the start of the medication, making it difficult to coach our patients to continue the medication in the first few weeks of therapy
  - SSRIs are used in pregnancy, but the risk versus the benefits need to be assessed on a case by case basis
  - SSRIs can decrease libido
- Monitoring: EKG, potassium and magnesium if the patient is at risk for QTc prolongation; sodium level if the patient is displaying symptoms of hyponatremia
- Drug and Diet Considerations:
  - Weight gain or weight loss can happen with SSRIs; monitor for changes over time once started, increased, reduced, or discontinued
  - Diarrhea can happen, but isn't common; assess fluid status, notify provider if the patient is reporting this side effect
  - If the patient has a prolonged QT interval, out of range electrolytes like potassium and magnesium could increase the risk for Torsades de Pointes
  - Low sodium can be a rare adverse effect
  - Can be taken with or without food
  - Alcohol has additive, unpredictable effects when used with SSRIs
  - St John's wort has additive effects on any drug that has serotonergic type activity

Esomeprazole (Nexium)

- Class: Proton pump inhibitor (PPI)
- Mechanism of Action: Inhibits proton pumps in the stomach leading to a less acidic environment
- Common Uses: Treatment of GERD, ulcer and Barrett's esophagus

- Memorable Side Effects: Generally well tolerated but long term use may cause: increased fracture risk, decreased B12 and magnesium levels, C. diff risk
- Clinical Pearls:
  - PPIs are the most potent acid blocker on the market
  - PPIs are generally dosed 30 minutes or so before meals – this is a recommendation, not an absolute (example if a patient likes to get up and eat right away upon rising, the medication will still likely be beneficial, but may not have a maximal effect)
  - For some patients PPIs may take a few days for maximal effect
  - For the above reason, as needed (PRN) PPIs can possibly be effective, but are generally not used
  - Use short term if possible due to increased risk of osteoporosis, low magnesium, and B12 deficiency when used long term
  - Most common primary outcome of PPI would be to improve symptoms likely heartburn and stomach from GERD, stomach ulcer, or other related conditions
  - Barrett's esophagus, high risk GI medications (i.e. NSAIDs, prednisone), or chronic GI bleed may require indefinite therapy
  - If GI bleed is problematic, monitoring hemoglobin and/or hemoccult is appropriate to assess possible blood loss
- Monitoring: Magnesium (chronic use), B12
- Drug and Diet Considerations:
  - When used chronically, it is a possible cause or contributing factor to B12 and magnesium deficiency
  - PPIs are typically best given at least 30-60 minutes before a meal
  - St. John's wort should be avoided as it can significantly reduce concentrations of the drug
  - Reduced stomach acid (high pH) may impair the absorption of iron supplements

Eszopiclone (Lunesta)

- Class: Sedative, "Z" Drug
- Mechanism of Action: Enhances activity of GABA, an inhibitory neurotransmitter that causes sedation
- Common Uses: Management of insomnia
- Memorable Side Effects: Sedation, confusion, fall risk, dizziness, abnormal sleep behaviors (sleep walking, eating, etc.)
- Clinical Pearls:
  - Often termed as a "Z" drug
  - Medications like eszopiclone are sedating; when medications are sedating we always have to be mindful of the morning after and make sure patients realize that driving and/or operating machinery can be extremely dangerous
  - It is recommended to try to use these medications only for short term if possible
  - Non-drug interventions such as sleep hygiene are the preferred treatment for insomnia
  - Before this type of medication is prescribed, keep an eye out for patients who may be on stimulating type medications or medications that can contribute to insomnia and make sure that these are assessed prior to giving a sleep medication – classic examples: methylphenidate, prednisone, too much levothyroxine, etc.

- o Eszopiclone is a controlled substance in the U.S.; there is a risk of addiction/dependence
- o Very similar effects to benzodiazepines
- o Can increase risk of falls in our elderly patients
- Monitoring: Routine lab work is not necessary
- Drug and Diet Considerations:
  - o Meals with a high fat content may delay absorption; typically not an issue as it is usually dosed at night long after a patient's evening meal
  - o Alcohol can exacerbate the CNS depressant effects
  - o Grapefruit juice may cause an increase in drug concentrations

Etanercept (Enbrel)
- Class: DMARD (antirheumatic), TNF blocker
- Mechanism of Action: Blocks tumor necrosis factor (TNF); TNF plays a role in the inflammatory process
- Common Uses: Treatment of rheumatoid arthritis and psoriasis/psoriatic arthritis
- Memorable Side Effects: Infection risk (suppresses immune system), injection site reaction
- Clinical Pearls:
  - o Watch for frequent or serious infections, due to a suppressed immune system
  - o Acts as a controller of inflammatory conditions, not immediate relief
  - o Expensive
  - o Injection
  - o Refrigerated; but may warm to room temp to make injection less painful
- Monitoring: Signs of infection, CBC, HBV and TB screening as necessary
- Drug and Diet Considerations:
  - o Avoid the use of the supplement, echinacea, as it may interfere with the immunosuppressive nature of the drug

Ethacrynic Acid (Edecrin)
- Class: Loop diuretic
- Mechanism of Action): Inhibits sodium and chloride reabsorption in the ascending "Loop" of Henle in the kidney
- Common Use: Treatment of edema, hypertension and heart failure
- Memorable Side Effects: Frequent urination, electrolyte depletion, low blood pressure, dehydration and renal impairment
- Clinical Pearls:
  - o While furosemide can cause significant reductions in magnesium, calcium, sodium, etc., potassium is one of the most important electrolytes to monitor and often patients require potassium supplementation; this can sometimes be offset by potassium sparing diuretics like spironolactone, ARBs, like losartan, and ACE inhibitors like lisinopril (all potentially increase potassium)
  - o Frequent urination can be significantly upsetting to patients and can greatly impact their wellbeing, including upsetting their sleep; if

117

possible, make sure these loop diuretics are not given too close to bedtime
- o Whenever you see a new Rx for a loop diuretic, be sure to look at the other medications the patient is taking to make sure that the edema is not a side effect; classic causes of edema include calcium channel blockers, pioglitazone, pregabalin, and NSAIDs.
- o Loops deplete volume in the body, so patients run the risk of not having adequate perfusion through the kidney; elevations in creatinine from baseline can help us monitor for this risk
- o Kidney function and electrolytes are going to be the primary labs to monitor
- o Urinary output and monitoring of weights can be very important patient factors to monitor and help assess the efficacy of the loop diuretic
- o Does not have a sulfa group in the event of allergic reaction from other loop diuretics
- Monitoring: Renal function and electrolytes (essentially can deplete all electrolytes), weights, blood pressure, hearing (when used at high doses)
- Drug and Diet Considerations:
  - o Potassium supplementation is usually required as bumetanide can cause significant hypokalemia
  - o Monitor for dehydration warning signs
  - o Give with food or milk

Ethambutol (Myambutol)

- Class: Anti-tuberculosis agent
- Mechanism of Action: Blocks arabinosyl transferase which blocks bacterial cell wall production
- Common Uses: Part of combination therapy for treatment of tuberculosis and MAC
- Memorable Side Effects: Dizziness, GI upset, hyperuricemia, ocular toxicities, hepatic toxicity
- Clinical Pearls:
  - o Routine eye exams are recommended
- Monitoring: Eye, renal function, LFTs
- Drug and Diet Considerations:
  - o May give with food if GI upset occurs
  - o Aluminum hydroxide may bind up the drug; separate by a minimum of 4 hours

Ethosuximide (Zarontin)

- Class: Antiepileptic
- Mechanism of Action: Reduces neuronal transmission in the CNS
- Common Uses: Treatment of seizures
- Memorable Side Effects: Sedation, dizziness, behavioral changes, GI upset, blood pressure variability (pediatrics), skin reactions (rare), CBC alterations (rare), Lupus exacerbation, hepatic dysfunction
- Clinical Pearls:
  - o Used specifically for absence seizures
- Monitoring: Weight, CBC, LFTs
- Drug and Diet Considerations:

- o Weight loss may be a potential adverse effect, monitor caloric intake and appetite
- o Give with food or milk as GI upset is common

Etodolac (Lodine)
- Class: NSAID, analgesic
- Mechanism of Action: Inhibits Cyclooxygenase-1 and 2 (COX-1 and COX-2); results in a reduction in prostaglandins which cause pain, fever, inflammation
- Common Uses: Management of pain, fever and inflammation
- Memorable Side Effects: GI ulcer, worsening kidney function, edema, hypertension, inhibits platelets which can exacerbate bleed risk
- Clinical Pearls:
  - o NSAIDs are one of the most common causes of GI bleeding; this risk increases in the elderly and those on medications that increase risk of bleeding (anticoagulants and antiplatelet medications)
  - o Due to effects on platelets, NSAIDs are typically held before/after surgery to reduce the risk of bleeding
  - o NSAIDs can contribute to edema and exacerbate CHF (congestive heart failure); have NSAIDs reassessed if you see a patient with a CHF exacerbation or a patient requiring increasing diuretics like furosemide
  - o NSAIDs can cause worsening kidney function (creatinine should be monitored); this risk can be greatly increased in patients on ACE inhibitors or ARBs and/or diuretics
  - o Due to above reasons on kidney function, GI bleed risk, and CHF, NSAIDs are not the safest medication in the elderly; acetaminophen is generally preferred for generalized pain with a few exceptions
  - o Although generally considered riskier in the elderly, a big advantage of NSAIDs over acetaminophen is that they can reduce inflammation
  - o Pregnancy category C/D when >30 weeks gestation; NSAIDs are generally avoided in pregnancy and especially after 30 weeks gestation
- Monitoring: Renal function, hemoglobin, platelets (contained within CBC), blood pressure, signs of bruising or bleeding, weight (risk for edema)
- Drug and Diet Considerations:
  - o Because of significant incidence of GI upset, it is recommended to give with food or milk
  - o Dehydration may exacerbate the risk for acute renal failure
  - o Excessive alcohol may increase GI bleed risk
  - o Vitamin E, Omega-3 fatty acids, gingko, garlic, ginseng, turmeric, and fish oil supplements have been purported to have antiplatelet type activity which, in theory, could increase the risk of bleed – clinical significance is questionable; the most common resolution is to discontinue the supplements if they are not necessary

Etoposide (Hycamtin)
- Class: Oncology agent, topoisomerase 2 inhibitor
- Mechanism of Action: Inhibits DNA/RNA synthesis by inhibiting topoisomerase 2
- Common Uses: Treatment of different types of metastatic cancer

- Memorable Side Effects: Myelosuppression, nausea, vomiting, diarrhea, hair loss, thrombocytopenia, infusion reaction
- Clinical Pearls:
    - Boxed warning for the risk of myelosuppression
    - Oral or IV administration
- Monitoring: CBC, renal function, LFTs, blood pressure
- Drug and Diet Considerations:
    - Weight loss and poor nutrition may result on account of nausea and vomiting adverse effects
    - Monitor hydration status

Evolocumab (Repatha)
- Class: Antilipemic, PCSK9 inhibitor
- Mechanism of Action: PCSK9 destroys LDL receptors in the liver; by inhibiting this protein, it allows LDL receptors to do their job and to remove circulating LDL from the blood stream, thus lowering LDL
- Common Uses: Decrease LDL and reduce the risk of cardiovascular events
- Memorable Side Effects: Injection site reactions, myopathy (lower risk than statins), fatigue
- Clinical Pearls:
    - Additional agent to consider in high risk patients where statins have been insufficient at lowering cholesterol (LDL)
    - Injection only
    - Very expensive and access often limited by insurance
- Monitoring: Lipids
- Drug and Diet Considerations:
    - Food does not affect the pharmacokinetics: it can be administered anytime in relation to dietary intake
    - Encourage a lipid lowering diet for any patient taking a cholesterol medication

Exenatide (Byetta, Bydureon)
- Class: Antidiabetic, GLP-1 agonist
- Mechanism of Action: Enhances glucose dependent insulin secretion, slows gastric emptying, and reduces post prandial glucagon to reduce blood sugars
- Common Uses: Treatment of type 2 diabetes
- Memorable Side Effects: Nausea, vomiting, hypoglycemia if taken in combination with insulin or a sulfonylurea, pancreatitis concerns exist, but are rare
- Clinical Pearls:
    - Long acting formulation is dosed once weekly
    - Short acting formulation needs to be dosed within 60 minutes of morning and evening meals
    - Boxed warning to avoid use in certain types of thyroid tumors
    - Promotes fullness, weight loss can be a beneficial effect
    - Typically better in HbA1c reduction than most oral diabetes medications
- Monitoring: Blood sugar, HbA1c, triglycerides, and renal function as clinically indicated
- Drug and Diet Considerations:
    - Short acting formulation needs to be dosed within 60 minutes of morning and evening meals

- o Long acting can be administered without regard to meals
- o Reduces appetite which can be helpful in obese type 2 diabetes patients
- o Implementation of a diabetic diet

Ezetimibe (Zetia)
- Class: Antilipemic
- Mechanism of Action: Inhibits intestinal absorption of cholesterol
- Common Uses: Reduction of cholesterol, particularly LDL
- Memorable Side Effects: Overall well tolerated, low risk of diarrhea, myopathy (when used in combination with statins)
- Clinical Pearls:
  - o May be used in combination with a statin
  - o Pretty well tolerated when used alone, but not nearly as potent at reducing LDL as statins
  - o Still fairly expensive at this time
  - o Can possibly increase the risk of rhabdomyolysis when added to statin therapy; monitor for muscle pain/soreness
  - o Convenient once daily dosing
- Monitoring: Lipids, LFTs if clinical parameters indicate
- Drug and Diet Considerations:
  - o Timing of administration isn't critical – with or without food is acceptable
  - o Encourage a lipid lowering diet for any patient taking a cholesterol medication

Famotidine (Pepcid)
- Class: H2 blocker
- Mechanism of Action: Blocks histamine 2 receptors, which results in reduced gastric acid secretion and a higher pH in the stomach
- Common Uses: Treatment of GERD, heartburn and GI bleed
- Memorable Side Effects: Well tolerated, watch out for CNS changes in elderly and/or patients with poor kidney function
- Clinical Pearls:
  - o H2 blockers are cleared by the kidney, so they can accumulate, in CKD and require dose adjustments
  - o Generally less effective at suppressing stomach acid than PPIs
  - o Available over the counter, inexpensive
  - o CNS effects likely more common in elderly, on higher doses, and in patients with kidney disease
  - o Generally used before PPIs if something more than Tums (calcium carbonate) is needed in pregnancy
- Monitoring: No routine lab work is typically necessary; LFTs, hemoglobin when clinically indicated
- Drug and Diet Considerations:
  - o Reduced stomach acid (high pH) may impair the absorption of iron supplements
  - o Associations with B12 deficiency in chronic users

121

Febuxostat (Uloric)

- Class: Anti-gout, xanthine oxidase inhibitor
- Mechanism of Action: Inhibits xanthine oxidase resulting in decreased production of uric acid
- Common Uses: Gout prophylaxis
- Memorable Side Effects: Rash, GI upset, liver function abnormalities (rare)
- Clinical Pearls:
  - Generally avoided due to boxed warning for CV death
  - Alternative to allopurinol for controlling uric acid levels in gout
  - NOT for treatment of acute flare
  - Keep an eye out for medications, particularly thiazides diuretics, that may exacerbate gout
  - Expensive alternative to allopurinol at this time
- Monitoring: Uric acid, LFTs as clinically indicated, CV risks
- Drug and Diet Considerations:
  - Adequate hydration is important to help flush uric acid out of the body; this can also be helpful in reducing the risk for uric acid based kidney stones
  - Alcohol, certain seafood (i.e. sardines, anchovies, shellfish, and tuna), liver, bacon, veal, and red meats have higher purine content and may increase the risk for gout flares; assess diet if a patient is having frequent attacks and requiring escalating doses of allopurinol and flare medications like NSAIDs and corticosteroids

Felodipine (Plendil)

- Class: Antihypertensive, calcium channel blocker
- Mechanism of Action: Blocks calcium ions from entering voltage smooth muscle, resulting in relaxation (vasodilation); dihydropyridine calcium channel blocker
- Common Uses: Treatment of hypertension
- Memorable Side Effects: Low blood pressure, edema, constipation
- Clinical Pearls:
  - Very important distinction: You will not see nifedipine used in atrial fibrillation, because its activity is primarily on the vessels; this differs from non-dihydropyridine calcium channel blockers like verapamil and diltiazem that act on the heart AND blood vessels; This also means that pulse monitoring will not be necessary with nifedipine
  - The higher you push the dose on these medications, the more likely you will see the side effect of edema
  - Keep an eye out for new diuretic prescriptions to treat the edema caused by the calcium channel blockers
  - Educate patients to get up slowly to minimize risk of orthostatic hypotension
- Monitoring: Blood pressure, weight (in association with edema risk)
- Drug and Diet Considerations:
  - May give with food if GI upset occurs
  - St. John's wort may reduce effectiveness
  - Standard calcium supplementation typically will not impact the effectiveness of amlodipine; excessive doses of calcium may have a higher likelihood of blunting the effects of amlodipine
  - Avoid grapefruit and its juice as they can raise concentrations

Fenofibrate (Tricor, Fenoglide, Triglide)

- Class: Antilipemic agent, fibric acid derivative
- Mechanism of Action: Activates lipoprotein lipase and reduces apoprotein C-3 production which leads to breaking down of fat and triglyceride rich particles
- Common Uses: Reduction of cholesterol, particularly triglycerides
- Memorable Side Effects: Dyspepsia (GI), rhabdomyolysis/myopathy possible especially when co-administered with statins
- Clinical Pearls:
    - Interacts with many of the statins, but sometimes used together
    - Important to educate patients, have heightened monitoring for adverse effects if using this medication with a statin
    - GI upset is usually the primary adverse effect
- Monitoring: Lipids, LFTs as clinically indicated
- Drug and Diet Considerations:
    - Encourage cholesterol lowering diet
    - To maximize absorption, give 30 minutes before meals

Fentanyl (Duragesic)

- Class: Opioid, analgesic
- Mechanism of Action: Binds opioid receptors inhibiting CNS pain pathways
- Common Uses: Management of pain disorders, both chronic (patches only for chronic pain) and acute
- Memorable Side Effects: Constipation, sedation, respiratory depression, CNS effects like confusion and delirium
- Clinical Pearls:
    - Fentanyl is a scheduled 2 controlled substance; risk of addiction and dependence
    - It is critical to educate/assess patients for constipation if they are taking scheduled opioids like fentanyl
    - Fentanyl patches are not recommended in patients who have never received an opioid before (opioid naïve patients)
    - Naloxone is reversal agent for opioids
    - Patches should never be used as needed; onset of pain relief is slow, taking hours to days
    - In most cases, flushing fentanyl patches is appropriate (risk of pets, children getting them out of garbage and overdosing)
    - They are very potent; 25 mcg patch is equivalent to approximately 60 mg of oral morphine per day
- Monitoring: Bowel movements, pain management, risk for addiction
- Drug and Diet Considerations:
    - Alcohol can exacerbate the CNS depressant effect
    - Encourage a constipation friendly diet consisting of fiber, fluids and exercise, as fentanyl can be very constipating

Ferrous Fumarate (Erretts, Ferrimin)

- Class: Iron Supplement
- Mechanism of Action: Replaces body's iron stores
- Common Uses: Prevention of iron deficiency anemia
- Memorable Side Effects: Constipation, black stools, GI pain

123

- Clinical Pearls:
  - Iron deficiency anemia is the most common use for iron supplements
  - In patients with CKD, anemia may likely be due to kidney disease versus iron deficiency (erythropoietin is produced in the kidney)
  - Educate patients regarding troublesome constipation and black stools
  - Restless legs can present as a possible symptoms of iron deficiency
  - Contains 33% elemental iron
- Monitoring: Iron related lab work including ferritin, hemoglobin
- Drug and Diet Considerations:
  - Any antacid medication (PPIs, H2 blockers, Tums, etc.) that reduces stomach acid can impair the absorption of oral iron
  - Iron can bind numerous drugs and reduce their effectiveness, examples include: bisphosphonates (i.e. alendronate), baloxavir, cefdinir, quinolone antibiotics, and tetracycline antibiotics
  - Numerous foods may reduce oral iron absorption, examples include: eggs, milk, fiber, cereals, tea, and coffee
  - While there can be many interactions that reduce iron absorption, we can monitor iron labs to assess if a patient is responding to iron replacement; if iron stores are increasing, we won't need to alter the way the patient is taking the supplement
  - Give on an empty stomach with water or juice; if GI upset occurs, it may be given with food
  - May be administered with vitamin C to create a more acidic environment in the stomach and aid in iron absorption

Ferrous Gluconate (Ferate)

- Class: Iron supplement
- Mechanism of Action: Replaces body's iron stores
- Common Uses: Prevention of iron deficiency anemia
- Memorable Side Effects: Constipation, black stools, GI pain
- Clinical Pearls:
  - Iron deficiency anemia is the most common use for iron supplements
  - In patients with CKD, anemia may likely be due to kidney disease versus iron deficiency (erythropoietin is produced in the kidney)
  - Educate patients regarding troublesome constipation and black stools
  - Restless legs can present as a possible symptom of iron deficiency
  - Contains 12% elemental iron
- Monitoring: Iron related lab work including ferritin, hemoglobin
- Drug and Diet Considerations:
  - Any antacid medication (PPIs, H2 blockers, Tums, etc.) that reduces stomach acid can impair the absorption of oral iron
  - Iron can bind numerous drugs and reduce their effectiveness, examples include: bisphosphonates (i.e. alendronate), baloxavir, cefdinir, quinolone antibiotics, and tetracycline antibiotics
  - Numerous foods may reduce oral iron absorption, examples include: eggs, milk, fiber, cereals, tea, and coffee
  - While there can be many interactions that reduce iron absorption, we can monitor iron labs to assess if a patient is responding to iron

replacement; if iron stores are increasing, we won't need to alter the way the patient is taking the supplement
- o Give on an empty stomach with water or juice; if GI upset occurs, it may be given with food
- o May be administered with vitamin C to create a more acidic environment in the stomach and aid in iron absorption

Ferrous Sulfate (Feosol)

- Class: Iron Supplement
- Mechanism of Action: Replaces body's iron stores
- Common Uses: Prevention of iron deficiency anemia
- Memorable Side Effects: Constipation, black stools, GI pain
- Clinical Pearls:
  - o Iron deficiency anemia is the most common use for iron supplements
  - o In patients with CKD, anemia may likely be due to kidney disease versus iron deficiency (erythropoietin is produced in the kidney)
  - o Educate patients regarding troublesome constipation and black stools
  - o Restless legs can present as a possible symptom of iron deficiency
  - o Contains 20% elemental iron
- Monitoring: Iron related lab work including ferritin, hemoglobin
- Drug and Diet Considerations:
  - o Any antacid medication (PPIs, H2 blockers, Tums, etc.) that reduces stomach acid can impair the absorption of oral iron
  - o Iron can bind numerous drugs and reduce their effectiveness, examples include: bisphosphonates (i.e. alendronate), baloxavir, cefdinir, quinolone antibiotics, and tetracycline antibiotics
  - o Numerous foods may reduce iron oral iron absorption, examples include: eggs, milk, fiber, cereals, tea, and coffee
  - o While there can be many interactions that reduce iron absorption, we can monitor iron labs to assess if a patient is responding to iron replacement; if iron stores are increasing, we generally won't need to alter the way the patient is taking the supplement
  - o May be administered with vitamin C to create a more acidic environment in the stomach and aid in iron absorption

Fesoterodine (Toviaz)

- Class: Bladder anticholinergic
- Mechanism of Action: Blocks muscarinic receptors in the bladder which increases urine volume in the bladder and potentially decreases frequency/urge
- Common Uses: Management of overactive bladder and bladder spasms
- Memorable Side Effects: dry mouth, dry eyes, urinary retention, constipation
- Clinical Pearls:
  - o Anticholinergic effects
  - o Fesoterodine is less likely to cause anticholinergic effects than older bladder agents like oxybutynin as it is more selective for the bladder
  - o Be sure to assess if the medication is working for incontinence/frequency

- - Keep an eye out for patients on diuretics; if frequency is the major issue, make sure that diuretics are at the minimum effective dose (not always possible to reduce diuretics with CHF history, etc.)
    - Frequency can be especially problematic in patients who have an active social life as well as at night when trying to sleep
- Monitoring: Renal function as clinically indicated, LFTs
- Drug and Diet Considerations:
  - Slows the motility of the GI tract which could increase the risk for constipation; maintain adequate fluids and non-constipating diet
  - If GI upset occurs, there are no issues in giving the drug with food
  - Dry mouth may increase thirst and alter taste/pleasure of food

Fexofenadine (Allegra)

- Class: Antihistamine (2nd generation)
- Mechanism of Action: Blocks histamine - 1 receptors
- Common Uses: Relief of allergic rhinitis and itching
- Memorable Side Effects: Sedation (much less than 1st generation antihistamines like diphenhydramine or hydroxyzine), mildly anticholinergic
- Clinical Pearls:
  - Fexofenadine is a newer generation antihistamine, so it will have less anticholinergic and sedative effects than older antihistamines like diphenhydramine
  - Generally well tolerated and available over the counter
  - Usually only needs to be dosed once daily which is an advantage over some of the older antihistamines
- Monitoring: No routine lab work is necessary
- Drug and Diet Considerations:
  - Modest CNS depressant effect may be exacerbated by alcohol
  - Grapefruit, apple, and orange juice may reduce the absorption of fexofenadine; patients may drink these juices, but recommend separation of 4-6 hours apart
  - Meals high in fat intake can reduce absorption of fexofenadine

Fidaxomicin (Dificid)

- Class: Macrolide antibiotic
- Mechanism of Action: Blocks the action of bacterial RNA polymerase which prevents protein synthesis
- Common Uses: Clostridium difficile infection
- Memorable Side Effects: Nausea, GI upset, anemia (rare), low WBC count (rare)
- Clinical Pearls:
  - Be aware of patients who have an allergy to macrolide antibiotics (i.e. azithromycin, erythromycin) as there may be a cross-reaction risk
- Monitoring: Minimal systemic absorption, so no routine monitoring is necessary
- Drug and Diet Considerations:
  - Monitor fluid and electrolyte status in patients with diarrhea

Filgrastim (Neupogen)

- Class: Colony stimulating factor (CSF)

- Mechanism of Action: Stimulates production of WBCs
- Common Uses: Prevention of neutropenia in chemo patients
- Memorable Side Effects: Ostealgia (bone pain), anaphylaxis (rare)
- Clinical Pearls:
    o Helps patients continue on chemotherapy by boosting the immune system
    o Bone pain is common due to its ability to stimulate bone marrow, which resides inside the bones
    o White blood cell count is incredibly important to monitor for response to treatment; always obtain CBC
    o Fever and signs of infection are also incredibly important to watch for in a patient on filgrastim
- Monitoring: CBC including white blood cell count and absolute neutrophil count
- Drug and Diet Considerations:
    o Some drug products will contain small amounts of sodium; typically not clinically significant

Finasteride (Proscar)
- Class: 5 alpha reductase inhibitor
- Mechanism of Action: Inhibits 5-alpha reductase which results in less dihydrotestosterone
- Common Uses: Treatment of BPH and hair loss in men
- Memorable Side Effects: Impotence, weakness
- Clinical Pearls:
    o Not for immediate relief of acute urinary retention
    o Takes weeks to months for clinical benefit
    o Well tolerated usually with impotence being most common
    o Hair growth
    o Keep an eye out for anticholinergics, they will exacerbate BPH
    o Women who may be pregnant or who are of childbearing age should absolutely not handle crushed or broken tables – fetal abnormalities of genitalia are possible
- Monitoring: Prostate specific antigen (PSA)
- Drug and Diet Considerations:
    o Can be given with or without food

Fluconazole (Diflucan)
- Class: Antifungal, azole
- Mechanism of Action: Ultimately inhibits formation in fungal cell membrane
- Common Uses: Treatment of fungal infections like candidiasis and Cryptococcus
- Memorable Side Effects: GI side effects most common, liver failure is very rare and more likely with chronic use
- Clinical Pearls:
    o Classically used to treat yeast infections (candidiasis) and many patients may only require one dose
    o Notorious cause of drug interactions via CYP3A4 inhibition; It can increase concentrations of statins, seizure medications, etc. (if you

see patients started on this medication, be sure to look up possible drug interactions)
- o Fungal infections are much more common in patients who are immunocompromised (i.e. AIDS, patient on immunosuppressant medications, etc.)
- o Can potentially cause prolonged QTc intervals especially in patients on other medications that prolong the QTc
- o Liver toxicity is rare, but should be monitored for especially if patients are receiving chronic therapy
- Monitoring: LFTs, renal function, potassium – only if clinically indicated or on chronic therapy
- Drug and Diet Considerations:
  - o Can be given with or without food
  - o Abnormal levels of potassium or magnesium could increase the risk of fluconazole causing QTc prolongation

Fluorouracil (Adrucil, 5-FU)

- Class: Oncology agent, antimetabolite
- Mechanism of Action: Pyrimidine antimetabolite that is incorporated into RNA and terminates extending of the strand and ultimately stops cell growth
- Common Uses: Treatment of numerous types of cancers including metastatic cancer
- Memorable Side Effects: Diarrhea, nausea and vomiting, stomatitis, elevated ammonia level, hand-foot syndrome, myelosuppression, neuropathy, photosensitivity
- Clinical Pearls:
  - o Lowest WBC count will typically occur around day 10 with some exceptions
  - o Patients with certain dihydropyrimidine dehydrogenase (DPD) gene mutations may be at higher risk for adverse effects
- Monitoring: CBC, LFTs, renal function, electrolytes, EKG (as clinically indicated), INR in patients on warfarin
- Drug and Diet Considerations:
  - o Monitor for adequate hydration particularly if the patient has diarrhea, vomiting or excessive fluid loss
  - o Thiamine replacement may be necessary
  - o Weight loss and poor nutrition may result on account of nausea and vomiting or stomatitis adverse effect

Fluoxetine (Prozac)

- Class: SSRI, antidepressant
- Mechanism of Action: selective serotonin reuptake inhibitor; increases serotonin in the brain
- Common Uses: Treatment of depression, anxiety and PTSD
- Memorable Side Effects: GI side effects (N/V/D), sedation or activation depending upon the patient, changes in mental status, hyponatremia (rare)
- Clinical Pearls:
  - o SSRIs are generally considered the first line medication to treat depression, they are generally well tolerated, and less risky than other antidepressants in the situation of attempted suicide through overdose

- o Boxed warning for an increased risk of suicidal thinking when first starting these medications
- o In most patients, fluoxetine tends to be more activating versus sedating
- o Although not terribly common, hyponatremia (low sodium) is a possible unique side effect with SSRIs and much more likely in patients already prone to hyponatremia; classic example would be patients who are taking diuretics, which can also lower sodium
- o Remember that these drugs are not an immediate fix; in most cases, SSRIs take weeks to months before a patient will start improving; however side effects can be apparent from the start of the medication, making it difficult to coach our patients to continue the medication in the first few weeks after starting it
- o SSRIs are used in pregnancy, but the risk versus the benefits need to be assessed on a case by case basis
- o SSRIs can decrease libido
- Monitoring: EKG, potassium and magnesium if the patient is at risk for QTc prolongation; sodium level if the patient is displaying symptoms of hyponatremia
- Drug and Diet Considerations:
  - o Weight gain or weight loss can happen with SSRIs; monitor for changes over time once started, increased, reduced, or discontinued
  - o Diarrhea can happen, but isn't common; assess fluid status, notify provider if the patient is reporting this side effect
  - o If the patient has a prolonged QT interval, out of range electrolytes like potassium and magnesium could increase the risk for Torsades de Pointes
  - o Low sodium can be a rare adverse effect
  - o Can be taken with or without food
  - o Alcohol has additive, unpredictable effects when used with SSRIs

Flurazepam (Dalmane)
- Class: Antianxiety, antiepileptic
- Mechanism of Action: Enhances activity of GABA; an inhibitory neurotransmitter that causes sedation
- Common Uses: Management of insomnia
- Memorable Side Effects: Sedation, confusion, fall risk, dizziness
- Clinical Pearls:
  - o The best way I remember benzodiazepines is that they are very close to "alcohol in a pill"
  - o Sedation, slurred speech, trouble walking (ataxia), etc. are all common with benzos/alcohol; they are also commonly used in alcohol withdrawal
  - o Be cautious with patients on higher doses of benzodiazepines to make sure they aren't abruptly stopped
  - o Educate patients on driving/operating machinery (remember that benzodiazepines are often used for sleep as well as anxiety)
  - o Fall risk in the elderly is a big downside to using these medications
  - o Benzos are a controlled substance; they can cause addiction and dependence
  - o Flumazenil is antidote in overdose

129

- Monitoring: Routine lab monitoring typically isn't necessary unless clinically indicated
- Drug and Diet Considerations:
  - Alcohol intake can have additive side effects of sedation, confusion, slurred speech, and other CNS depressant effects
  - Grapefruit juice may increase drug levels and the risk for adverse effects

Fluticasone (Flonase)

- Class: Nasal corticosteroid
- Mechanism of Action: Nasal steroid that helps to reduce inflammation
- Common Uses: Relief of allergy symptoms
- Memorable Side Effects: Well tolerated, nasal irritation and possible nose bleeds
- Clinical Pearls:
  - Gently shake the product before each use for nasal inhalation
  - Prime the nasal delivery device before using the first time and after 1 or more weeks of non-use
  - There is also an oral inhalation product that is used for asthma/COPD (Flovent)
  - Educate patients that it may not work right away, it may take a few hours or up to a day or two to start working (because of this, it may not be ideal to use this as needed, but it may be tried)
  - It may only be necessary to use this medication seasonally based upon timing and duration of allergy symptoms
  - Be sure to educate patients to clean the tip of the nasal delivery device as it can get pretty nasty
- Monitoring: No lab work is necessary; minimal systemic absorption
- Drug and Diet Considerations:
  - No notable issues with diet

Fluticasone (Flovent, Arnuity Ellipta)

- Class: Inhaled corticosteroid
- Mechanism of Action: Inhaled steroid that helps to reduce inflammation
- Common Uses: Treatment of asthma and COPD
- Memorable Side Effects: Well tolerated, thrush, rhinitis, cough, systemic corticosteroid effects are possible, but not likely, as absorption is low (see prednisone for adverse effects)
- Clinical Pearls:
  - Educate patients that it is not meant to provide emergency relief of symptoms
  - Rinse mouth after administration
- Monitoring: FEV1, peak-flow, growth in pediatric patients
- Drug and Diet Considerations:
  - Certain formulations main contain lactose which could cause a reaction in patients with milk protein allergy

Fluticasone and Salmeterol (Advair, Wixela, AirDuo)

- Class: Inhaled corticosteroid and long acting beta-agonist

- Mechanism of Action: Provides anti-inflammatory effects through fluticasone and stimulates beta-2 receptors leading to relaxation of smooth muscle and opening of airways
- Common Uses: Treatment of asthma and COPD
- Memorable Side Effects: Thrush, tachycardia, tremor, anxiousness; rare effects include: reduced bone mineral density, HPA suppression, hypokalemia and hyperglycemia
- Clinical Pearls:
  - Inhaled corticosteroids have a very low rate of systemic absorption, so issues such as reduced bone mineral density, hyperglycemia, and HPA suppression are unlikely to be clinically significant
- Monitoring: Frequency of use, FEV1, peak-flow, pulse, blood pressure, and potassium (usually only necessary in high dosages), glucose (rarely clinically significant
- Drug and Diet Considerations:
  - Assess potassium intake and blood levels of potassium if the patient is using a beta agonist frequently or has a history of hypokalemia
  - Be aware of caffeine intake in combination with a beta-agonist as it can have an additive effect on blood pressure and heart rate
  - Monitor diabetes patients for elevations in blood sugar

Fluticasone and Vilanterol (Breo Ellipta)
- Class: Inhaled corticosteroid and long acting beta-agonist
- Mechanism of Action: Provides anti-inflammatory effects through fluticasone and stimulates beta-2 receptors leading to relaxation of smooth muscle and opening of airways
- Common Uses: Treatment of asthma and COPD
- Memorable Side Effects: Thrush, tachycardia, anxiousness, tremor; rare effects include: reduced bone mineral density, HPA suppression, hypokalemia and hyperglycemia
- Clinical Pearls:
  - Inhaled corticosteroids have a very low rate of systemic absorption, so issues such as reduced bone mineral density, hyperglycemia, and HPA suppression are unlikely to be clinically significant
- Monitoring: Frequency of use, FEV1, peak-flow, pulse, blood pressure, and potassium (usually only necessary in high dosages), glucose (rarely clinically significant
- Drug and Diet Considerations:
  - Assess potassium intake and blood levels of potassium if the patient is using a beta agonist frequently or has a history of hypokalemia
  - Be aware of caffeine intake in combination with a beta-agonist as it can have an additive effect on blood pressure and heart rate
  - Monitor diabetes patients for elevations in blood sugar

Fluvastatin (Lescol)
- Class: Statin, antilipemic
- Mechanism of Action: HMG Co-A reductase inhibitor
- Common Uses: Reduction of cholesterol, particularly LDL
- Memorable Side Effects: Muscle aches, rhabdomyolysis (rare, but serious)
- Clinical Pearls:

- Statins, like atorvastatin, are one of the mainstays of therapy to reduce cholesterol, and more particularly LDL (bad cholesterol)
- The most notable side effect with statins that you will likely hear patients complain about is myopathy (muscle aches/pain)
- Usually muscle aches are all over which can help you differentiate from other pain conditions or pain/soreness from an injury or overuse
- Contraindicated in pregnancy
- Patients who do not tolerate atorvastatin, may try another statin as long as adverse effects aren't too severe (i.e. rhabdomyolysis); if you notice that the patient had an allergy or intolerance, you need to clarify with the provider
- CPK will be the primary lab to test for rhabdomyolysis, breakdown of muscle; this elevation in CPK may eventually lead to kidney failure
- Patients usually will present with myopathy when the medication is first started or increased, but be on the lookout for new medications that can interact with statins like CYP3A4 inhibitor drug interactions with medications like fluconazole or erythromycin; these interactions will cause atorvastatin concentrations in the body to go up, potentially leading to toxicity
- Gemfibrozil is a cholesterol medication that also interacts with atorvastatin and dual use should be addressed with the primary provider
- For many statins it is "recommended" to give them at night; the theory is cholesterol production happens at night
- Monitoring: Lipids, LFTs, CPK if experiencing muscle pain (myopathy)
- Drug and Diet Considerations:
  - Liver toxicity risk from alcohol (usually in excess) may be increased if used in combination with statins
  - Low, not clinically significant, risk of elevating blood sugars in patients with diabetes
  - Can be taken with or without food
  - Encourage a lipid lowering diet for any patient taking a cholesterol medication

Fluvoxamine (Luvox)

- Class: SSRI, antidepressant
- Mechanism of Action: Selective serotonin reuptake inhibitor; increases serotonin in the brain
- Common Uses: Treatment of depression, anxiety and PTSD
- Memorable Side Effects: GI side effects (N/V/D), sedation or activation depending upon the patient, changes in mental status, hyponatremia (rare)
- Clinical Pearls:
  - Fluvoxamine is not a typical first line agent as it has numerous drug interactions
  - Boxed warning for an increased risk of suicidal thinking when first starting these medications)
  - Although not terribly common, hyponatremia (low sodium) is a possible unique side effect with SSRIs and much more likely in patients already prone to hyponatremia; a classic example would be patients who are taking diuretics, which can also lower sodium

- o Remember that these drugs are not an immediate fix; SSRIs take weeks to months before a patient will start improving; however side effects can be apparent from the start of the medication, making it difficult to coach our patients to continue the medication in the first few weeks after starting it
  - o SSRIs can decrease libido
- Monitoring: EKG, potassium and magnesium if the patient is at risk for QTc prolongation; sodium level if the patient is displaying symptoms of hyponatremia
- Drug and Diet Considerations:
  - o Weight gain or weight loss can happen with SSRIs; monitor for changes over time once started, increased, reduced, or discontinued
  - o Diarrhea can happen, but isn't incredibly common; assess fluid status, notify provider if the patient is reporting this side effect
  - o If the patient has a prolonged QT interval, out of range electrolytes like potassium and magnesium could increase the risk for Torsades de Pointes
  - o Low sodium can be a rare adverse effect
  - o Can be taken with or without food
  - o Alcohol has additive, unpredictable effects when used with SSRIs

Folic Acid
- Class: Folic acid supplement
- Mechanism of Action: Replacement of dietary folic acid
- Common Uses: Pregnancy, patients on methotrexate or other meds that cause low folic acid levels and in folate-deficiency anemia
- Memorable Side Effects: GI upset if anything, but virtually no side effects
- Clinical Pearls:
  - o Deficiency can lead to anemia
  - o Found in nearly all multivitamins
  - o Added to certain foods per FDA requirements
  - o Water soluble, won't accumulate in the body
- Monitoring: Hemoglobin and folate levels
- Drug and Diet Considerations:
  - o Methotrexate, trimethoprim, triamterene, sulfasalazine, and pyrimethamine can all reduce levels of folic acid
  - o Folic acid supplementation is recommended in pregnancy to minimize risk of neural tube defects
  - o No preference as to with or without food
  - o Folic acid may modestly reduce phenytoin and primidone levels

Formoterol (Foradil, Perforomist)
- Class: Long acting beta-agonist
- Mechanism of Action: Stimulates beta-2 receptors leading to relaxation of smooth muscle and opening of airways
- Common Uses: Treatment of COPD and prevention of asthma attacks and exercise-induced bronchospasm
- Memorable Side Effects: Tachycardia, tremor, anxiousness, hypokalemia (rare), hyperglycemia (rare)
- Clinical Pearls:

133

- o Increased risk of asthma death in patients who take long acting beta agonists as monotherapy
- o Perforomist is a nebulized formulation
- o Available in combination with inhaled budesonide as brand name Symbicort
- Monitoring: Frequency of use, FEV1, peak-flow, pulse, blood pressure, and potassium (usually only necessary in high dosages), glucose (rarely clinically significant
- Drug and Diet Considerations:
  - o Assess potassium intake and blood levels of potassium if the patient is using a beta agonist frequently or has a history of hypokalemia
  - o Be aware of caffeine intake in combination with a beta-agonist as it can have an additive effect on blood pressure and heart rate
  - o Monitor diabetes patients for elevations in blood sugar

Fosfomycin (Monurol)
- Class: Antibiotic
- Mechanism of Action: Fosfomycin deactivates pyruvyl transferase which is necessary for bacterial cell wall synthesis
- Common Uses: Treatment of uncomplicated urinary tract infections
- Memorable Side Effects: GI upset is common, rarely may cause elevated LFTs and hypersensitivity reactions
- Clinical Pearls:
  - o Comes as a 3 gram packet
  - o Typically done as a one-time dose
  - o If the patient has any potential systemic symptoms indicating upper UTI (kidney infection) this drug should not be used as it only has activity in the lower urinary tract
- Monitoring: For short term use, lab work is not typically necessary
- Drug and Diet Considerations:
  - o Mix oral agent with 90-120 mls of cool water prior to administration
  - o May be given with or without food

Fosinopril (Monopril)
- Class: Antihypertensive, ACE inhibitor
- Mechanism of Action: Inhibits angiotensin converting enzyme which prevents the production of angiotensin 2 and leads to lower BP; angiotensin 2 is a potent vasoconstrictor
- Common Uses: Treatment of hypertension, acute MI and heart failure
- Memorable Side Effects: Cough, kidney impairment, low blood pressure, hyperkalemia, angioedema
- Clinical Pearls:
  - o ACE inhibitors are notoriously known for causing a dry chronic cough
  - o Angiotensin Receptor Blockers (ARBs) are the cousins to the ACE Inhibitors and are the first line substitute to a patient who has had a cough with an ACE inhibitor
  - o ACE inhibitors can exacerbate kidney impairment as well as contribute to acute renal failure especially in patients who are already on other potential renal toxic medications (i.e. diuretics,

NSAIDs, etc.) even though in conditions like heart failure, diuretics and ACE inhibitors are often used together
- ○ ACE inhibitors can cause elevated potassium levels; if your patient has hyperkalemia, you must make sure the ACE inhibitor has been addressed
- ○ In some cases, patients of African descent may not respond to ACE inhibitors as well as other ethnicities
- ○ ACE inhibitors should not be used in combination with an ARB
- ○ ACE inhibitors and ARBs are frequently used in patients with hypertension and a history of diabetes, stroke, CAD, CKD, or CHF
- ○ Angioedema (swelling of the lips/airway) is classically caused by ACE inhibitors; it is an extremely rare, but very serious reaction requiring immediate discontinuation
- • Monitoring: Renal function, potassium, blood pressure
- • Drug and Diet Considerations:
  - ○ Be cautious and monitor potassium closely in patients with high dietary intake of potassium as this could contribute to hyperkalemia in combination with this medication
  - ○ Administer with or without food

Frovatriptan (Frova)
- • Class: Anti-migraine, triptan
- • Mechanism of Action: Serotonin 5HT agonist which causes vasoconstriction and reduction in inflammation associated with migraine
- • Common Uses: Acute relief of migraine
- • Memorable Side Effects: Dizziness, changes in CNS
- • Clinical Pearls:
  - ○ Meant for acute relief of migraine, not prophylaxis
  - ○ Be sure to assess frequent use; if using frequently, need to have control of migraines assessed and have controller medication added (valproic acid, propranolol, topiramate, etc.)
  - ○ Often used with NSAIDs (i.e. naproxen) in migraine treatment
  - ○ Does have serotonin activity so could potentially contribute to serotonin syndrome (higher risk in patients already on SSRIs, tramadol, etc.)
- • Monitoring: Blood pressure, EKG when clinically indicated to assess risk for QTc prolongation
- • Drug and Diet Considerations:
  - ○ Given as needed for migraine, so administration at any point is fine with regards to food

Furosemide (Lasix)
- • Class: Loop diuretic
- • Mechanism of Action: Inhibit sodium and chloride reabsorption in the ascending "Loop" of Henle in the kidney
- • Common Use: Treatment of edema, hypertension and heart failure
- • Memorable Side Effects: Frequent urination, electrolyte depletion, low blood pressure, dehydration and renal impairment
- • Clinical Pearls:
  - ○ While furosemide can cause significant reductions in magnesium, calcium, sodium, etc., potassium is one of the most important

135

electrolytes to monitor and often patients require potassium supplementation; this can sometimes be offset by potassium sparing diuretics like spironolactone, ARBs, like losartan, and ACE inhibitors like lisinopril (all potentially increase potassium)

- o Frequent urination can be significantly upsetting to patients and can greatly impact their wellbeing; if possible, make sure these loop diuretics are not given too close to bedtime and disrupting their sleep
- o Whenever you see a new Rx for a loop diuretic, be sure to look at the other medications the patient is taking to make sure that the edema is not a side effect; classic causes of edema include calcium channel blockers, pioglitazone, pregabalin, and NSAIDs.
- o Loops deplete volume in the body, so patients run the risk of not having adequate perfusion through the kidney; elevations in creatinine from baseline can help us monitor for this risk
- o Kidney function and electrolytes are going to be the primary labs to monitor
- o Urinary output and monitoring of weights can be very important patient factors to monitor and help assess the efficacy of how well the loop diuretics working

- Monitoring: Renal function and electrolytes (essentially can deplete all electrolytes), weights, blood pressure, hearing (when used at high doses)
- Drug and Diet Considerations:
  - o Potassium supplementation is usually required as furosemide can cause significant hypokalemia
  - o Monitor for dehydration warning signs
  - o With or without food is acceptable

Gabapentin (Neurontin)

- Class: Antiepileptic
- Mechanism of Action: Not very clear, but may modulate excitatory neurotransmitters
- Common Uses: Relief of various types of nerve pain, seizures, anxiety
- Memorable Side Effects: Sedation, dizziness, edema
- Clinical Pearls:
  - o Generally classified as an anti-seizure medication, but most often used for neuropathy
  - o Keep an eye out for patients with kidney disease who may be experiencing side effects, this drug can accumulate in patients with poor renal function
  - o Watch out for dizziness and sedation in our elderly patients as this can potentially contribute to falls
  - o Weight gain in the form of edema may potentially happen with gabapentin; be on the lookout for patients with a history CHF and edema issues, as well as those who may already be receiving diuretics like furosemide
  - o Pregabalin in general has a very similar mechanism of action to gabapentin, so it may also potentially be used, although currently more expensive
- Monitoring: Renal function (dose adjustments need to be made based upon kidney function)
- Drug and Diet Considerations:
  - o Alcohol can have additive CNS depressant effects

- o With or without food is acceptable for the immediate release product

Galantamine (Razadyne, Razadyne ER)
- Class: Dementia agent, acetylcholinesterase inhibitor
- Mechanism of Action: Inhibits acetylcholinesterase which increases acetylcholine in the CNS
- Common Uses: Treatment of Alzheimer's dementia
- Memorable Side Effects: GI (N/V/D), weight loss, insomnia, dizziness, bradycardia
- Clinical Pearls:
  - o One of the more common drug causes of weight loss in the elderly
  - o Likely will NOT reverse dementia symptoms, but may help with some symptom improvement
  - o Dementia medications in general can contribute to behavioral changes (good or bad)
- Monitoring: Weight, GI adverse effects, pulse
- Drug and Diet Considerations:
  - o Significant cause of weight loss and poor appetite
  - o Assess for GI upset and loose stools
  - o Giving with food is preferable but not necessary

Ganciclovir (Cytovene)
- Class: Antiviral
- Mechanism of Action: Inhibits DNA synthesis and viral replication
- Common Uses: Cytomegalovirus prophylaxis
- Memorable Side Effects: Diarrhea, weight loss, GI upset, blood dyscrasias, neuropathy
- Clinical Pearls:
  - o Boxed warning for carcinogenicity and teratogenicity
  - o Boxed warning for the risk of granulocytopenia, thrombocytopenia, anemia, or pancytopenia
- Monitoring: Renal function, CBC, pregnancy testing
- Drug and Diet Considerations:
  - o Assess dietary intake while taking this medication due to the risk of anorexia

Gemfibrozil (Lopid)
- Class: Antilipemic agent, fibric acid derivative
- Mechanism of Action: Not well understood, ultimately decreases cholesterol, particularly used for triglycerides
- Common Uses: Treatment of elevated triglycerides
- Memorable Side Effects: Dyspepsia , rhabdomyolysis/myopathy possible especially when co-administered with statins
- Clinical Pearls:
  - o Interacts with many of the statins, but sometimes used together
  - o Important to educate patients and have heightened monitoring for statin adverse effects if using gemfibrozil with a statin
  - o Usually dosed twice daily, 30 minutes prior to breakfast and dinner
  - o GI upset is usually the primary adverse effect

137

- Monitoring: Lipids, LFTs as clinically indicated
- Drug and Diet Considerations:
    - Encourage cholesterol lowering diet
    - To maximize absorption, give 30 minutes before meals

Gentamicin
- Class: Aminoglycoside, antibiotic
- Mechanism of Action: Blocks bacterial protein synthesis
- Common Uses: Treatment of UTIs, sepsis and skin infections caused by gram negative bacteria
- Memorable Side Effects: CNS changes, diarrhea, kidney impairment, changes in hearing
- Clinical Pearls:
    - Nephrotoxic drug, kidney function monitoring is critical
    - Monitoring of drug levels important
    - Usual trough target is less than 2mcg/mL
    - Ototoxicity is more likely with prolonged use
    - Peak sample usually drawn 30 minutes after infusion complete and trough right before next dose
- Monitoring: Renal function, drug levels, hearing test in patients on long-term therapy, electrolytes
- Drug and Diet Considerations:
    - Dehydration may exacerbate the risk of renal impairment caused by gentamicin
    - Supplementation of certain electrolytes might be considered if clinically indicated (potassium, magnesium, or calcium)
    - Monitor for anorexia risk with long term use

Glimepiride (Amaryl)
- Class: Anti-diabetic agent, sulfonylurea
- Mechanism of Action: Stimulates pancreatic cells to produce/release insulin
- Common Uses: Treatment of diabetes
- Memorable Side Effects: Hypoglycemia, weight gain
- Clinical Pearls:
    - Via its mechanism of action, whenever you increase insulin, hypoglycemia is of highest concern
    - Blood sugars may bottom out in the early morning upon awakening, due to lack of dietary intake overnight
    - Elderly can be especially at risk for hypoglycemia and severe complication from an event
    - Weight gain can be problematic in type 2 patients as many likely struggle with metabolic syndrome/weight control already
- Monitoring: HbA1c, blood glucose, risk for hypoglycemia
- Drug and Diet Considerations:
    - Be very cautious of the risk of hypoglycemia if there is a significant reduction in dietary intake (i.e. acute illness, nausea/vomiting)
    - Rarely, alcohol could cause a disulfiram or flushing type reaction when combined with the drug
    - Be attentive to appetite changes or new diabetes medications and monitor for hypoglycemia
    - Generally given with the first meal of the day

- o Patient without caloric intake will likely have to hold this medication (i.e. before surgery)

Glipizide (Glucotrol)
- Class: Anti-diabetic agent, sulfonylurea
- Mechanism of Action: Stimulates pancreatic cells to produce/release insulin
- Common Uses: Management of diabetes
- Memorable Side Effects: Hypoglycemia, weight gain
- Clinical Pearls:
  - o Via its mechanism of action, whenever you increase insulin, hypoglycemia is of highest concern
  - o Be attentive to appetite changes or new diabetes medications and monitor for hypoglycemia
  - o Blood sugars may bottom out in the early morning upon awakening, due to lack of dietary intake overnight
  - o Elderly can be especially at risk for hypoglycemia
  - o Weight gain can be problematic in type 2 patients as many likely struggle with metabolic syndrome/weight control already
- Monitoring: HbA1c, blood glucose, risk for hypoglycemia
- Drug and Diet Considerations:
  - o Be very cautious of the risk of hypoglycemia if there is a significant reduction in dietary intake (i.e. acute illness, nausea/vomiting)
  - o Immediate release tablets should be administered 30 minutes before meals; extended release can be given with breakfast
  - o Rarely, alcohol could cause a disulfiram or flushing type reaction when combined with the drug
  - o Patient without caloric intake will likely have to hold this medication (i.e. before surgery)

Glucagon
- Class: Hypoglycemia antidote
- Mechanism of Action: Stimulates adenylate cyclase which results in increased glucose production causing an increase in blood sugar
- Common Uses: Treatment of hypoglycemia
- Memorable Side Effects: Hyperglycemia, change in BP/Pulse, GI
- Clinical Pearls:
  - o Be sure patients are educated on how/when to use glucagon
  - o If alert without any mental status change, most cases should be able to use oral glucose vs. glucagon
  - o Risk of aspiration exists if try to give oral glucose gel (or other source of sugar) to a patient who is in and out of consciousness – so give glucagon in this case
  - o Intranasal administration now available
- Monitoring: Blood glucose, pulse, blood pressure, cognition
- Drug and Diet Considerations:
  - o Glucagon will pull from glycogen stores which will reduce them over time; frequent use of glucagon is unlikely in clinical practice as it is primarily an emergency medication
  - o Replacement with carbohydrates is still going to be necessary following glucagon use

Glyburide (Micronase, Diabeta)

- Class: Antidiabetic agent, sulfonylurea
- Mechanism of Action: Stimulates pancreatic cells to produce/release insulin
- Common Uses: Diabetes management
- Memorable Side Effects: Hypoglycemia, weight gain
- Clinical Pearls:
    - Glipizide is usually preferred over glyburide in the elderly if a sulfonylurea is used
    - Via its mechanism of action, whenever you increase insulin, hypoglycemia is of highest concern
    - Be attentive to appetite changes or new diabetes medications and monitor for hypoglycemia
    - Blood sugars may bottom out in the early morning upon awakening, due to lack of dietary intake overnight
    - Elderly can be especially at risk for hypoglycemia
    - Weight gain can be problematic in type 2 patients as many likely struggle with metabolic syndrome/weight control already
- Monitoring: HbA1c, blood glucose, risk for hypoglycemia
- Drug and Diet Considerations:
    - Be very cautious for the risk of hypoglycemia if there is a significant reduction in dietary intake (i.e. acute illness, nausea/vomiting)
    - Take with meals
    - Rarely, alcohol could cause a disulfiram or flushing type reaction when combined with the drug
    - Patient without caloric intake will likely have to hold this medication (i.e. before surgery)

Glycopyrrolate (Robinul)

- Class: Anticholinergic
- Mechanism of Action: Blocks acetylcholine receptors which relaxes parasympathetic smooth muscle, dries secretions and can provide motion sickness and nausea and vomiting relief
- Common Uses: Reduce secretions
- Memorable Side Effects: Anticholinergic effects (can't spit, see, pee or poop)
- Clinical Pearls:
    - Oral and IV dosage forms are available
    - Tachycardia is a rare, dose dependent complication
- Monitoring: Pulse
- Drug and Diet Considerations:
    - Alcohol can exacerbate the CNS depressant effect
    - The side effect of dry mouth could affect eating habits
    - Give 1 hour before or 2 hours after food to maximize absorption

Glycopyrrolate (Seebri, Lonhala Magnair)

- Class: Inhaled anticholinergic
- Mechanism of Action: Inhaled anticholinergic can open up airways and decrease secretions
- Common Uses: Treatment of COPD

- Memorable Side Effects: Dry mouth, cough, irritation to the lungs, minimal systemic absorption and usually well tolerated
- Clinical Pearls:
  - It is long acting and meant to be used as a controller medication
  - It will not provide acute relief from respiratory distress, not meant to be a rescue inhalation product
  - Often by using this medication in COPD, our goal is likely to improve respiratory status, but also to reduce the amount of as needed albuterol and/or albuterol/ipratropium (Duoneb or Combivent)
  - With the delivery device, it is imperative to assess if patients are able to adequately coordinate how to use the device as well as if they are able to inhale quickly and forcefully enough to get the drug into their lungs
  - Systemic anticholinergic effects (can't spit, see, pee or poop) are usually not a concern as systemic absorption is low
  - Nebulized formulation
- Monitoring: FEV1, peak flow
- Drug and Diet Considerations:
  - Inhaled, local medication
  - Dry mouth may impact dietary/fluid intake

Glycopyrronium and Formoterol (Bevespi)
- Class: Inhaled anticholinergic and long acting beta-agonist
- Mechanism of Action: Provides anti-cholinergic effects and stimulates beta-2 receptors leading to relaxation of smooth muscle and opening of airways
- Common Uses: Long term maintenance and treatment of COPD
- Memorable Side Effects: Tachycardia, tremor, anxiousness and dry mouth, rarely, hypokalemia and hyperglycemia
- Clinical Pearls:
  - See Glycopyrrolate for further information on this medication
- Monitoring: Frequency of use, FEV1, peak-flow, pulse, blood pressure, and potassium (usually only necessary in high dosages), glucose (rarely clinically significant
- Drug and Diet Considerations:
  - Assess potassium intake and blood levels of potassium if the patient is using a beta agonist frequently or has a history of hypokalemia
  - Be aware of caffeine intake in combination with a beta-agonist as it can have an additive effect on blood pressure and heart rate
  - Monitor diabetes patients for elevations in blood sugar
  - See Glycopyrrolate for further information on this medication

Goserelin (Zoladex)
- Class: Oncology agent, GnRH (LHRH) agonist
- Mechanism of Action: Ultimately leads to a blockade of gonadotropin secretion which can lower gonadotropin (LH) and follicle stimulating hormone activity (FSH) and subsequently reduce testosterone and estrogen production
- Common Uses: Treatment of prostate cancer, endometriosis and breast cancer
- Memorable Side Effects: Flushing, weight changes, injection site reaction, edema, sweating, reduced libido, CNS changes, GI upset, reduce bone mineral density, blood sugar elevations, hyperlipidemia

141

- Clinical Pearls:
  - Injection only
- Monitoring: Hormonal levels depending upon indication, bone mineral density, cardiovascular risk factors such as lipids and blood pressure, HbA1C in at risk diabetes patients, renal function
- Drug and Diet Considerations:
  - Assess calcium and vitamin D intake due to reduced bone mineral density risks
  - Ensure adequate electrolyte levels
  - Lipid and diabetes friendly diet may be appropriate in at risk patients

Granisetron (Sustol, Sancuso)
- Class: Antiemetic, serotonin receptor antagonist
- Mechanism of Action: Blocks serotonin at 5HT3 receptors; acts centrally in the chemoreceptor trigger zone
- Common Uses: Prevention of nausea and vomiting in association with chemotherapy or radiation
- Memorable Side Effects: Constipation, sedation, QTc prolongation is a risk, but rare unless the patient is on other drugs that can contribute to QTc prolongation or has risk factors
- Clinical Pearls:
  - Frequently used in patients undergoing chemotherapy (nausea/vomiting common with chemo)
  - Can be used as needed or scheduled
  - Can cause QTc prolongation especially when used in combo with other QTc prolonging agents
  - Has serotonin activity, be on the lookout for other serotonergic medications (like SSRIs, tramadol etc.)
- Monitoring: Assessment for QTc prolongation and associated risk factors such as EKG, magnesium, and potassium
- Drug and Diet Considerations:
  - With or without food is acceptable (oral, IV formulation)
  - Typically timed before chemotherapy

Griseofulvin (Gris-PEG)
- Class: Antifungal
- Mechanism of Action: Blocks mitosis of fungal cells
- Common Uses: Treatment of resistant infections such as Athlete's Foot, toe nail infections, ringworm
- Memorable Side Effects: Sedation, dizziness, skin reactions, GI upset
- Clinical Pearls:
  - Drug of choice for tinea capitis
  - Lab work is typically not done unless the patient is on chronic therapy
- Monitoring: CBC, LFTs, renal function
- Drug and Diet Considerations:
  - A high fat meal is recommended to increase absorption; taking with food will also reduce the risk of GI upset
  - Alcohol intake may cause a disulfiram reaction when taking this medication

Guaifenesin (Mucinex, Tussin, Mucus Relief, and Multiple Other Names)

- Class: Mucous expectorant
- Mechanism of Action: Possibly increases amount of liquid in respiratory tract thereby has an expectorant effect
- Common Uses: Promote loosening of mucus
- Memorable Side Effects: Pretty well tolerated overall
- Clinical Pearls:
    - Some argue that guaifenesin is not an effective expectorant
    - Found in many OTC cough and cold preparations
    - There is an immediate release and extended release product
    - Always important with over the counter medications to educate patients on factors that may help guide them on when to seek medical attention with common cold symptoms (symptoms greater than 7 days, continually worsening symptoms, significant fever, rash, underlying respiratory condition, high risk for complications, etc.)
    - Common combination product guaifenesin and codeine (brand names: Robitussin AC, Cheratussin)
- Monitoring: No routine lab work is necessary
- Drug and Diet Considerations:
    - No significant concerns with diet changes

Guaifenesin and Codeine (Robitussin AC, Cheratussin)

- Class: Mucous expectorant, cough suppressant
- Mechanism of Action: See individual agents (codeine/APAP, and guaifenesin)

Guanfacine (Tenex)

- Class: Antihypertensive, alpha-2 agonist
- Mechanism of Action: Centrally acting alpha-2 agonist which results in decreased sympathetic activity and drop in blood pressure
- Common Uses: Treatment of hypertension and symptoms associated with ADHD and anxiety
- Memorable Side Effects: Drowsiness, dizziness, dry mouth
- Clinical Pearls:
    - Mainly used in hypertension, but occasionally will see it used off-label for various psych issues
    - Low blood pressure and pulse is possible
    - Sedating which can be a significant problem especially in the elderly
    - Rebound hypertension is a risk if abruptly discontinued
- Monitoring: Blood pressure, pulse
- Drug and Diet Considerations:
    - Alcohol can exacerbate the CNS depressant effect
    - Can be given with or without food
    - Grapefruit juice can raise concentrations

Haloperidol (Haldol)

- Class: 1st generation antipsychotic
- Mechanism of Action: Blocks dopamine receptors

- Common Uses: Management of schizophrenia and bipolar disorder symptoms; off label to treat dementia-related behaviors like aggression, hallucinations and delusions
- Memorable Side Effects: Sedation, fall risk, orthostatic BP changes, EPS, metabolic syndrome
- Clinical Pearls:
  - Haloperidol is a first generation antipsychotic and has a very high rate of EPS (movement disorder side effects)
  - Usually higher doses are required for younger patients with schizophrenia and/or bipolar disorder while lower doses can and should be used in the elderly
  - Antipsychotic medications block dopamine and can exacerbate conditions where there is a shortage of dopamine, like Parkinson's disorder (remember that we use dopamine to treat Parkinson's – i.e. carbidopa/levodopa)
  - Sedation, orthostatic hypotension and movement disorder side effects can all increase the risk of falls especially in our elderly patients
  - NMS (neuroleptic malignant syndrome) is a very rare but very serious complication with antipsychotic medications; a few symptoms of NMS include: fever, hyperreflexia, confusion, delirium and tremor
  - Antipsychotics increase risk of metabolic syndrome (diabetes, elevated lipids, weight gain, etc.); it is important to periodically monitor for this, especially in younger patients with schizophrenia and/or bipolar disorder who may be likely to require long term use of higher doses
  - Anticholinergic effects are possible as well with antipsychotics, dry eyes, dry mouth, exacerbation of urinary retention (i.e. BPH), constipation (SLUD – can't salivate, lacrimate, urinate or defecate)
  - Antipsychotics can contribute to QTc prolongation, which can be especially problematic in patients who are already on antiarrhythmic medications and at risk
- Monitoring: Weight, BMI, lipids, HbA1c, blood sugars, EKG as clinically appropriate, electrolytes (potassium and magnesium important if the patient is at risk for QTc prolongation)
- Drug and Diet Considerations:
  - Increased appetite and risk for metabolic syndrome
  - Increased blood sugars can result in our diabetes patients, monitor blood sugars closely with acute changes in the drug
  - Alcohol may exacerbate the CNS depressant effect
  - Can be administered with or without meals

Heparin
- Class: Anticoagulant
- Mechanism of Action: Primarily inactivates thrombin, may also have effects on other clotting factors
- Common Uses: Treatment and prevention of clots, also used in PCI, and to prevent clotting/flush IV lines
- Memorable Side Effects: Bleeding, thrombocytopenia, HIT (rare)
- Clinical Pearls:
  - Bleed risk is top monitoring parameter

- o Risk of thrombocytopenia (heparin induced thrombocytopenia – "HIT"); platelets are very important to monitor
- o Used to flush IV lines and prevent clotting
- o Many concentrations available (scary for medication error risk)
- Monitoring: CBC, platelets, PT, aPTT, anti-Factor Xa, bleed risk, renal function, potassium (not likely to be done in short term use unless clinical circumstances dictate)
- Drug and Diet Considerations:
  - o Vitamin E, Omega-3 fatty acids, gingko, garlic, ginseng, turmeric, and fish oil supplements have been purported to have antiplatelet type activity which in theory could increase the risk of bleed – clinical significance is questionable; the most common resolution is to discontinue the supplements if they are not necessary
  - o Alcohol may have an additive antiplatelet type effect and increase the risk of GI bleed
  - o Very rare risk for hyperkalemia, be aware of any diet contributions as well as other medications if the patient's potassium is elevated

Hydralazine (Apresoline)
- Class: Vasodilator, antihypertensive
- Mechanism of Action: Directly dilates arteries and arterioles to decrease BP
- Common Uses: Treatment of hypertension
- Memorable Side Effects: Low BP, CNS changes, exacerbate/contribute to lupus (rare)
- Clinical Pearls:
  - o Fall/orthostatic blood pressure risk
  - o Can exacerbate lupus
  - o Dosed multiple times per day so difficult for patients to adhere to medication regimen
- Monitoring: Blood pressure, ANA (if Lupus-type reaction is suspected), pulse, CBC as clinically indicated
- Drug and Diet Considerations:
  - o Consistent administration with respect to food is recommended, however, that can be challenging due to multiple daily doses

Hydrochlorothiazide (Hydrodiuril)
- Class: Antihypertensive, thiazide diuretic
- Mechanism of Action: Inhibits sodium/chloride transporter in the distal tubules
- Common Use: Treatment of hypertension, edema and heart failure
- Memorable Side Effects: Similar to loop diuretics, they increase urine output and decrease amount of volume in the body which can lead to frequent urination, electrolyte depletion, low blood pressure, and increased risk of kidney failure, photosensitivity
- Clinical Pearls:
  - o One of the major differences between loops and thiazides are that thiazides can INCREASE serum calcium while loops will reduce it
  - o While loop diuretics can cause hyperuricemia (elevated uric acid possibly contributing to or exacerbating gout), thiazides are classically known to do this; be on the lookout for hydrochlorothiazide when gout medications are being added or patients are reporting gout flares

145

- o Hydrochlorothiazide (HCTZ) is used in many medication combinations for hypertension: Triamterene/HCTZ, Lisinopril/HCTZ, etc. This can often confuse patients and they may not realize that they are actually receiving two medications
  - o Kidney function and electrolytes are going to be the primary labs to monitor; potassium supplementation is common in patients taking diuretics
  - o Watch the timing of diuretics like hydrochlorothiazide; evening doses may cause frequent nighttime urination
- Monitoring: Renal function, electrolytes, blood pressure, uric acid (in patients with gout)
- Drug and Diet Considerations:
  - o A low potassium or low magnesium diet could increase the risk for deficiency in combination with the drug
  - o Hypercalcemia is possible; be aware of calcium and vitamin D intake
  - o This drug is dehydrating so be aware of acute renal failure risk in patients who have reduced fluid intake (i.e. acutely ill, geriatric patients, etc.)
  - o Alcohol may exacerbate low blood pressure and urinary frequency
  - o Modest increases in glucose may happen in our diabetes patients (typically not clinically significant)
  - o Possible cause of weight loss

Hydrochlorothiazide and Spironolactone (Aldactazide)
- See individual agents hydrochlorothiazide and spironolactone

Hydrocodone/acetaminophen (Norco, Lortab)
- Class: Opioid analgesic – also see acetaminophen
- Mechanism of Action: Binds opioid receptors to inhibit CNS pain pathways and cause pain relief; acetaminophen is believed to inhibit prostaglandin production, but does not have anti-inflammatory effects like NSAIDs
- Common Uses: Management of pain disorders, both chronic and acute
- Memorable Side Effects: Constipation, sedation, respiratory depression, CNS effects like confusion, delirium, etc., itch, liver toxicity (acetaminophen in large doses >4 grams/day)
- Clinical Pearls:
  - o With continuous use of opioid-type medication, we have to assess constipation and patients will likely require the use of laxatives
  - o Be extremely cautious with acetaminophen use and make sure our patient is aware that this product has acetaminophen in it; accidental overdose is a significant problem as acetaminophen is in literally hundreds of over the counter and other prescription products
  - o In general, a 3,000 mg (3 gram) max is recommended; 4,000 mg is generally considered safe, and you may see it utilized under certain controlled situations in adults
  - o Naloxone is reversal agent for opioids
  - o Oxycodone and hydrocodone are not interchangeable
- Monitoring: Bowel movements, pain management, risk for addiction
- Drug and Diet Considerations:
  - o Alcohol can exacerbate the CNS depressant effect from hydrocodone
  - o Giving with food and water can reduce the risk of GI upset

- o Encourage a constipation friendly diet including fiber, fluids and exercise as hydrocodone can be very constipating
- o See acetaminophen for information on that medication

Hydromorphone (Dilaudid)
- Class: Opioid analgesic
- Mechanism of Action: Binds opioid receptors to inhibit CNS pain pathways and cause pain relief
- Common Uses: Management of pain disorders, both chronic and acute
- Memorable Side Effects: Constipation, sedation, CNS effects like confusion, delirium, etc., respiratory depression
- Clinical Pearls:
  - o Hydromorphone is a scheduled 2 controlled substance; risk of addiction and dependence
  - o It is critical to educate/assess patients for constipation if they are taking frequent opioids like hydromorphone
  - o Naloxone is reversal agent for opioids
  - o Driving/working machinery is certainly risky when using opioids as they can cause significant sedation; less sedation occurs with chronic use
- Monitoring: Bowel movements, pain management, risk for addiction
- Drug and Diet Considerations:
  - o Alcohol can exacerbate the CNS depressant effect from hydromorphone
  - o Giving with food and water can reduce the risk of GI upset
  - o Encourage a constipation friendly diet including fiber, fluids and exercise, as opioids can be very constipating

Hydroxychloroquine (Plaquenil)
- Class: Disease modifying antirheumatic drug, antimalarial, aminoquinoline
- Mechanism of Action: Inhibits dihydroorotate dehydrogenase which has an important role in synthesis of uridine monophosphate; uridine monophosphate is necessary for DNA/RNA production – leads to an immunosuppressive type effect
- Common Uses: Treatment of rheumatoid arthritis, lupus and malaria
- Memorable Side Effects: GI side effects, hair loss, ocular toxicity, anemia, myopathy, agranulocytosis, elevations in LFTs
- Clinical Pearls:
  - o Can cause birth defects, contraindicated in pregnancy
  - o QTc prolongation risk
- Monitoring: LFTs, CBC, eye exams, EKG as clinically indicated, electrolytes
- Drug and Diet Considerations:
  - o Administer with food

Hydroxyzine (Atarax, Vistaril)
- Class: Antihistamine, anticholinergic
- Mechanism of Action: Blocks muscarinic (anticholinergic) receptors and also has antihistamine effects
- Common Uses: Relief of itching caused by allergies, also short-term use to treat anxiety and insomnia

147

- Memorable Side Effects: Anticholinergic effects such as dry mouth, dry eyes, urinary retention, constipation, sedation, confusion
- Clinical Pearls:
  - Avoid, minimize use in geriatric patients
  - May have paradoxical insomnia reaction in pediatrics
- Monitoring: No routine lab work is typically necessary
- Drug and Diet Considerations:
  - Slows the motility of the GI tract which could increase the risk for constipation; maintain adequate fluids and non-constipating diet
  - Alcohol may exacerbate CNS depressant effects
  - Dry mouth may increase thirst and alter taste/pleasure of food
  - May be given with or without food

Hyoscyamine (Levsin)
- Class: GI antispasmodic, anticholinergic
- Mechanism of Action: Blocks acetylcholine receptors (anticholinergic) which relaxes smooth muscle
- Common Uses: Treatment of irritable bowel syndrome
- Memorable Side Effects: Anticholinergic effects (can't spit, see, pee or poop), sedation, confusion, increase in fall risk
- Clinical Pearls:
  - Primary use is to help relieve GI spasms/pain due to irritable bowel syndrome
  - Anticholinergic side effects can be prominent especially in the elderly population
  - Usually dosed multiple times throughout the day
  - If diarrhea is an issue associated with a patient's IBS, the anticholinergic effect of constipation can contribute to the patient's benefit
- Monitoring: No routine lab work is recommended
- Drug and Diet Considerations:
  - Alcohol can exacerbate the CNS depressant effect
  - The side effect of dry mouth could affect eating habits
  - Typically administered before a meal, but can still have benefits if administered with meals

Ibandronate (Boniva)
- Class: Bisphosphonate
- Mechanism of Action: Inhibits osteoclasts (osteoclasts break down bone)
- Common Uses: Treatment of osteoporosis
- Memorable Side Effects: Esophageal ulceration (administration procedure important to decrease this risk), GI side effects are most common
- Clinical Pearls:
  - Timing of administration is critical; take on an empty stomach in the morning, 60 minutes before first food, with 6-8 ounces of plain water)
  - Have patient remain sitting or standing upright for 60 minutes to reduce the risk of esophageal irritation/ulceration
  - Absorption will be limited and drug will not be effective if taken with food or other medications

- o After 5 years of bisphosphonate use, some lower risk patients may be able to have the medication reassessed for ongoing need and possibly discontinued
- o Osteonecrosis (destruction or dying) of bone in the jaw is extremely rare; patients may be at increased risk if recently had an invasive dental procedure
- o Be cautious with oral bisphosphonates in patients who already have esophageal or GI related concerns like a GI bleed or ulcer history
- o Once monthly dosing
- Monitoring: Bone mineral density, calcium, vitamin D levels
- Drug and Diet Considerations:
  - o Ensure the patient has adequate vitamin D and calcium intake of at least 1,200 mg per day of calcium and 1,000 units of vitamin D in females with osteoporosis
  - o Esophagitis and GI upset are possible which could cause changes in appetite and weight loss
  - o The drug must be taken in the morning prior to breakfast with 6-8 ounces of plain water and nothing else
  - o Wait at least 60 minutes prior to eating anything
  - o If taken with food, juice, or other medications, the absorption and effectiveness of the drug will be reduced

Ibuprofen (Motrin, Advil)

- Class: NSAID, antipyretic, analgesic
- Mechanism of Action: Inhibits Cyclooxygenase-1 and 2 (COX-1 and COX-2); results in a reduction in prostaglandins which cause pain, fever and inflammation
- Common Uses: Relief of pain, fever and inflammation
- Memorable Side Effects: GI ulcer, worsening kidney function, edema, hypertension and platelet inhibition, which can exacerbate bleed risk
- Clinical Pearls:
  - o NSAIDs are one of the most common causes of GI bleeding; this risk increases in the elderly and those on medications that increase risk of bleeding (anticoagulants and antiplatelet medications)
  - o Because of the side effects of GI upset/bleeding, NSAIDs should be taken with food
  - o Ibuprofen does have a relatively shorter half-life compared to other NSAIDs and usually needs to be dosed more frequently
  - o Due to effects on platelets, NSAIDs are typically held before/after surgery to reduce the risk of bleeding
  - o NSAIDs can contribute to edema and exacerbate CHF (congestive heart failure); be on the lookout and have NSAIDs reassessed if you see a patient with a CHF exacerbation or a patient requiring increasing diuretics, like furosemide
  - o NSAIDs can cause worsening kidney function (creatinine should be monitored); this risk can be greatly increased in patients on ACE inhibitors or ARBs and/or diuretic type medications
  - o Due to above reasons on kidney function, GI bleed risk, and CHF, NSAIDs are not the safest medication in the elderly; acetaminophen is generally preferred for generalized pain with a few exceptions

- o Although generally considered riskier in the elderly, a big advantage of NSAIDs over acetaminophen is that they can reduce inflammation
- o Pregnancy category C/D when >30 weeks gestation; NSAIDs are generally avoided in pregnancy and especially after 30 weeks gestation
- Monitoring: Renal function, hemoglobin, platelets (contained within CBC), blood pressure, signs of bruising or bleeding, weight (risk for edema)
- Drug and Diet Considerations:
  - o Because of significant incidence of GI upset, it is recommended to give with food or milk
  - o Dehydration coupled with ibuprofen may increase the risk for acute renal failure
  - o Excessive alcohol may increase GI bleed risk
  - o Vitamin E, Omega-3 fatty acids, gingko, garlic, ginseng, turmeric, and fish oil supplements have been purported to have antiplatelet type activity which in theory could increase the risk of bleed – clinical significance is questionable; the most common resolution is to discontinue the supplements if they are not necessary

Ifosfamide (Ifex)

- Class: Oncology agent, nitrogen mustard, alkylating agent
- Mechanism of Action: Prevents DNA cross-linking which ultimately prevents proliferation and growth of cells
- Common Uses: Treatment of numerous types of cancers
- Memorable Side Effects: Hemorrhagic cystitis, bladder toxicity, CNS toxicity, psychiatric changes, diarrhea, nausea and vomiting, hyponatremia, myelosuppression, hair loss, acidosis, renal toxicity
- Clinical Pearls:
  - o Mesna may be used in combination to reduce the risk for bladder toxicity
  - o IV hydration may also reduce the risk for bladder toxicity
- Monitoring: CBC, LFTs, renal function, electrolytes, urinalysis and output, EKG (as clinically indicated),
- Drug and Diet Considerations:
  - o Monitor for adequate hydration to reduce the risk for bladder complications
  - o Weight loss and poor nutrition may result on account of nausea and vomiting adverse effects

Iloperidone (Fanapt)

- Class: Antipsychotic
- Mechanism of Action: Blocks dopamine receptors
- Common Uses: Treatment of schizophrenia and bipolar disorder, and off label treatment of dementia-related behaviors like aggression, hallucinations and delusions
- Memorable Side Effects: Sedation, fall risk, orthostatic BP changes, EPS, metabolic syndrome
- Clinical Pearls:
  - o Usually higher doses are required for younger patients with schizophrenia and/or bipolar disorder while lower doses can and should be used in the elderly

- o Remember with antipsychotic medications that they block dopamine and can exacerbate conditions where there is a shortage of dopamine, like Parkinson's disorder (remember that we use dopamine to treat Parkinson's – i.e. carbidopa/levodopa or pramipexole)
- o Sedation, orthostatic hypotension, movement disorder side effects can all increase the risk of falls especially in our elderly patients
- o NMS (neuroleptic malignant syndrome) is a very rare but very serious complication with antipsychotic medications; a few symptoms of NMS include: fever, hyperreflexia, confusion, delirium and tremor
- o Antipsychotics increase risk of metabolic syndrome (diabetes, elevated lipids, weight gain, etc.); it is important to periodically monitor for this, especially in younger patients with schizophrenia and/or bipolar who may be likely to require long term use of higher doses
- o Anticholinergic effects are possible as well with antipsychotics: dry eyes, dry mouth, exacerbation of urinary retention (i.e. BPH), constipation (SLUD – can't salivate, lacrimate, urinate or defecate)
- o Antipsychotics can contribute to QTC prolongation, which can be especially problematic in patients who are already at risk (i.e. on antiarrhythmic medications)
- Monitoring: Weight, lipids, HbA1c, blood sugars
- Drug and Diet Considerations:
  - o Increased appetite and risk for metabolic syndrome
  - o Increased blood sugars can happen in our diabetes patients, monitor blood sugars closely with acute changes in the drug
  - o Can be administered with or without meals
  - o Alcohol may exacerbate CNS depressant effect

Imipenem/cilastatin (Primaxin)
- Class: Carbapenem, antibiotic
- Mechanism of Action: Binds penicillin-binding proteins and inhibits production of the bacterial cell wall; cilastatin blocks elimination of the drug by inhibiting dehydropeptidase in the renal tubules
- Common Uses: Broad spectrum antibiotic used in may resistant, severe infections, like complicated UTIs involving resistant organisms
- Memorable Side Effects: Reduction in hemoglobin and hematocrit, elevated liver enzymes, diarrhea, GI upset, lowers seizure threshold
- Clinical Pearls:
  - o Usually reserved for very severe, resistant infections
  - o Known for its coverage of Pseudomonas
  - o Good coverage for gram positive and gram negatives
    - Generally they do not cover MRSA
- Monitoring: Renal function, CBC, LFTs (as clinically indicated)
- Drug and Diet Considerations:
  - o Minimal concerns with shorter term use
  - o Monitor fluid and electrolyte status if diarrhea is problematic

Imipramine (Tofranil)
- Class: Tri-cyclic antidepressant (TCA)

- Mechanism of Action: Inhibits reuptake of serotonin and possibly norepinephrine
- Common Uses: Treatment of depression, neuropathy, pain syndromes, anxiety and PTSD
- Memorable Side Effects: Confusion, fall risk in elderly
- Clinical Pearls:
    - Old TCA generally not recommended in the elderly due to anticholinergic effects
    - Highly anticholinergic (can't spit, see, pee, or sh*t and increases confusion/fall risk) which can be especially problematic in geriatric patients – avoid if possible
    - In addition, cognitive impairment is not a good thing in the elderly due to possibility of preexisting dementia
    - TCAs may have some benefit in neuropathy, generally much cheaper than SNRIs, like duloxetine, which can also be beneficial in neuropathy
    - Not a good first line choice for sleep or depression; other agents exist that are much safer
    - Look out for TCAs causing the prescribing cascade; addition of artificial tears for dry eyes, constipation medications, BPH medications like tamsulosin, dementia medications, or artificial saliva will be a red flag
    - Often dosed in the evening due to the adverse effect of sedation
- Monitoring: EKG, and possibly electrolytes in at risk patients (especially in overdose), behavioral changes, weight, sodium (in patients with signs of hyponatremia),
- Drug and Diet Considerations:
    - Weight gain is possible and may be problematic
    - Slows the motility of the GI tract which could increase the risk for constipation; maintain adequate fluids and non-constipating diet
    - If GI upset occurs, no issues in giving the drug with food
    - Dry mouth may increase thirst and alter taste/pleasure of food
    - Poor intake may place the patient at higher risk for complications from electrolyte abnormalities (i.e. hyponatremia, hypokalemia, or hypomagnesemia)
    - Alcohol may exacerbate sedative adverse effect

Indacaterol (Arcapta Neohaler)

- Class: Long acting beta-agonist
- Mechanism of Action: Stimulates beta-2 receptors leading to relaxation of smooth muscle and opening of airways
- Common Uses: Long-term maintenance of COPD
- Memorable Side Effects: Tachycardia, tremor, anxiousness, hypokalemia (rare), hyperglycemia (rare)
- Clinical Pearls:
    - Increased risk of asthma death in patients who take long acting beta agonists as monotherapy
- Monitoring: Frequency of use, FEV1, peak-flow, pulse, blood pressure, and potassium (usually only necessary in high dosages), glucose (rarely clinically significant
- Drug and Diet Considerations:

- o Assess potassium intake and blood levels of potassium if the patient is using a beta agonist frequently or has a history of hypokalemia (rare)
- o Be aware of caffeine intake in combination with a beta-agonist as it can have an additive effect on blood pressure and heart rate
- o Monitor diabetes patients for elevations in blood sugar (rare)

Indapamide (Lozol)
- Class: Antihypertensive, thiazide-like diuretic
- Mechanism of Action: Inhibits sodium/chloride transporter in the distal tubules
- Common Use: Treatment of hypertension, edema and heart failure
- Memorable Side Effects: Similar to loop diuretics, they are going to increase urine output and decrease amount of volume in the body which can lead to frequent urination, electrolyte depletion, low blood pressure, and increased risk of kidney failure, photosensitivity
- Clinical Pearls:
  - o One of the major differences between loops and thiazides are that thiazides (and thiazide-like) can INCREASE serum calcium while loops will reduce it
  - o While loop diuretics can cause hyperuricemia (elevated uric acid possibly contributing to or exacerbating gout), thiazides are classically known to do this; be on the lookout for hydrochlorothiazide when gout medications are being added or patients are reporting gout flares
  - o Watch the timing of diuretics; evening doses can cause frequent nighttime urination
- Monitoring: Renal function, electrolytes, blood pressure, weight, uric acid (in patients with gout)
- Drug and Diet Considerations:
  - o A low potassium or low magnesium diet could increase the risk for deficiency in combination with the drug
  - o Hypercalcemia is possible; be aware of calcium and vitamin D intake
  - o This drug is dehydrating so be aware of acute renal failure risk in patients who have reduced fluid intake (i.e. acutely ill, geriatric patients, etc.)
  - o Alcohol may exacerbate low blood pressure and urinary frequency
  - o Modest increases in glucose may happen in our diabetes patients (typically not clinically significant)
  - o Possible cause of weight loss

Indinavir (Crixivan)
- Class: Protease inhibitor, antiretroviral
- Mechanism of Action: Binds to site where protein cleavage occurs and prevents protease from releasing essential proteins
- Common Uses: HIV treatment
- Memorable Side Effects: Buffalo hump, fat redistribution, metabolic effects like increased cholesterol and hyperglycemia, hepatotoxicity, skin reaction, nausea, vomiting, diarrhea, kidney stones
- Clinical Pearls:

- o Metabolic risks are a significant downside to long term use in younger populations
- o Not a preferred agent
- Monitoring: Lipids, glucose, HIV parameters (i.e. viral load and CD4 count), LFTs, CBC
- Drug and Diet Considerations:
  - o Essential to maintain hydration as there is a risk for renal stones with this medication; do not drink less than 48 ounces (approximately 1,500 milliliters)
  - o Monitor hyperglycemia risk; may need to adjust diet accordingly
  - o Lipid-lowering diet could help reduce the adverse effect of hypercholesterolemia
  - o Ideal to take on an empty stomach to maximize absorption; if stomach upset occurs, give with a small meal/snack

Indomethacin (Indocin)

- Class: NSAID, analgesic
- Mechanism of Action: Inhibits Cyclooxygenase-1 and 2 (COX-1 and COX-2); results in a reduction in prostaglandins which cause pain, fever, inflammation
- Common Uses: Treatment of gout flare, pain, fever and inflammation
- Memorable Side Effects: GI ulcer, worsening kidney function, edema, hypertension, inhibits platelets (can exacerbate bleed risk)
- Clinical Pearls:
  - o NSAIDs are one of the most common causes of GI bleeding; this risk increases in the elderly and those on medications that increase risk of bleeding (anticoagulants and antiplatelet medications)
  - o Due to effects on platelets, NSAIDs are typically held before/after surgery to reduce the risk of bleeding
  - o NSAIDs can contribute to edema and exacerbate CHF (congestive heart failure); be on the lookout and have NSAIDs reassessed if you see a patient with a CHF exacerbation or a patient requiring increasing diuretics, like furosemide
  - o NSAIDs can cause worsening kidney function (creatinine should be monitored); this risk can be greatly increased in patients on ACE inhibitors or ARBs and/or diuretic type medications
  - o Due to above reasons on kidney function, GI bleed risk, and CHF, NSAIDs are not the safest medication in the elderly; acetaminophen is generally preferred for generalized pain with a few exceptions
  - o Although generally considered riskier in the elderly, a big advantage of NSAIDs over acetaminophen is that they can reduce inflammation
  - o Pregnancy category C/D when >30 weeks gestation; NSAIDs are generally avoided in pregnancy and especially after 30 weeks gestation
- Monitoring: Renal function, hemoglobin, platelets (contained within CBC), blood pressure, signs of bruising or bleeding, weight (risk for edema)
- Drug and Diet Considerations:
  - o Because of significant incidence of GI upset, it is recommended to give with food or milk
  - o Dehydration may exacerbate the risk for acute renal failure
  - o Excessive alcohol may increase GI bleed risk
  - o Vitamin E, Omega-3 fatty acids, gingko, garlic, ginseng, turmeric, and fish oil supplements have been purported to have antiplatelet

type activity which in theory could increase the risk of bleed – clinical significance is questionable; the most common resolution is to discontinue the supplements if they are not necessary

Infliximab (Remicade)

- Class: Antirheumatic, TNF blocker
- Mechanism of Action: Blocks tumor necrosis factor (TNF); TNF plays a role in the inflammatory process
- Common Uses: Treatment of rheumatoid arthritis, psoriasis/psoriatic arthritis, Crohn's disease and ulcerative colitis
- Memorable Side Effects: Infection risk (suppresses immune system), injection site reaction
- Clinical Pearls:
  - Boxed warning for increased risk of serious infections
  - Boxed warning for malignancy
  - Increased risk of elevated LFTs especially if used with methotrexate
  - Infusion related side effects
- Monitoring: TB and hepatitis B screening, signs of cancer or infection, CBC, LFTs as clinically indicated
- Drug and Diet Considerations:
  - GI upset is possible but not incredibly common

Insulin Aspart (Novolog)

- Class: Rapid acting insulin analog
- Mechanism of Action: Rapid acting insulin causes reduction in blood glucose
- Common Uses: Treatment of diabetes
- Memorable Side Effects: Weight gain, hypoglycemia, injection site issues (rotating sites usually alleviates this problem)
- Clinical Pearls:
  - Rapid acting insulin used to quickly bring down blood sugar, compared to the long acting insulins like detemir and glargine
  - Sliding scale insulin is not ideal for diabetes management as you often end up "chasing" blood sugars
  - When giving rapid acting insulin like aspart, remember to be aware of hypoglycemia protocols (juice, glucose gel, saltine crackers, etc., or glucagon if patient is incapable of taking oral food/liquid)
  - In many type 2 diabetes patients uncontrolled by oral medications, a combination of long acting once daily with rapid acting insulin with meal(s) is often used
  - With insulin products, some providers will use hold orders on insulin if blood sugars are below a certain value (i.e. 100 mg/dL)
  - Keep an eye out for patients who have a change in appetite as they may require a reduction or increase in insulin based upon their dietary intake
  - Can be given acutely to manage hyperkalemia (lowers potassium levels)
- Monitoring: Blood sugar, HbA1c, weight, kidney function, eye exams, potassium
- Drug and Diet Considerations:
  - Greater risk for hypoglycemia with short acting agents versus long acting insulins

155

- Patient education about blood sugar, diet and the function of insulin is critical to avoid hypo and hyperglycemia
- When patients are using both long acting and short acting, the ratio of both is typically split approximately 50/50
- Targets post prandial increases in blood sugar

Insulin degludec (Tresiba)

- Class: Long acting insulin
- Mechanism of Action: Long acting insulin causes reduction in blood glucose
- Common Uses: Treatment of diabetes
- Memorable Side Effects: Weight gain, hypoglycemia, injection site issues (rotating sites usually alleviates this problem)
- Clinical Pearls:
  - Degludec is a long acting, sometimes called "peakless" or "basal" insulin
  - Degludec has a much longer duration of action than detemir/glargine; be careful with increasing dose to quickly as it takes longer to get to steady state
    - May have to wait longer before increasing (up to 5-7 days versus 2-3 days for glargine/detemir)
  - Typically target about 10% increases in dose for patients not at goal
  - The intent with long acting insulin is to mimic the consistent low level output of insulin by the pancreas
  - Basal insulin in Type 2 diabetes is often (but doesn't have to be) used after patients have tried oral medications without successful decrease in HbA1c
  - Hypoglycemia is always a concern with any insulin product
  - May have a lower risk of nocturnal hypoglycemia and larger fasting glucose reduction than glargine
- Monitoring: Blood sugar, HbA1c, weight, kidney function, eye exams, potassium as clinically indicated
- Drug and Diet Considerations:
  - Patient education about blood sugar, diet and the function of insulin is critical to avoid hypo and hyperglycemia
  - When patients are using both long acting and short acting, the ratio of both is typically split approximately 50/50
  - Targets fasting blood sugars, so this is what dose adjustments are usually based off of

Insulin Detemir (Levemir)

- Class: Long acting insulin
- Mechanism of Action: Long acting insulin causes reduction in blood glucose
- Common Uses: Treatment of diabetes
- Memorable Side Effects: Weight gain, hypoglycemia, injection site issues (rotating sites usually alleviates this problem)
- Clinical Pearls:
  - Detemir is a long acting, sometimes called "peakless" or "basal" insulin
  - Typically target about 10% increases in dose for patients not at goal
  - The intent with long acting insulin is to mimic the consistent low level output of insulin by the pancreas

- o Usually dosed once daily, but providers may be more likely to try to do twice daily as the dose increases; downside of more injections for the patient
- o Basal insulin in type 2 diabetes is often, but doesn't have to be, used after patients have tried oral medications without a successful decrease in HbA1c
- o Hypoglycemia is always a concern with any insulin product
- Monitoring: Blood sugar, HbA1c, weight, kidney function, eye exams, potassium as clinically indicated
- Drug and Diet Considerations:
  - o Patient education about blood sugar, diet and the function of insulin is critical to avoid hypo and hyperglycemia
  - o When patients are using both long acting and short acting, the ratio of both is typically split approximately 50/50
  - o Targets fasting blood sugars

Insulin Glargine (Lantus, Basaglar, Toujeo)

- Class: Long acting insulin
- Mechanism of Action: Long acting insulin causes reduction in blood glucose
- Common Uses: Treatment of diabetes
- Memorable Side Effects: Weight gain, hypoglycemia, injection site issues (rotating sites usually alleviates this problem)
- Clinical Pearls:
  - o Glargine is a long acting, sometimes called "peakless" or "basal" insulin
  - o Toujeo product contains 300 units/mL versus Lantus and Basaglar which contain 100 units/mL
  - o Typically target about 10% increases in dose for patients not at goal
  - o The intent with long acting insulin is to mimic the consistent low level output of insulin by the pancreas
  - o Usually dosed once daily, but providers may be more likely to try to do twice daily as the dose increases; downside of more injections for the patient
  - o Basal insulin in type 2 diabetes is often, but doesn't have to be, used after patients have tried oral medications without successful decrease in HbA1c
  - o Hypoglycemia is always a concern with any insulin product
- Monitoring: Blood sugar, HbA1c, weight, kidney function, eye exams, potassium as clinically indicated
- Drug and Diet Considerations:
  - o Patient education about blood sugar, diet and the function of insulin is critical to avoid hypo and hyperglycemia
  - o When patients are using both long acting and short acting, the ratio of both is typically split approximately 50/50
  - o Targets fasting blood sugars

Insulin glulisine (Apidra)

- Class: Rapid acting insulin analog
- Mechanism of Action: Rapid acting insulin causes reduction in blood glucose
- Common Uses: Treatment of diabetes

157

- Memorable Side Effects: Weight gain, hypoglycemia, injection site issues (rotating sites usually alleviates this problem)
- Clinical Pearls:
    - Rapid acting insulin used to quickly bring down blood sugar, compared to the long acting insulins like detemir and glargine
    - Sliding scale insulin is not ideal for diabetes management as you often end up "chasing" blood sugars
    - When giving rapid acting insulin like glulisine, be aware of hypoglycemia protocols (juice, glucose gel, saltine crackers, etc., or glucagon if patient is incapable of taking oral food/liquid)
    - In many type 2 diabetes patients uncontrolled by oral medications, a combination of long acting once daily with rapid acting insulin with meal(s) is often used
    - With insulin products, some providers will use hold orders on insulin if blood sugars are below a certain value (i.e. 100 mg/dL)
    - Keep an eye out for patients who have a change in appetite as they may require a reduction or increase in insulin based upon their dietary intake
    - Can be given acutely to manage hyperkalemia (lowers potassium levels)
- Monitoring: Blood sugar, HbA1c, weight, kidney function, eye exams, potassium
- Drug and Diet Considerations:
    - Greater risk for hypoglycemia with short acting agents versus long acting insulins
    - Patient education about blood sugar, diet and the function of insulin is critical to avoid hypo and hyperglycemia
    - When patients are using both long acting and short acting, the ratio of both is typically split approximately 50/50
    - Targets post prandial increases in blood sugar

Insulin Lispro (Humalog)

- Class: Rapid acting insulin
- Mechanism of Action: Rapid acting insulin causes reduction in blood glucose
- Common Uses: Treatment of diabetes used via sliding scale
- Memorable Side Effects: Weight gain, hypoglycemia, injection site issues (rotating sites usually alleviates this problem)
- Clinical Pearls:
    - Rapid acting insulin used to quickly bring down blood sugar, compared to the long acting insulins like detemir and glargine
    - Sliding scale insulin is not ideal for diabetes management as you often end up "chasing" blood sugars
    - When giving rapid acting insulin like lispro, remember to be aware of hypoglycemia protocols (juice, glucose gel, saltine crackers, etc., or glucagon if patient is incapable of taking oral food/liquid)
    - In many type 2 diabetes patients uncontrolled by oral medications, a combination of long acting once daily with rapid acting insulin with meal(s) is often used
    - With insulin products, some providers will use hold orders on insulin if blood sugars are below a certain value (i.e. 100 mg/dL)
    - Keep an eye out for patients who have a change in appetite as they may require a reduction or increase in insulin based upon their dietary intake

- Monitoring: Blood sugar, HbA1c, weight, kidney function, eye exams, potassium
- Drug and Diet Considerations:
    - Greater risk for hypoglycemia with short acting agents versus long acting insulins
    - Patient education about blood sugar, diet and the function of insulin is critical to avoid hypo and hyperglycemia
    - When patients are using both long acting and short acting, the ratio of both is typically split approximately 50/50
    - Targets post prandial increases in blood sugar

Insulin NPH (Humulin N, Novolin N)

- Class: Intermediate acting insulin
- Mechanism of Action: Intermediate acting insulin causes reduction in blood glucose
- Common Uses: Treatment of diabetes
- Memorable Side Effects: Weight gain, hypoglycemia, injection site issues (rotating sites usually alleviates this problem)
- Clinical Pearls:
    - Rarely used due to better predictability of long acting agents
    - Potential situations for use; a patient who has been stable on this medication for a long time or doesn't have adequate insurance to cover longer acting insulin costs
    - May be used in combination with rapid acting insulin and dosed twice daily for those who have difficulty with basal/bolus regimens
    - Dosed two or three times daily
    - Hypoglycemia is always a concern with any insulin product
- Monitoring: Blood sugar, HbA1c, weight, kidney function, eye exams, potassium as clinically indicated
- Drug and Diet Considerations:
    - Patient education about blood sugar, diet and the function of insulin is critical to avoid hypo and hyperglycemia
    - When patients are using both long acting and short acting, the ratio of both is typically split approximately 50/50
    - Targets fasting blood sugars

Insulin regular (Humulin R, Novolin R)

- Class: Rapid acting insulin analog
- Mechanism of Action: Short acting insulin causes reduction in blood glucose
- Common Uses: Treatment of diabetes
- Memorable Side Effects: Weight gain, hypoglycemia, injection site issues (rotating sites usually alleviates this problem)
- Clinical Pearls:
    - Short acting insulin used to quickly bring down blood sugar, compared to the long acting insulins like detemir and glargine
    - Sliding scale insulin is not ideal for diabetes management as you often end up "chasing" blood sugars
    - Take slightly longer than rapid acting insulin analogs to have effects; typically administered 15-30 minutes before a meal

- o Less expensive, but more challenging to time the administration than rapid acting agents
- o Available without a prescription
- o Keep an eye out for patients who have a change in appetite as they may require a reduction or increase in insulin based upon their dietary intake
- o Can be given acutely to manage hyperkalemia (lowers potassium levels)
- • Monitoring: Blood sugar, HbA1c, weight, kidney function, eye exams, potassium
- • Drug and Diet Considerations:
    - o Greater risk for hypoglycemia with short acting agents versus long acting insulins
    - o Patient education about blood sugar, diet and the function of insulin is critical to avoid hypo and hyperglycemia
    - o When patients are using both long acting and short acting, the ratio of both is typically split approximately 50/50
    - o Targets post prandial increases in blood sugar

Ipratropium (Atrovent)

- • Class: Inhaled anticholinergic, nasal anticholinergic
- • Mechanism of Action: Short acting inhaled anticholinergic can open up airways and decrease secretions
- • Common Uses: Management of COPD
- • Memorable Side Effects: Dry mouth, cough, irritation to the lungs; usually well tolerated due to minimal systemic absorption
- • Clinical Pearls:
    - o It will not provide acute relief from respiratory distress, not meant to be a rescue inhalation product
    - o Often by using this medication in COPD, our goal is likely to improve respiratory status, but also to reduce the amount of as needed albuterol and/or albuterol/ipratropium (Duoneb or Combivent)
    - o With the delivery device, it is imperative to assess if patients are able to adequately coordinate how to use the device as well as if they are able to inhale quickly and forcefully enough to get the drug into their lungs
    - o Systemic anticholinergic effects (can't spit, see, pee or poop) are usually not a concern as systemic absorption is low
    - o Nebulized formulation
- • Monitoring: FEV1, peak flow
- • Drug and Diet Considerations:
    - o Inhaled, local medication
    - o Dry mouth may impact dietary/fluid intake

Irbesartan (Avapro)

- • Class: Antihypertensive, ARB
- • Mechanism of Action: Blocks the angiotensin 2 receptor, preventing vasoconstriction, aldosterone release, etc.
- • Common Uses: Treatment of hypertension and heart failure
- • Memorable Side Effects: Hyperkalemia, exacerbate/worsen kidney function, low blood pressure

160

- Clinical Pearls:
  - When you think of ARBs and ACE inhibitors, you can lump the side effects together as they are overall the same
  - One major exception to the above rule is the side effect of cough; cough usually doesn't happen with ARBs, and in many patients, you will see patients who develop cough on an ACE inhibitor be transitioned to an ARB
  - Kidney function changes and monitoring of potassium is critical when doses are changed or an ARB is initiated
  - This worsening kidney function risk increases in patients who may be taking NSAIDs and/or diuretics
  - As with any medication used to treat hypertension, we need to educate our patients to rise slowly when getting up to minimize risk of orthostatic (sometimes called postural) hypotension
- Monitoring: Renal function, potassium, blood pressure
- Drug and Diet Considerations:
  - Be cautious and monitor potassium closely in patients with high dietary intake of potassium as this could contribute to hyperkalemia in combination with this medication
  - Administer with or without food

Irinotecan (Camptosar)

- Class: Oncology agent, topoisomerase 1 inhibitor
- Mechanism of Action: Inhibits topoisomerase 1 which blocks the formation of the DNA strand
- Common Uses: Treatment of colorectal cancer, off-label for numerous types of other cancers
- Memorable Side Effects: Diarrhea, myelosuppression, nausea, vomiting, cholinergic syndrome (see clinical pearls), hair loss, anemia, thrombocytopenia, altered liver function enzymes, pulmonary toxicity, weakness, fever
- Clinical Pearls:
  - Boxed warning for the risk of myelosuppression and diarrhea
  - Dosing may be altered based upon genetic variation of UGT1A1*28
  - Pretreatment with atropine may be considered if patient experiences excessive salivation, sweating, diarrhea, abdominal pain or other cholinergic symptoms
- Monitoring: CBC, renal function, electrolytes, LFTs
- Drug and Diet Considerations:
  - Diarrhea can cause substantial fluid loss and electrolyte deficiencies, monitor and replace as appropriate
  - Weight loss and poor nutrition may result on account of nausea and vomiting adverse effects

Iron sucrose (Venofer)

- Class: Iron supplement
- Mechanism of Action: Restoration of iron stores
- Common Uses: Treatment of iron deficiency anemia
- Memorable Side Effects: Hypotension, GI, anaphylaxis (rare, but serious)
- Clinical Pearls:
  - Risk of anaphylaxis from infusion is a significant risk

- o Ferritin and hemoglobin are important labs to monitor
- o May cause hypotension, monitor BP
- Monitoring: Ferritin, iron, transferring saturation, total iron-binding capacity, hemoglobin, blood pressure
- Drug and Diet Considerations:
  - o IV administration – no notable administration concerns with regards to diet

Isocarboxazid (Marplan)

- Class: Monoamine oxidase inhibitor, antidepressant
- Mechanism of Action: Inhibits the action of monoamine oxidase which increases the CNS neurotransmitters serotonin, norepinephrine, and epinephrine
- Common Uses: Treatment of depression
- Memorable Side Effects: Nausea, dizziness, blood pressure fluctuations, hypertension (with tyramine), hypotension, tachycardia, unusual behavior, SIADH (hyponatremia), serotonin syndrome
- Clinical Pearls:
  - o Boxed warning for increased risk of suicidal thoughts in pediatric patients and young adults
  - o Avoid use of other serotonergic agents (i.e. SSRIs)
  - o Not a first line agent in depression due to adverse effect profile, diet interactions, and drug interactions
- Monitoring: Blood pressure, pulse, electrolytes (as clinically indicated), renal function, LFTs
- Drug and Diet Considerations:
  - o Patch may be administered consistently without regard to meals while oral disintegrating table is typically given before breakfast
  - o Alcohol should be avoided as it may increase risk for toxicity
  - o MAOI/Tyramine interaction is less likely than traditional MAOIs
    - Foods high in tyramine: fermented, cured, aged foods such as cheese, smoked meats/fish, beer
    - Reaction: Tachycardia, N/V, headache
    - Risk of reaction increases as the dose of the medication increases
  - o Food and beverages with large amounts of caffeine, tyrosine, phenylalanine, dopamine, or tryptophan may also cause elevated blood pressure

Isoniazid (Nydrazid, INH)

- Class: Anti-tuberculosis agent
- Mechanism of Action: Peroxidative activation of isoniazid by bacterial enzymes creates a reactive compound that ultimately inhibits nucleic acid and lipid synthesis
- Common Uses: Treatment and prevention of tuberculosis
- Memorable Side Effects: Neuropathy, liver toxicity (boxed warning), skin reaction, CNS changes
- Clinical Pearls:
  - o Be aware of liver toxic agents, like acetaminophen, that may have additive effects
- Monitoring: LFTs, renal function
- Drug and Diet Considerations:

- o   Avoid alcohol as it may exacerbate liver failure risk
- o   Administer on an empty stomach
- o   Pyridoxine (vitamin B6) supplementation can help prevent isoniazid-induced peripheral neuropathy
- o   Recommended to increase intake of folate, magnesium, and niacin when taking this medication
- o   Mild MAOI activity could increase the risk for tyramine-like reactions; consuming large quantities of aged cheeses, certain wines, cured meats could increase the risk of this reaction
- o   Foods with a high amount of histamine may increase the risk of a reaction that can result in tachycardia, flushing, itching, sweating, and hypotension; examples of foods that contain larger amounts of histamine include alcohol, canned foods, pickled foods, aged cheeses, smoked meats, and shellfish

Isosorbide Dinitrate (Dilatrate, Isordil)
- • Class: Antihypertensive, antianginal, nitrate
- • Mechanism of Action: Direct acting vasodilation by nitric oxide which causes smooth muscle relaxation and reduction in blood pressure
- • Common Uses: Treatment or prevention of angina (chest pain)
- • Memorable Side Effects: Low BP, headache, dizziness
- • Clinical Pearls:
  - o   Tolerance can develop without a break in drug therapy during the day
  - o   An 8-12 hour off period is recommended to reduce the risk of tolerance
  - o   Isosorbide dinitrate combined with hydralazine may be used as an alternative in heart failure patients who cannot tolerate or don't benefit from an ACE inhibitor or ARB
  - o   Avoid combination with PDE-5 inhibitors for erectile dysfunction (i.e. sildenafil)
- • Monitoring: Blood pressure, pulse
- • Drug and Diet Considerations:
  - o   Alcohol could exacerbate low blood pressure risk
  - o   Grapefruit juice may increase concentrations

Isosorbide Mononitrate (Imdur)
- • Class: Antihypertensive, antianginal, nitrate
- • Mechanism of Action: Direct acting vasodilation by nitric oxide which causes smooth muscle relaxation and reduction in blood pressure
- • Common Uses: Treatment or prevention of angina (chest pain)
- • Memorable Side Effects: Low BP, headache, dizziness
- • Clinical Pearls:
  - o   Tolerance can develop without a break in drug therapy during the day
  - o   An 8-12 hour off period is recommended to reduce the risk of tolerance
  - o   Isosorbide mononitrate combined with hydralazine may be used as an alternative in heart failure patients who cannot tolerate or don't benefit from an ACE inhibitor or ARB

- o Avoid combination with PDE-5 inhibitors for erectile dysfunction (i.e. sildenafil)
- Monitoring: Blood pressure, pulse
- Drug and Diet Considerations:
  - o Alcohol could exacerbate low blood pressure risk
  - o Grapefruit juice may increase concentrations

Isotretinoin (Accutane, Claravis)
- Class: Retinoid, acne agent
- Mechanism of Action: Activates retinoic acid receptors which can help create immunomodulatory and anti-inflammatory activity
- Common Uses: Treatment of acne
- Memorable Side Effects: Sun sensitivity, dry lips, hair thinning, CNS effects, skin reactions, GI upset, reduced bone mineral density
- Clinical Pearls:
  - o Birth defect risk
  - o Special REMS program
    - ▪ iPLEDGE
    - ▪ Required pregnancy test being negative before issuing the medication every month
    - ▪ Only allowed to dispense within a given window
- Monitoring: Pregnancy testing, lipids, LFTs, CBC, glucose
- Drug and Diet Considerations:
  - o Administer with food
  - o Avoid use of products that have vitamin A
  - o Can add to hypertriglyceridemia, may require an alteration in diet to reduce the risk for elevated cholesterol
  - o Monitor diabetes patients as blood sugar may be raised

Isradipine (Dynacirc)
- Class: Antihypertensive, dihydropyridine calcium channel blocker
- Mechanism of Action: Blocks calcium ions from entering voltage smooth muscle, resulting in relaxation (vasodilation)
- Common Uses: Treatment of hypertension
- Memorable Side Effects: Low blood pressure, edema, constipation
- Clinical Pearls:
  - o Very important distinction: You will not see nifedipine used in atrial fibrillation, because its activity is primarily on the vessels; this differs from non-dihydropyridine calcium channel blockers like verapamil and diltiazem that act on the heart AND blood vessels; this also means that pulse monitoring will not be necessary with nifedipine
  - o The higher you push the dose on these medications, the more likely you will see the side effect of edema
  - o Keep an eye out for new requirement of diuretic prescriptions to treat the edema caused by the calcium channel blockers
  - o Educate our patients to get up slowly to minimize risk of orthostatic hypotension
- Monitoring: Blood pressure, weight (in association with edema risk)
- Drug and Diet Considerations:
  - o May be given with or without food
  - o St. John's wort may reduce effectiveness

- o Standard calcium supplementation typically will not impact the effectiveness of amlodipine; excessive doses of calcium may have a higher likelihood of blunting the effects of amlodipine
- o Avoid grapefruit and its juice as they can raise concentrations

Itraconazole (Sporanox)
- Class: Antifungal, azole
- Mechanism of Action: Ultimately inhibits formation of the fungal cell membrane
- Common Uses: Treatment of fungal infections like candidiasis, blastomycosis and aspergillosis
- Memorable Side Effects: GI upset, diarrhea, liver failure (very rare, more likely with chronic use)
- Clinical Pearls:
  - o Notorious cause of drug interactions via CYP3A4 inhibition; it can increase concentrations of statins, seizure medications, etc. (if you see patients started on this medication, be sure to look up possible drug interactions)
  - o Fungal infections are much more common in patients who are immunocompromised (i.e. AIDS, patient on immunosuppressant medications, etc.)
  - o Can potentially cause prolonged QTc intervals especially in patients on other medications that prolong the QTc
  - o Liver toxicity is rare, but should be monitored for especially if patients are receiving chronic therapy
- Monitoring: LFTs, renal function, potassium – only if clinically indicated or on chronic therapy
- Drug and Diet Considerations:
  - o Capsule/tablet should be given with food
  - o Oral solution should be given on an empty stomach
  - o Abnormal levels of potassium or magnesium could increase the risk of itraconazole causing QTc prolongation
  - o Grapefruit juice may alter drug concentrations, encourage consistent intake or avoidance
  - o Increasing the acidity in the stomach may increase absorption

Ketoconazole
- Class: Antifungal, azole
- Mechanism of Action: Ultimately inhibits formation of the fungal cell membrane
- Common Uses: Treatment of fungal infections
- Memorable Side Effects: GI upset, liver failure
- Clinical Pearls:
  - o Notorious cause of drug interactions via CYP3A4 inhibition; It can increase concentrations of statins, seizure medications, etc. (if you see patients started on this medication, be sure to look up possible drug interactions)
  - o Fungal infections are much more common in patients who are immunocompromised (i.e. AIDS, patient on immunosuppressant medications, etc.)

- o Boxed warning for hepatotoxicity, avoid use in non-serious fungal infections, and QT prolongation risk
- Monitoring: LFTs, renal function, potassium – only if clinically indicated or on chronic therapy
- Drug and Diet Considerations:
  - o Alcohol may increase the risk for liver complication
  - o Abnormal levels of potassium or magnesium could increase the risk of ketoconazole causing QTc prolongation
  - o Grapefruit juice may alter drug concentrations, encourage consistent intake or avoidance
  - o Acidic drinks, like soda, can increase absorption

Ketorolac (Toradol)

- Class: NSAID, analgesic
- Mechanism of Action: Inhibits Cyclooxygenase-1 and 2 (COX-1 and COX-2); results in a reduction in prostaglandins which cause pain, fever and inflammation
- Common Uses: Reduction of pain, fever and inflammation
- Memorable Side Effects: GI ulcer, worsening kidney function, edema, hypertension, inhibits platelets (can exacerbate bleed risk)
- Clinical Pearls:
  - o Injectable available
  - o One of the highest risk NSAIDs for GI bleed; this risk increases in the elderly and those on medications that increase risk of bleeding (anticoagulants and antiplatelet medications)
  - o Due to effects on platelets, NSAIDs are typically held before/after surgery to reduce the risk of bleeding
  - o NSAIDs can contribute to edema and exacerbate congestive heart failure (CHF); be on the lookout and have NSAIDs reassessed if you see a patient with a CHF exacerbation or a patient requiring increasing diuretics like furosemide
  - o NSAIDs can cause worsening kidney function and creatinine should be monitored; this risk can be greatly increased in patients on ACE inhibitors or ARBs and/or diuretic type medications
  - o Due to above reasons of kidney function, GI bleed risk, and CHF, NSAIDs are not the safest medication in the elderly, acetaminophen is generally preferred for generalized pain with a few exceptions
  - o Pregnancy category C/D when >30 weeks gestation; NSAIDs are generally avoided in pregnancy and especially after 30 weeks gestation
- Monitoring: Renal function, hemoglobin, platelets (contained within CBC), blood pressure, signs of bruising or bleeding, weight (risk for edema)
- Drug and Diet Considerations:
  - o Because of significant incidence of GI upset when taken orally, it is recommended to give with food or milk
  - o Dehydration coupled with ketorolac may increase the risk for acute renal failure
  - o Excessive alcohol may increase GI bleed risk
  - o Vitamin E, Omega-3 fatty acids, gingko, garlic, ginseng, turmeric, and fish oil supplements have been purported to have antiplatelet type activity which in theory could increase the risk of bleed – clinical significance is questionable; the most common resolution is to discontinue the supplements if they are not necessary

Labetalol (Trandate)

- Class: Antihypertensive, beta-blocker with alpha blocking activity
- Mechanism of Action: Blocks beta and alpha receptors leading to lower pulse/BP
- Common Uses: Treatment of hypertension and atrial fibrillation
- Memorable Side Effects: Low pulse, low BP, fatigue
- Clinical Pearls:
  - The trick to remembering beta receptors: You have 1 heart and 2 lungs (beta-1 is primarily on the heart and beta-2 primarily in the lungs). You will see beta receptors again with respiratory medications. If beta-1 is stimulated, heart rate increases. If beta-1 is blocked, heart rate decreases.
  - Often in practice, providers will place a hold order on beta-blockers if the pulse is too low. This is obviously done to reduce the risk of significant bradycardia; clinically it may depend upon the situation, but in an ambulatory setting, you may see the order set to hold the beta blocker when pulse is less than 55 or 60.
  - Potential option in pregnancy
- Monitoring: Pulse, blood pressure, EKG as clinically indicated (i.e. acute atrial fibrillation)
- Drug and Diet Considerations:
  - While food may increase concentrations, it may be given with or without food (consistency will help maintain steady concentrations)

Lacosamide (Vimpat)

- Class: Antiepileptic
- Mechanism of Action: Causes stabilization of neuronal membranes by increasing slow inactivation of sodium channels which prevents repetitive firing of the neurons
- Common Uses: Treatment of seizures
- Memorable Side Effects: Sedation, dizziness, GI upset, tachycardia
- Clinical Pearls:
  - Be cautious in patients with a history of cardiac arrhythmias or those who are taking antiarrhythmics
- Monitoring: EKG
- Drug and Diet Considerations:
  - Alcohol can have additive CNS depressant effects
  - May be given with or without food

Lactulose (Enulose, Generlac)

- Class: Osmotic laxative, ammonia reducer
- Mechanism of Action: Bacteria breakdown ammonia in the gut which creates an acidic environment; the acidic environment causes NH_3 to be converted to NH_4+ which doesn't allow ammonia to get into the blood stream; as a laxative, it works by pulling water into the gut which promotes motility and bowel movements
- Common Uses: Treatment of constipation and hyperammonemia
- Memorable Side Effects: Diarrhea, abdominal cramps, GI upset, hypokalemia, dehydration

- Clinical Pearls:
  - Aggressiveness of dosing usually depends upon tolerability
  - Target dose to around 3 loose stools per day if possible in the management of hyperammonemia
- Monitoring: Ammonia levels (in patients with hyperammonemia), bowel movements, electrolytes, fluid status, blood pressure
- Drug and Diet Considerations:
  - Assess fluid status
  - Ensure adequate potassium intake and monitor lab work
  - May elevate sodium levels, adjust diet accordingly as lab work indicates
  - May cause increases in blood sugar levels as the solution contains sugars

Lamivudine (Epivir, 3TC)
- Class: Antiretroviral, nucleoside reverse transcriptase inhibitor (NRTI)
- Mechanism of Action: Converted to active triphosphate forms which competes with natural substrates to inhibit reverse transcriptase; the HIV virus uses the enzyme reverse transcriptase to convert RNA into DNA
- Common Uses: Treatment of HIV and hepatitis B
- Memorable Side Effects: Lactic acidosis/fatty liver boxed warning, osteoporosis, GI adverse effects, elevation in cholesterol, fatigue, neuropathy
- Clinical Pearls:
  - In combination products such as Combivir
  - Different dosage forms may contain varying amounts of drug, patients with HIV should only receive dosage forms for HIV
  - Rare reports of pancreatitis
- Monitoring: Liver function, HIV and/or Hepatitis B parameters such as viral load and CD4 count
- Drug and Diet Considerations:
  - Monitor cholesterol and implement cholesterol lowering diet in patients who may have elevated levels due to the adverse effects of the drug
  - May be given with or without meals

Lamotrigine (Lamictal)
- Class: Antiepileptic
- Mechanism of Action: Inhibits release of glutamate, an excitatory neurotransmitter, and inhibits sodium channels
- Common Uses: Management of seizures and bipolar disorder symptoms
- Memorable Side Effects: GI, CNS (drowsiness, dizziness), rash (can be very serious)
- Clinical Pearls:
  - Very slow dosing titration
  - If increase dose too fast, one of the major risks is Steven Johnson's syndrome (very severe, potentially life threatening rash)
  - Does have interactions with other seizure medications; use lower starting dose with valproic acid, higher with enzyme inducers like phenytoin
  - Blood levels usually aren't routinely taken
- Monitoring: Skin reaction, LFTs and renal function as clinically indicated
- Drug and Diet Considerations:

168

- o Taking with food is acceptable if patients develop nausea or GI upset

Lansoprazole (Prevacid)
- Class: PPI
- Mechanism of Action: Inhibits proton pumps in the stomach leading to a less acidic environment
- Common Uses: GERD, ulcer and Barrett's esophagus
- Memorable Side Effects: Well tolerated; when used long term there is a possibility to increase fracture risk, decrease B12 levels, C. diff risk, low magnesium
- Clinical Pearls:
  - o PPIs are the most potent acid blocker on the market
  - o PPIs are generally dosed 30 minutes before meals; this is a recommendation, not an absolute. If a patient likes to get up and eat right away upon rising, the medication will still likely be beneficial, but may not have a maximal effect
  - o For some patients PPIs may not work very quickly, it might take a few days for maximal effect
  - o For the above reason, as needed (PRN) PPIs can possibly be effective, but are generally not recommended
  - o Use short term if possible due to increased risk of osteoporosis, low magnesium, and B12 deficiency if used long term
  - o Most common primary outcome of PPI would be to improve symptoms, likely heartburn and stomach from GERD, stomach ulcer, or other related condition
  - o Barrett's esophagus, high risk GI medications (i.e. NSAIDs, prednisone), or chronic GI bleed may require indefinite therapy
  - o If GI bleed is problematic, monitoring hemoglobin and/or hemoccult might be appropriate to assess possible blood loss
- Monitoring: Magnesium (chronic use), B12
- Drug and Diet Considerations:
  - o When it is used chronically, it is a possible cause or contributing factor to B12 and magnesium deficiency
  - o PPIs are typically best given at least 30-60 minutes before a meal
  - o St. John's wort should be avoided as it can significantly reduce concentrations of the drug
  - o Reduced stomach acid (high pH) may impair the absorption of iron supplements

Latanoprost (Xalatan)
- Class: Prostaglandin analog
- Mechanism of Action: Decreases intraocular pressure
- Common Uses: Treatment of glaucoma
- Memorable Side Effects: Change in eye color, eye irritation
- Clinical Pearls:
  - o Generally dosed in the evening for glaucoma
  - o Change in eye color may be permanent (change to brown)
  - o Many glaucoma patients will be on multiple eye drops; at least 5 minutes is the appropriate amount of time to wait between drops

169

- o Expires in 42 days once removed from the fridge (REFRIGERATE until needed)
- Monitoring: Eye exams, intraocular pressure
- Drug and Diet Considerations:
  - o No notable concerns

Ledipasvir/sofosbuvir (Harvoni)
- Class: Hepatitis C antiviral, polymerase inhibitor
- Mechanism of Action: Ledipasvir causes inhibition of NS5A which is a viral phosphoprotein necessary for replication, assembly, and viral secretion; sofosbuvir is incorporated into the RNA chain which ends the chain and leads to stoppage in replication processes
- Common Uses: Treatment of hepatitis C
- Memorable Side Effects: Fatigue, asthenia, myalgia, nausea, diarrhea
- Clinical Pearls:
  - o Potential association with new onset diabetes
  - o Boxed warning for risk of hepatitis B reactivation
  - o Very high cure rates (~95%)
  - o Duration of treatment ranges from 8 to 24 weeks, but typically 12 weeks
- Monitoring: CBC, liver function, renal function, INR, cardiac monitoring if using it with amiodarone
- Drug and Diet Considerations:
  - o Calcium supplements and antacids may reduce the absorption, separate by at least 4 hours
  - o May be given with or without food
  - o May alter blood sugars, monitor in patients with diabetes

Leflunomide (Arava)
- Class: Disease modifying antirheumatic drug
- Mechanism of Action: Inhibits dihydroorotate dehydrogenase which has an important role in synthesis of uridine monophosphate, which is necessary for DNA/RNA production, this leads to an immunosuppressive-type effect
- Common Uses: Treatment of rheumatoid arthritis
- Memorable Side Effects: GI side effects, hair loss, rash, elevated LFTs, hypertension
- Clinical Pearls:
  - o Can cause birth defects, contraindicated in pregnancy
  - o Boxed warning for hepatotoxicity
- Monitoring: LFTs, renal function, blood pressure, TB screening, and CBC; pregnancy test as clinically indicated
- Drug and Diet Considerations:
  - o Administer with or without food
  - o Avoidance of alcohol would be recommended

Letrozole (Femara)
- Class: Aromatase inhibitor, antineoplastic
- Mechanism of Action: Prevents formation of estrogen which ultimately helps induce ovulation and also can manage cancers dependent upon estrogen for growth

170

- Common Uses: Treatment of breast cancer and induction of ovulation in infertility
- Memorable Side Effects: Flushing, fatigue, hypercholesterolemia, arthralgia, reduced bone mineral density
- Clinical Pearls:
    - Increases chance of having multiples (twins, triplets, etc.)
- Monitoring: Lipids, bone mineral density, pregnancy (as appropriate), LFTs
- Drug and Diet Considerations:
    - May be administered with or without food
    - Supplementation with calcium and vitamin D may be recommended
    - Implement a lipid lowering diet as necessary

Leucovorin (Folinic Acid)
- Class: Reversal agent, vitamin
- Mechanism of Action: Active folic acid metabolite that is necessary for DNA production, it "rescues" normal cells from chemotherapy toxicity
- Common Uses: Rescue from methotrexate and fluorouracil treatment
- Memorable Side Effects: Adverse effects are typically caused by the chemotherapy agents leucovorin is being used with, hypercalcemia with higher dose IV administration, infusion reaction
- Clinical Pearls:
    - Accumulation may be possible in renal failure
    - Intrathecal administration is contraindicated
- Monitoring: CBC, electrolytes (other labs as indicated by chemotherapy drugs that are being used in combination)
- Drug and Diet Considerations:
    - Contains calcium, be cautious with rate of infusion and accumulation (no more than 160mg/minute)
    - Oral absorption is limited to 25 mg at a time; must use IV if need higher doses

Leuprolide (Lupron)
- Class: Oncology agent, GnRH agonist
- Mechanism of Action: Ultimately leads to a blockade of gonadotropin secretion which can lower LH and FSA and subsequently reduce testosterone and estrogen production
- Common Uses: Treatment of prostate cancer and endometriosis
- Memorable Side Effects: Flushing, weight changes, injection site reaction, edema, sweating, reduced libido, CNS changes, GI upset, reduced bone mineral density, blood sugar elevations, hyperlipidemia
- Clinical Pearls:
    - Injection only
- Monitoring: Hormonal levels (depending upon indication), bone mineral density, cardiovascular risk factors such as lipids and blood pressure, HbA1c in at risk diabetes patients, renal function
- Drug and Diet Considerations:
    - Assess calcium and vitamin D intake due to reduced bone mineral density risks
    - Ensure adequate electrolyte levels

171

- o Lipid and diabetes friendly diet may be appropriate in at risk patients

Levalbuterol (Xopenex)
- Class: Beta-agonist
- Mechanism of Action: Stimulates beta-2 receptors leading to relaxation of smooth muscle and opening of airways
- Common Uses: Acute relief of respiratory distress in asthma and COPD
- Memorable Side Effects: Tachycardia, tremor, anxiousness, hypokalemia (rare), hyperglycemia (rare)
- Clinical Pearls:
  - o Remember that levalbuterol, a beta agonist, will have opposite effects of beta-blockers. Instead of reduced pulse, you could see tachycardia
  - o Too much beta-agonist can also be a potential cause of tremor/shakiness
  - o In patients who are taking multiple inhaled respiratory medications at the same time, albuterol will be done first to help open up the airways
  - o With patients who are frequently using their albuterol inhaler (or nebs) or presenting to the emergency room, make sure that they are reassessed to have their controller (usually inhaled corticosteroids) medication adjusted
- Monitoring: Frequency of use, FEV1, peak-flow, pulse, blood pressure, and potassium (usually only necessary in high dosages), glucose (rarely clinically significant
- Drug and Diet Considerations:
  - o Assess potassium intake and blood levels of potassium if the patient is using a beta agonist frequently or has a history of hypokalemia
  - o Be aware of caffeine intake in combination with a beta-agonist as it can have an additive effect on blood pressure and heart rate
  - o Monitor diabetes patients for elevations in blood sugar

Levetiracetam (Keppra)
- Class: Antiepileptic
- Mechanism of Action: Binds to SV2A, inhibits presynaptic calcium channels and theorized to reduce neurotransmitter release
- Common Uses: Treatment of seizures
- Memorable Side Effects: Sedation, dizziness, behavioral changes, GI upset, blood pressure variability (pediatrics), skin reactions (rare), CBC alterations (rare)
- Clinical Pearls:
  - o Levels typically not done
    - Possibly checked to assure adherence
  - o Watch accumulation with poor kidney function
  - o Titrate dose based upon seizures/signs of adverse effects versus drug levels
  - o Lower risk for drug interactions compared to other agents like phenytoin and carbamazepine
- Monitoring: CBC, drug levels (likely for adherence only)
- Drug and Diet Considerations:
  - o Alcohol can have additive CNS depressant effects

172

o   May be given with or without food

Levofloxacin (Levaquin)
- Class: Quinolone, antibiotic
- Mechanism of Action: Inhibits bacterial DNA synthesis
- Common Uses: Treatment of pneumonia, UTIs and complicated skin infections
- Memorable Side Effects: GI side effects, QTc prolongation (rare)
- Clinical Pearls:
    o   Commonly used for both UTIs and pneumonia
    o   Watch out for binding interactions that can decrease absorption, like co-administration with calcium or iron
    o   May increase QTc prolongation risk especially in patients already on antiarrhythmic medications or other meds that may prolong QTc interval
    o   Spontaneous tendon rupture has been reported (extremely rare)
- Monitoring: In the short term, lab monitoring is typically not necessary; in long term therapy, renal function, LFTs, CBC, and risk for hypoglycemia in diabetes may be assessed as clinically indicated
- Drug and Diet Considerations:
    o   Antacids, iron, calcium, zinc, magnesium, aluminum, and dairy products can interfere with the absorption of this drug; administer oral levofloxacin 2 hours before or up to 6 hours after any of the above listed products
    o   The interaction with dairy is less severe if the patients are eating an entire meal with other food while taking the medication

Levothyroxine (Synthroid)
- Class: Hypothyroid replacement
- Mechanism of Action: Synthetic T4 hormone, converted to active T3 metabolite
- Common Uses: Replacement hormone for patients with hypothyroidism
- Memorable Side Effects: Anxiety, tachycardia, weight loss, decreased bone mineral density, insomnia, GI side effects
- Clinical Pearls:
    o   Remember that in patients with hypothyroidism, they will have a lack of energy, fatigue, possible weight gain and many symptoms that might mimic depression
    o   If hypothyroidism causes fatigue and lethargy symptoms, remember that giving too much levothyroxine will cause the opposite, ramping up the patient putting them at risk for tachycardia, anxiety, etc.
    o   In practice, I commonly see ½ tabs, and possibly alternating daily doses which can increase risk for errors and confusion
- Monitoring: TSH is the major monitoring parameter for levothyroxine dosing. Remember that dosing is counterintuitive, when TSH is high, it indicates that levothyroxine should be increased; the reason for this is due to a negative feedback loop; tachycardia, blood pressure, bone mineral density in older females
- Drug and Diet Considerations:
    o   With administration of levothyroxine, it is generally recommended to give early in the morning prior to other meds or food,

HOWEVER if a patient is stabilized (TSH is normal) and doesn't take it this way, it is ok – consistency is the key!
- o Use of calcium supplements is extremely common, giving calcium and levothyroxine together will significantly block the absorption of the levothyroxine requiring an increase in the levothyroxine dose, recommend separating by at least 4 hours
- o Iron, fiber, certain nuts, grapefruit juice, and soy may alter GI absorption; consistency is key along with monitoring TSH

Linagliptin (Tradjenta)
- Class: Antidiabetic, DDP-4 inhibitor
- Mechanism of Action: Inhibits DPP-4, which increases incretin levels; incretin increases insulin and decreases glucagon in the body and also might help patients' stomachs "feel full"
- Common Uses: Treatment of type 2 diabetes
- Memorable Side Effects: Hypoglycemia if taken in combination with insulin or sulfonylurea, pancreatitis concerns exist, but are rare
- Clinical Pearls:
  - o Usually fairly well tolerated, once daily dosing is nice for a diabetes medication
  - o No dose adjustment necessary in CKD
- Monitoring: Blood sugar, HbA1c, and renal function as clinically indicated
- Drug and Diet Considerations:
  - o Administer with or without food
  - o Implementation of a diabetic diet

Linezolid (Zyvox)
- Class: Oxazolidinone, antibiotic
- Mechanism of Action: Inhibition of bacterial protein synthesis by bind to 23s subunit as part of the 50s subunit
- Common Uses: Treatment of gram positive, resistant infections, alternative to vancomycin in many situations
- Memorable Side Effects: Diarrhea, risk of myelosuppression, lactic acidosis, neuropathy
- Clinical Pearls:
  - o MRSA and VRE coverage
  - o MAOI activity so may need to hold or adjust antidepressants that can increase serotonin syndrome risk (SSRIs, TCAs, SNRIs, etc.)
  - o Oral and IV available
- Monitoring: CBC, WBC
- Drug and Diet Considerations:
  - o Can be given with or without food
  - o MAOI/Tyramine interaction
    - ▪ Foods high in tyramine: fermented, cured, aged foods such as cheese, smoked meats/fish, beer
    - ▪ Reaction: tachycardia, N/V, headache
  - o Alcohol should be avoided as it may increase risk for toxicity

Liraglutide (Victoza)
- Class: Antidiabetic, GLP-1 agonist

174

- Mechanism of Action: Glucagon-like peptide 1 agonists enhance glucose dependent insulin secretion, slows gastric emptying, and reduces post prandial glucagon to reduce blood sugars
- Common Uses: Treatment of type 2 diabetes and weight loss
- Memorable Side Effects: Nausea, vomiting, hypoglycemia if taken in combination with insulin or sulfonylurea, increase in heart rate, pancreatitis concerns exist, but are rare
- Clinical Pearls:
  - Has an indication for weight loss; dosing is higher for this indication compared to diabetes
  - Boxed warning to avoid medication in certain types of thyroid tumors
  - Promotes fullness, weight loss can be a beneficial effect
  - Typically better in HbA1c reduction than most oral diabetes medications
- Monitoring: Blood sugar, HbA1c, triglycerides, and renal function as clinically indicated
- Drug and Diet Considerations:
  - Administer with or without food
  - Reduces appetite which can be helpful in obese type 2 diabetes patients
  - Implementation of a diabetic diet

Lisdexamfetamine (Vyvanse)
- Class: CNS stimulant
- Mechanism of Action: Causes release of dopamine and norepinephrine and may also block reuptake of norepinephrine and dopamine leading to CNS stimulation
- Common Uses: Management of ADHD symptoms and may be off-label to treat depression/fatigue
- Memorable Side Effects: Anxiety, insomnia, poor appetite, weight loss, hypertension, pulse, emotional lability
- Clinical Pearls:
  - Remembering that this medication ramps you up (stimulant) will help you remember its side effects of anxiety, insomnia, weight loss, poor appetite, increased BP, increased pulse, etc.
  - When used in pediatrics, poor appetite can be a significant problem and should be something that should be assessed
  - BP and pulse monitoring is important
  - Be cautious in patients who may have cardiovascular risk (hypertension, etc.)
  - Schedule 2 controlled substance, highly addictive
- Blood pressure, pulse, weight, cardiac monitoring (in patients with preexisting cardiac condition or at risk for cardiac complications) and growth in pediatric patients
- Drug and Diet Considerations:
  - Food should have minimal impact on overall effectiveness, with or without food is ok
  - Use caution with other foods/supplements that may have additive effects to heart rate, blood pressure, and insomnia (i.e. caffeine)

175

- o Vitamin C may reduce the effectiveness by acidifying the urine which can enhance renal elimination of the drug; this is usually not clinically significant, but often we can discontinue the vitamin C supplement in patients who have a relatively normal diet
- o Assessing appetite and risk for anorexia is important

Lisinopril (Zestril, Prinivil)
- Class: Antihypertensive, ACE inhibitor
- Mechanism of Action: Inhibits angiotensin converting enzyme which prevents the production of angiotensin 2 and leads to lower BP; angiotensin 2 is a potent vasoconstrictor
- Common Uses: Treatment of hypertension, acute MI and heart failure
- Common Side Effects: Cough, kidney impairment, low blood pressure, and hyperkalemia
- Clinical Pearls:
    - o ACE inhibitors are notoriously known for causing a dry chronic cough; if you ever have a patient with a chronic cough, you must assess if they are on an ACE inhibitor
    - o Angiotensin Receptor Blockers (ARBs) are the cousins to the ACE inhibitors, and are the first line substitute to a patient who has had a cough with an ACE inhibitor
    - o ACE inhibitors can exacerbate kidney impairment as well as contribute to acute renal failure especially in patients who are already on other potential renal toxic medications (i.e. diuretics, NSAIDs, etc.) even though in conditions like heart failure, diuretics and ACE inhibitors are often used together
    - o ACE inhibitors are a classic cause of elevated potassium levels; if your patient has hyperkalemia, you must make sure the ACE inhibitor has been addressed
    - o In some cases, patients of African descent may not respond to ACE inhibitors as well as other ethnicities
    - o A common mistake I've seen clinicians make is using an ACE inhibitor with and ARB; this is generally not recommended
    - o ACE inhibitors (and ARBs) are frequently used in patients with hypertension and a history of diabetes, stroke, CAD, CKD, and CHF
    - o Angioedema (swelling of the lips/airway) is classically caused by ACE inhibitors; it is an extremely rare, but very serious adverse reaction requiring immediate discontinuation
- Monitoring: Renal function, potassium, blood pressure
- Drug and Diet Considerations:
    - o Be cautious and monitor potassium closely in patients with high dietary intake of potassium as this could contribute to hyperkalemia in combination with this medication
    - o Administer with or without food

Lithium (Lithobid)
- Class: Mood stabilizer, antimanic agent
- Mechanism of Action: Not well understood
- Common Uses: Acute and maintenance treatment for bipolar disorder
- Memorable Side Effects: Ataxia, GI, tremor, hypothyroid
- Clinical Pearls:

176

- o Early toxicity signs are nausea, vomiting, sedation, weakness, difficulty walking or coordinating movements, tremor
- o Risk of seizure/coma with very high levels
- o Kidney function very important to monitor
- o Can impact thyroid function; monitor TSH
- o Drug interactions with NSAIDs, ACE inhibitors and diuretics
- o Usually therapeutic level considered 0.5-1.2 mEq/L
- Monitoring: Lithium levels, renal function, thyroid function, electrolytes, weight
- Drug and Diet Considerations:
  - o Giving with food may help with GI upset
  - o Caffeine may lower drug levels
  - o Consistent hydration is recommended to reduce the risk of toxicity and variable levels
  - o Significant changes in sodium chloride intake may alter levels, more intake equates to lower lithium levels

Loperamide (Imodium)
- Class: Antidiarrheal
- Mechanism of Action: Acts on opioid receptors on intestines and slows peristalsis (GI movement)
- Common Uses: Treatment of diarrhea
- Memorable Side Effects: Constipation, abdominal pain
- Clinical Pearls:
  - o Over-the-counter availability
  - o Make sure to have patients who use this chronically on their own assessed for other problems (IBS, infection, etc.)
  - o Can be used as needed
  - o Rarely, you may see this medication abused, really high doses give an opioid-type effect
- Monitoring: Bowel movement frequency
- Drug and Diet Considerations:
  - o Assess benefit of medication and if the patient continues to have diarrhea concerns, monitor fluid and electrolytes

Loratadine (Claritin, Alavert, Allergy Relief)
- Class: Second generation antihistamine
- Mechanism of Action: Blocks Histamine-1 receptors
- Common Uses: Relief of allergic rhinitis and itching
- Memorable Side Effects: Sedation (much less than 1st generation antihistamines like diphenhydramine or hydroxyzine), mildly anticholinergic
- Clinical Pearls:
  - o Second generation H1 blockers like loratadine are generally preferred for seasonal allergies as they are more tolerable than first generation antihistamines
  - o Generally less sedating and less anticholinergic effects than first generation
  - o Often with antihistamines, if one doesn't work, patients may try another one from the same class (cetirizine, loratadine, fexofenadine, etc.)
  - o Over-the-counter availability

177

- Monitoring: No routine lab work is necessary
- Drug and Diet Considerations:
    - Absorption may be slightly increased with food, but it is likely not clinically significant so can give with or without food
    - It has mild anticholinergic side effects so dry mouth could potentially alter taste and desire to eat
    - Alcohol may exacerbate mild sedative effects

Lorazepam (Ativan)

- Class: Antianxiety, benzodiazepine
- Mechanism of Action: Enhances activity of GABA, an inhibitory neurotransmitter that causes sedation
- Common Uses: Treatment of anxiety, seizure and insomnia
- Memorable Side Effects: Sedation, confusion, fall risk, dizziness
- Clinical Pearls:
    - The best way I remember benzodiazepines is that they are very close to "alcohol in a pill"
    - Sedation, slurred speech, trouble walking (ataxia) etc. are all common with benzos/alcohol; they are also commonly used in alcohol withdrawal
    - Be cautious with patients on higher doses of benzodiazepines to make sure they aren't abruptly stopped
    - Educate patients on driving/operating machinery; remember that benzodiazepines are often used for sleep as well as anxiety
    - Unlike SSRIs for anxiety, a great advantage of benzos is that they work quickly and can be used as needed
    - Fall risk in the elderly is a big downside to using these medications
    - Benzos are a controlled substance; they can cause addiction and dependence
    - Can be used for acute behavioral issues as well as seizure
    - Flumazenil is antidote in overdose
- Monitoring: Routine lab monitoring typically isn't necessary unless clinically indicated
- Drug and Diet Considerations:
    - Alcohol intake can have additive side effects of sedation, confusion, slurred speech, and other CNS depressant effects

Losartan (Cozaar)

- Class: Antihypertensive, ARB
- Mechanism of Action: Block the angiotensin 2 receptor preventing vasoconstriction, aldosterone release, etc. (remember aldosterone antagonists can raise potassium just like ARBs and ACE inhibitors)
- Common Uses: Treatment of hypertension and heart failure
- Memorable Side Effects: Hyperkalemia, exacerbate/worsen kidney function, low blood pressure
- Clinical Pearls:
    - When you think of ARBs and ACE inhibitors, you can lump the side effects together, they are overall the same
    - One major exception to the above rule is the side effect of cough; cough usually doesn't happen with ARBs, and in many situations, you will see patients who develop cough on an ACE inhibitor be transitioned to an ARB

- o Kidney function changes and monitoring of potassium is critical when doses are changed or an ARB is initiated
- o This worsening kidney function risk increases in patients who may be taking NSAIDs and/or diuretics
- o As with any medication used to treat hypertension, we need to educate our patients to rise slowly when getting up to minimize risk of orthostatic (sometimes called postural) hypotension
- Monitoring: Renal function, potassium, blood pressure
- Drug and Diet Considerations:
  - o Be cautious and monitor potassium closely in patients with high dietary intake of potassium as this could contribute to hyperkalemia in combination with this medication
  - o Administer with or without food
  - o Possible reduction in concentration when using St. John's wort

Lovastatin (Mevacor)
- Class: Antilipemic, statin
- Mechanism of Action: HMG Co-A reductase inhibitor which leads to a decrease in LDL
- Common Uses: Reduction of cholesterol, particularly LDL
- Memorable Side Effects: Muscle aches, rhabdomyolysis (rare but serious)
- Clinical Pearls:
  - o Statins, like lovastatin, are one of the mainstays of therapy to reduce cholesterol, and more particularly LDL (bad cholesterol)
  - o The most notable side effect with statins that you will likely hear patients complain about is myopathy (muscle aches/pain)
  - o Usually muscle aches are all over which can help you differentiate from other pain conditions or pain/soreness from an injury or overuse
  - o Contraindicated in pregnancy
  - o Patients who do not tolerate lovastatin, may try another statin as long as adverse effects aren't too severe (i.e. rhabdomyolysis); if you notice that the patient had an allergy or intolerance, you need to clarify with the provider
  - o CPK will be the primary lab to test for rhabdomyolysis due to breakdown of muscle; this elevation in CPK may eventually lead to kidney failure
  - o Patients usually will present with myopathy when the medication is first started or increased, but be on the lookout for new medications that can interact with statins like CYP3A4 inhibitor drug interactions with classic medications like fluconazole or erythromycin
  - o For most statins it is "recommended" to give them at night; this is not an absolute, but the drugs ideally work the best when given at night
  - o Lovastatin is used less frequently because it doesn't reduce LDL as much as newer statins like atorvastatin, simvastatin, and rosuvastatin
- Monitoring: Lipids, LFTs, CPK if experiencing muscle pain (myopathy)
- Drug and Diet Considerations:
  - o Liver toxicity risk from alcohol (usually in excess) may be increased if used in combination with statins

- o Low, often not clinically significant, risk of elevating blood sugars in patients with diabetes
- o Grapefruit juice can significantly increase the concentrations of lovastatin, generally avoid using grapefruit juice
- o Can be taken with or without food
- o St. John's wort can lower concentrations of lovastatin
- o Encourage a lipid lowering diet for any patient taking a cholesterol medication

Lubiprostone (Amitiza)

- Class: Laxative, calcium channel activator
- Mechanism of Action: Calcium channel activator, which promotes fluid entry and secretion into the intestine
- Common Uses: Treatment of constipation
- Memorable Side Effects: Nausea
- Clinical Pearls:
  - o Expensive treatment option at this time in comparison to other agents
- Monitoring: Bowel movements
- Drug and Diet Considerations:
  - o Give with food and water

Lurasidone (Latuda)

- Class: Antipsychotic
- Mechanism of Action: Blocks dopamine receptors
- Common Uses: Treatment of schizophrenia, bipolar disorder and off-label to treat dementia related behaviors like aggression, hallucinations and delusions
- Memorable Side Effects: Sedation, fall risk, orthostatic BP changes, EPS, metabolic syndrome
- Clinical Pearls:
  - o Usually higher doses are required for younger patients with schizophrenia and/or bipolar disorder while lower doses can and should be used in the elderly
  - o Remember with antipsychotic medications that they block dopamine and can exacerbate conditions where there is a shortage of dopamine like Parkinson's disorder (remember that we use dopamine to treat Parkinson's – i.e. carbidopa/levodopa or pramipexole)
  - o Sedation, orthostatic hypotension, movement disorder side effects can all increase the risk of falls especially in our elderly patients
  - o NMS (neuroleptic malignant syndrome) is a very rare but very serious complication with antipsychotic medications; a few symptoms of NMS include: fever, hyperreflexia, confusion, delirium, tremor
  - o Antipsychotics increase risk of metabolic syndrome (diabetes, elevated lipids, weight gain, etc.); it is important to periodically monitor for this, especially in younger patients with schizophrenia and/or bipolar disorder who may be likely to require long term use of higher doses
  - o Anticholinergic effects are possible as well with antipsychotics, dry eyes, dry mouth, exacerbation of urinary retention (i.e. BPH), constipation (SLUD – can't salivate, lacrimate, urinate or defecate)

- o Antipsychotics can contribute to QTc prolongation, which can be especially problematic in patients who are already at risk (i.e. on antiarrhythmic medications)
- Monitoring: Weight, BMI, lipids, HbA1c, blood sugars, EKG as clinically appropriate, electrolytes (potassium and magnesium important if the patient is at risk for QTc prolongation)
- Drug and Diet Considerations:
  - o Increased appetite and risk for metabolic syndrome
  - o Increased blood sugars can result in our diabetes patients, monitor blood sugars closely with acute changes in the drug
  - o Alcohol may exacerbate the CNS depressant effect
  - o Give with food (at least 350 calories)
  - o Grapefruit juice can increase concentrations, avoid use

Magnesium (Mag-Oxide)

- Class: Electrolyte
- Mechanism of Action: Important in enzymatic reactions, carbohydrate breakdown, protein synthesis, and skeletal-muscular functioning
- Common Uses: Deficiency, antacid, constipation (see Milk of Magnesia)
- Memorable Side Effects: Diarrhea
- Clinical Pearls:
  - o Accumulation is more likely in patients with renal impairment
  - o RDA 310-420 mg/day (range varies based upon age, pregnancy, lactation)
- Monitoring: Magnesium levels (usual range 1.5-2.5 mg/dL)
- Drug and Diet Considerations:
  - o Drugs that may cause deficiency include PPIs, loop diuretics, certain oncology agents (cisplatin), immunosuppressives (tacrolimus, cyclosporine), amphotericin B
  - o May bind common antibiotics such as quinolones, certain cephalosporins, and tetracycline derivatives (reduces concentrations); separate medication by at least 2 hours
  - o Bisphosphonates, baloxavir, and integrase inhibitors (HIV medications) may have concentrations reduced by magnesium: separate medication by at least 2 hours

Magnesium Hydroxide (Milk of Magnesia)

- Class: Osmotic laxative, antacid
- Mechanism of Action: It works by pulling water into the gut which promotes motility and bowel movements
- Common Uses: Treatment of constipation and used as a bowel prep prior to colonoscopy
- Memorable Side Effects: Diarrhea, abdominal cramps, GI upset
- Clinical Pearls:
  - o Caution with kidney impairment
    - ▪ Usually not an issue with as needed/seldom use
  - o Higher risk of magnesium accumulation in kidney disease with frequent use
  - o Levothyroxine, quinolone and tetracycline antibiotics can have their effectiveness reduced
  - o Over-the-counter availability

181

- o Ensure that patients are educated to consult a healthcare professional if use is needed for longer than 1-2 weeks
- Monitoring: Renal function, magnesium levels as clinically indicated, bowel movements
- Drug and Diet Considerations:
  - o Excessive dietary intake of magnesium may exacerbate risk for hypermagnesemia
  - o Some products may contain propylene glycol which could be toxic in neonates
  - o Drink a glass of water following administration
  - o May reduce iron absorption

Meclizine (Antivert)

- Class: Antiemetic, antihistamine, dopamine blocker
- Mechanism of Action: Blocks dopamine receptors as well as H1 receptors
- Common Uses: Treatment of vertigo (chronic dizziness), nausea/vomiting and motion sickness
- Memorable Side Effects: Sedation, fall risk, orthostatic BP changes, EPS, metabolic syndrome
- Clinical Pearls:
  - o Whenever you see an order for meclizine to treat dizziness, be sure to assess other medications (sleepers, psych meds, opioids, antihypertensives, etc.) to make sure they aren't causing or worsening dizziness
  - o Can be given as needed
  - o Blocks H1 receptors, so sedation will be common
  - o Anticholinergic effects, but probably not a major deal if used infrequently at low doses
- Monitoring: EKG, and possibly electrolytes, in at risk patients (especially in overdose)
- Drug and Diet Considerations:
  - o Slows the motility of the GI tract which could increase the risk for constipation, maintain adequate fluids and non-constipating diet
  - o If GI upset occurs, no issues in giving the drug with food
  - o Dry mouth may increase thirst and alter taste/pleasure of food
  - o With or without food is acceptable
  - o CNS depressant activity which could be exacerbated by alcohol

Medroxyprogesterone (Provera, Depo-Provera)

- Class: Progestin
- Mechanism of Action: Blocks the action of the pituitary and the release of gonadotropins which prevents ovulation and stimulates endometrial thinning
- Common Uses: Alteration in menstrual bleeding, weight fluctuation, hot flashes, GI upset
- Clinical Pearls:
  - o Boxed warning on reduced bone mineral density (injection – Depo-Provera)
  - o Not recommended for birth control for longer than 2 years
- Monitoring: Bone mineral density, weight
- Drug and Diet Considerations:
  - o Oral administration is typically given with food, but acceptable to give on an empty stomach
  - o Possible weight gain

- o Because of the potential reduced bone mineral density, encourage adequate calcium and vitamin D intake

Megestrol (Megace)
- Class: Progestin, appetite stimulant, antineoplastic agent
- Mechanism of Action: Progestin action can block the effects of estrogen and have anti-tumor activities; may block the effects of cytokines which is theorized to help stimulate appetite
- Common Uses: Appetite stimulation and treatment of breast and endometrial cancer
- Memorable Side Effects: Hypertension, edema, blood clot risk, elevated glucose levels, Cushing's syndrome-type effects
- Clinical Pearls:
  - o Recommended to avoid use in geriatric patients
  - o Evidence for weight gain, appetite stimulation is weak in geriatric (non-AIDS, non-cancer) patients
- Monitoring: Blood pressure, blood sugar, weight
- Drug and Diet Considerations:
  - o Assess and adjust dietary intake and blood sugars accordingly in diabetes patients who may experience hyperglycemia

Melatonin
- Class: Sedative
- Mechanism of Action: Binds to MT1 and MT2 (melatonin receptors) which help stimulate and regulate the sleep/wake cycle
- Common Uses: Treatment of insomnia and sleep-wake cycle regulation
- Memorable Side Effects: Confusion, sedation, headache, alterations in sleep pattern, psychological changes, elevated prolactin, hypothermia (all adverse effects more likely as dose escalates)
- Clinical Pearls:
  - o Available over-the-counter
  - o Naturally produced and secreted in the body
  - o Use cautiously in patients taking other sedating agents
- Monitoring: No routine lab work is typically recommended
- Drug and Diet Considerations:
  - o Typically dosed in the evening without regard to food
  - o Although rare, and not typically clinically significant, it may alter blood sugar levels

Meloxicam (Mobic)
- Class: NSAID, analgesic
- Mechanism of Action: Inhibits cyclooxygenase-1 and 2 (COX-1 and COX-2); results in a reduction in prostaglandins which cause pain, fever and inflammation
- Common Uses: Reduction of pain, fever and inflammation
- Memorable Side Effects: GI ulcer, worsening kidney function, edema, hypertension, inhibits platelets (can exacerbate bleed risk)
- Clinical Pearls:

- NSAIDs are one of the most common causes of GI bleeding; this risk increases in the elderly and those on medications that increase risk of bleeding (anticoagulants and antiplatelet medications)
- Because of the side effects of GI upset/bleeding, NSAIDs should be taken with food
- Due to effects on platelets, NSAIDs are typically held before/after surgery to reduce the risk of bleeding
- NSAIDs can contribute to edema and exacerbate CHF (congestive heart failure); be on the lookout and have NSAIDs reassessed if you see a patient with a CHF exacerbation or a patient requiring increasing diuretics like furosemide
- NSAIDs can cause worsening kidney function (creatinine should be monitored); this risk can be greatly increased in patients on ACE inhibitors or ARBs and/or diuretic type medications
- Due to above reasons on kidney function, GI bleed risk, and CHF, NSAIDs are not the safest medication in the elderly; acetaminophen is generally preferred for generalized pain with a few exceptions
- Although generally considered riskier in the elderly, a big advantage of NSAIDs over acetaminophen is that they can reduce inflammation
- Pregnancy category C/D when >30 weeks gestation; NSAIDs are generally avoided in pregnancy and especially after 30 weeks gestation
- Monitoring: Renal function, hemoglobin, platelets (contained within CBC), blood pressure, signs of bruising or bleeding, weight (risk for edema)
- Drug and Diet Considerations:
  - Because of significant incidence of GI upset, it is recommended to give with food or milk
  - Dehydration coupled with ibuprofen may increase the risk for acute renal failure
  - Excessive alcohol may increase GI bleed risk
  - Vitamin E, Omega-3 fatty acids, gingko, garlic, ginseng, turmeric, and fish oil supplements have been purported to have antiplatelet type activity which in theory could increase the risk of bleed – clinical significance is questionable; the most common resolution is to discontinue the supplements if they are not necessary

Melphalan (Alkeran, Evomela)

- Class: Oncology agent, nitrogen mustard
- Mechanism of Action: Prevents DNA cross-linking which ultimately prevents proliferation and growth of cells
- Common Uses: Treatment of numerous types of cancers
- Memorable Side Effects: Nausea, vomiting, diarrhea, fatigue, hypokalemia, hypophosphatemia, edema, anemia, thrombocytopenia, myelosuppression, hypersensitivity reactions
- Clinical Pearls:
  - Boxed warnings for the risk of hypersensitivity reactions, malignancy, and myelosuppression
- Monitoring: CBC, renal function, electrolytes, LFTs, uric acid
- Drug and Diet Considerations:
  - Given on an empty stomach (oral dosage form) as food can block absorption

184

- o Weight loss and poor nutrition may result on account of nausea and vomiting adverse effects
- o Assess for diet implications on hyperuricemia risk

Memantine (Namenda)
- Class: Anti-dementia, NMDA antagonist
- Mechanism of Action: Blocks NMDA receptors
- Common Uses: Management of symptoms associated with Alzheimer's dementia
- Memorable Side Effects: Changes in behavior, worsening confusion, dizziness
- Clinical Pearls:
  - o Remember that medications used for dementia only help with symptoms management; they do NOT reverse dementia
  - o Memantine has dose adjustments in kidney disease, so keep an eye out for our patients who may have worsening kidney function (rising creatinine) as the drug may begin to accumulate
  - o There is both an extended release and immediate release product available now
  - o Memantine has a different mechanism of action from other dementia medications, like. donepezil, galantamine and rivastigmine, so it can be used in combination
- Monitoring: Cognition and function; routine lab work is not necessary
- Drug and Diet Considerations:
  - o No concerns with regards to diet

Meperidine (Demerol)
- Class: Opioid, analgesic
- Mechanism of Action: Binds opioid receptors inhibiting CNS pain pathways and causing pain relief
- Common Uses: Management of pain disorders
- Memorable Side Effects: Constipation, sedation, CNS effects like confusion, delirium, etc., respiratory depression
- Clinical Pearls:
  - o Meperidine is a scheduled 2 controlled substance; risk of addiction and dependence
  - o Very frequently used short term for pain and post-op procedures
  - o It is critical to educate/assess patients for constipation if they are taking frequent opioids like morphine
  - o Driving/working machinery is certainly risky when using opioids as they can cause significant sedation (usually patients get used to this side effect if they take the medication chronically)
  - o Naloxone is reversal agent for opioids
  - o Boxed warning on 3A4 drug interactions that may increase concentrations and risk for overdose
  - o Do not use in the elderly
  - o Risk of CNS effects including seizure
- Monitoring: Bowel movements, pain management, risk for addiction
- Drug and Diet Considerations:
  - o Alcohol can exacerbate the CNS depressant effect from meperidine
  - o Giving with food and water can reduce the risk of GI upset

- o Encourage a constipation friendly diet including fiber, fluids, and exercise as the medication can be very constipating

Mercaptopurine (Purixan, 6-mercaptopurine)
- Class: Immunosuppressant, oncology agent
- Mechanism of Action: Acts as a purine antagonist that blocks DNA production by becoming incorporated into DNA and RNA strands
- Common Uses: Treatment of leukemia and inflammatory bowel disease (Crohn's, Ulcerative Colitis)
- Memorable Side Effects: Rash, fever, hair loss, photosensitivity, skin pigmentation changes, GI upset, weight loss, bone marrow suppression, liver toxicity, renal toxicity, immunosuppression
- Clinical Pearls:
  - o TPMT, NUDT15 genetic testing can be done to identify patients at risk for toxicity
- Monitoring: CBC, LFTs, renal function
- Drug and Diet Considerations:
  - o Ensure adequate hydration
  - o Give 1 hour prior to meals or 2 hours after
  - o Monitor weight and assess for anorexia risk and nutritional deficiency

Meropenem/vaborabactam (Vabomere)
- Class: Carbapenem and beta-lactamase inhibitor, antibiotic
- Mechanism of Action: Binds penicillin-binding proteins and inhibits production of the bacterial cell wall; vaborabactam blocks bacterial beta-lactamases, and carbapenemases, which can help prolong the activity of meropenem
- Common Uses: Broad spectrum antibiotic used in may resistant, severe infections (mainly gram-negative Enterobacteriaceae)
- Memorable Side Effects: Diarrhea, GI upset, headache, infusion reaction, lowers seizure threshold
- Clinical Pearls:
  - o Usually reserved for very severe, resistant infections
  - o Good coverage for most gram negatives
    - ▪ Generally this drug does not cover MRSA
- Monitoring: Renal function
- Drug and Diet Considerations:
  - o Minimal concerns with shorter term use
  - o Monitor fluid and electrolyte status if diarrhea is problematic

Mesalamine (Asacol, Canasa, Pentasa)
- Class: 5-aminosalicylic acid derivative (5-ASA compound)
- Mechanism of Action: Not well understood, but likely reduces inflammation by impacting leukotrienes
- Common Uses: Treatment of inflammatory bowel disease
- Memorable Side Effects: GI upset, belching
- Clinical Pearls:
  - o Slow onset to beneficial effects
  - o Multiple daily doses required
  - o Closely related to sulfasalazine in structure
- Monitoring: LFTs, CBC, and renal function as clinically indicated

- Drug and Diet Considerations:
  - Can give with or without food in most cases
    - Asacol HD – empty stomach
    - Lialda – with meals
    - Pentasa – with meals
  - Supplements that have an antacid effect (i.e. calcium carbonate) may reduce effectiveness of the medication
  - Different brand names may have alternative administration recommendations

Metformin (Glucophage)
- Class: Antidiabetic, biguanide
- Mechanism of Action: Decreases hepatic glucose production (doesn't stimulate production of insulin which is why it is not likely to cause hypoglycemia when used alone)
- Common Uses: Diabetes treatment
- Memorable Side Effects: N/V/D most common, B12 deficiency possible, lactic acidosis (very rare, more common in patients with poor kidney function)
- Clinical Pearls:
  - Metformin is the first line medication for type 2 diabetes
  - Metformin is contraindicated in patients with poor kidney function (serum creatinine >1.4 in females and >1.5 in males); if you know a patient has a history of chronic kidney disease (CKD) make sure use of this medication is reassessed
  - The risk of lactic acidosis increases as this medication is used in the elderly and those with poor kidney function
  - The most common side effect of metformin is GI upset; be on the lookout for patient complaints of this adverse effect and new medication use like PPIs, like omeprazole, or other medications that are used to relieve stomach symptoms
  - Administration with a meal is recommended and can really help minimize GI upset
  - Metformin does not cause weight gain compared to other diabetes medications, which is nice since many of our type 2 diabetes patients are overweight
- Monitoring: Blood sugar, HbA1c, B12 and hemoglobin as clinically indicated, renal function
- Drug and Diet Considerations:
  - Administer with food due to a high incidence of GI upset
  - Significant alcohol intake can increase the risk for lactic acidosis
  - B12 replacement may be necessary

Methadone (Methadose, Dolophine)
- Class: Opioid, analgesic
- Mechanism of Action: Binds opioid receptors inhibiting CNS pain pathways and causing pain relief
- Common Uses: Management of pain disorders, both chronic and acute, opioid detoxification
- Memorable Side Effects: Constipation, sedation, CNS effects like confusion, delirium etc., respiratory depression
- Clinical Pearls:

- - - Methadone is a scheduled 2 controlled substance; risk of addiction and dependence
    - Used in methadone maintenance programs for treatment of opioid addiction
    - It is critical to educate/assess patients for constipation if they are taking frequent opioids like methadone
    - Naloxone is reversal agent for opioids
    - Driving/working machinery is certainly risky when using opioids as they can cause significant sedation (usually patients get used to this side effect if they take the medication chronically)
    - QTc prolongation is a risk especially with other medications that can contribute to QTc prolongation (amiodarone, etc.)
  - Monitoring: Bowel movements, pain management, risk for addiction, QTc prolongation risk, EKG
  - Drug and Diet Considerations:
    - Alcohol can exacerbate the CNS depressant effect
    - Giving with food and water can reduce the risk of GI upset
    - Encourage a constipation friendly diet including fiber, fluids and exercise as methadone can be very constipating
    - Grapefruit juice can raise concentrations

Methimazole (Tapazole)

- Class: Antithyroid
- Mechanism of Action: Inhibits thyroid synthesis by interfering with oxidation of iodine; this is done via inhibition of the peroxidase enzyme
- Common Uses: Treatment of hyperthyroidism
- Memorable Side Effects: GI upset, hepatitis, agranulocytosis, anemia, lupus reaction
- Clinical Pearls:
  - Possible link with pancreatitis
  - Pay attention to symptoms of hyperthyroid and hypothyroid as these may indicate under-dosing or overdosing
  - Once daily dosing is an advantage over propylthiouracil
  - Typically, it will take a little while for the drug to work
- Monitoring: Thyroid function (TSH, T4, T3), LFTs, CBC
- Drug and Diet Considerations:
  - Under-dosing may result in weight loss
  - Overdosing may result in weight gain
  - May give with or without food

Methotrexate (Rheumatrex)

- Class: DMARD (disease modifying antirheumatic drug), antineoplastic agent
- Mechanism of Action: Binds dihydrofolate reductase; in treatment of rheumatoid arthritis, likely benefit is from suppressing the immune system
- Common Uses: Treatment of rheumatoid arthritis, psoriasis and certain cancers (much higher doses used in cancer treatment)
- Memorable Side Effects: Low WBC or platelet count, increased liver enzymes
- Clinical Pearls:
  - DMARDs are first line for rheumatoid arthritis
  - Usually dosed once weekly
  - Need to supplement folic acid when using chronically

- o Likely will not be beneficial in acute flare of inflammation (NSAIDs or prednisone typically used for acute RA flare)
- o Suppresses immune system so WBC and infection monitoring is important
- o LFTs should also be monitored
- Monitoring: CBC, LFTs, platelets, renal function
- Drug and Diet Considerations:
    - o Folic acid supplementation is necessary
    - o Alcohol can exacerbate liver toxicity risk
    - o Oral formulation can be taken with or without food

Methylcellulose (Citrucel)
- Class: Bulk-forming laxative, fiber supplement
- Mechanism of Action: Fiber and fiber like substances absorb water and keep it in the gut lumen which helps stimulate peristalsis and bowel movements
- Common Uses: Treatment of constipation
- Memorable Side Effects: Cramping, diarrhea, obstruction risk
- Clinical Pearls:
    - o May cause swallowing issues in at risk patients (elderly, Parkinson's, swallowing disorders, etc.) particularly if not taken with adequate fluids
- Monitoring: No routine monitoring is necessary
- Drug and Diet Considerations
    - o Encourage adequate fluid intake at time of administration (at least 240 mls of water) and all throughout the day
    - o Review specific product as there may be additional ingredients/electrolytes (typically not clinically significant)
    - o Phenylalanine may be an ingredient in some formulations

Methyldopa (Aldomet)
- Class: Antihypertensive, alpha-2 agonist
- Mechanism of Action: Centrally acting alpha-2 agonist which results in decreased sympathetic activity and drop in blood pressure
- Common Uses: Treatment of hypertension and management of ADHD symptoms
- Memorable Side Effects: Drowsiness, dizziness, dry mouth
- Clinical Pearls:
    - o Not the best in the elderly (on Beer's list)
    - o Can be considered an option in pregnant patients with hypertension
    - o Low blood pressure and pulse is possible
    - o Sedating which can be a significant problem especially in the elderly
    - o Rebound hypertension is a risk if abruptly discontinued
- Monitoring: Blood pressure, pulse, CBC, and LFTs as clinically indicated
- Drug and Diet Considerations:
    - o Can be given with or without food
    - o May reduce B12 and folate levels, consider supplementation

Methylphenidate (Ritalin, Concerta)
- Class: CNS stimulant

189

- Mechanism of Action: Blocks reuptake of norepinephrine and dopamine leading to CNS stimulation
- Common Uses: Treatment of ADHD and off-label for depression/fatigue
- Memorable Side Effects: Anxiety, insomnia, poor appetite, weight loss, hypertension, elevated pulse, emotional lability
- Clinical Pearls:
  - Remembering that this medication ramps you up (stimulant) will help you remember its side effects of anxiety, insomnia, weight loss, poor appetite, increased BP, increased pulse etc.
  - When used in pediatrics, poor appetite can be a significant problem and should be something that is assessed
  - BP and Pulse monitoring important
  - Be cautious in patients who may have cardiovascular risk (hypertension etc.)
  - Schedule 2 controlled substance, highly addictive
- Monitoring: Blood pressure, pulse, weight, cardiac monitoring (in patients with preexisting cardiac condition or at risk for cardiac complications) and growth in pediatric patients
- Drug and Diet Considerations:
  - Recommended to give 30-45 minutes before a meal as food can increase concentrations
  - Use caution with other foods/supplements that may have additive effects to heart rate, blood pressure, and insomnia (i.e. caffeine)
  - Vitamin C may reduce the effectiveness by acidifying the urine which can enhance renal elimination of the drug (usually not clinically significant, but often we can discontinue the vitamin C supplement in patients who have a relatively normal diet)
  - Assessing appetite and risk for anorexia is important
  - Alcohol can increase absorption with some formulations
  - Caffeine may increase stimulant effects

Methylprednisolone (Medrol)
- Class: Corticosteroid
- Mechanism of Action: Suppresses leukocytes and ultimately reduces inflammation, suppresses adrenal function and the immune system
- Common Uses: Suppression of acute inflammatory states (dermatitis, arthritis flare, Crohn's, pneumonia, asthma exacerbation, etc.)
- Memorable Side Effects: GI side effects, insomnia, hyperglycemia, long term use; suppress immune system, increase osteoporosis risk as well as cause adrenal insufficiency
- Clinical Pearls:
  - Most common use I've seen is a Medrol Dose Pak which is used for relief of short term inflammation related issues
  - Be sure to take steroids with food as they can be pretty hard on the GI tract
  - Long term corticosteroid use can lead to increased risk of Cushing's (moon face), diabetes, and osteoporosis; make sure long term use is assessed frequently to minimize length and dose of steroids
  - In patients on long term use, they should be assessed if vitamin D and/or calcium and bisphosphonates should be added to reduce osteoporosis risk
  - Insomnia is common in the short term, but may resolve as short term use goes to long term use

- o Short "bursts" (3 days to 1-2 weeks) are often used to relieve acute inflammatory states causing patient distress (asthma, rheumatoid arthritis, etc.)
        - o Corticosteroids, especially long term and higher doses, can suppress the immune system
        - o Antacids may lower concentrations
- Monitoring: Blood sugar (in diabetes patients), blood pressure, bone mineral density (longer term use), HPA suppression, weight, development (pediatric patients)
- Drug and Diet Considerations:
        - o Give with food as it can cause GI upset
        - o In patients with diabetes, educate them that a fluctuation in blood sugars may occur when starting, changing doses, or discontinuing this medication due to the adverse effect of hyperglycemia
        - o May reduce effectiveness of calcitriol (active vitamin D)
        - o Long term use may increase the need for certain nutrients and vitamins such as folic acid, calcium, phosphorus, vitamin C, and vitamin D
        - o Potassium and sodium may be elevated due to corticosteroids

Metoclopramide (Reglan)
- Class: Antiemetic, prokinetic
- Mechanism of Action: Blocks dopamine and serotonin receptors (in CRZ – chemoreceptor zone, lends to relief of nausea/vomiting)
- Common Uses: Treatment of gastroparesis (often caused by diabetes) and nausea/vomiting
- Memorable Side Effects: Extrapyramidal symptoms
- Clinical Pearls:
        - o Has dopamine blocking activity like antipsychotics, so it can cause movement disorders like EPS and tardive dyskinesia
        - o As above with dopamine blocking activity, it is not a great choice in a patient with a preexisting movement disorder (i.e. Parkinson's)
        - o Most commonly used for gastroparesis (slow moving GI tract); be on the lookout for anticholinergic medications which can worsen gastroparesis
        - o Usually dosed 3-4 times per day
- Monitoring: No routine lab work is necessary
- Drug and Diet Considerations:
        - o Give on an empty stomach, 30 minutes before meals, and before bedtime

Metolazone (Zaroxolyn)
- Class: Antihypertensive, thiazide diuretic
- Mechanism of Action: Inhibits sodium/chloride transporter in the distal tubules
- Common Use: Treatment of hypertension, edema and heart failure
- Memorable Side Effects: Photosensitivity, similar to loop diuretics, they increase urine output and decrease amount of volume in the body which can lead to frequent urination, electrolyte depletion, low blood pressure, and increased risk of kidney failure
- Clinical Pearls:

191

- One of the major differences between loops and thiazides are that thiazides (and thiazide-like) can INCREASE serum calcium while loops will reduce it
- While loop diuretics can cause hyperuricemia (elevated uric acid possibly contributing to or exacerbating gout), thiazides are classically known to do this; be on the lookout for metolazone use when gout medications are being added or patients are reporting gout flares
- Watch the timing of diuretics, too close to evening can cause frequent nighttime urination
- Monitoring: Renal function, electrolytes, blood pressure, weight, uric acid (in patients with gout)
- Drug and Diet Considerations:
  - A low potassium or low magnesium diet could increase the risk for deficiency in combination with the drug
  - Hypercalcemia is possible, be aware of calcium and vitamin D intake
  - This drug is dehydrating so be aware of acute renal failure risk in patients who have reduced fluid intake (i.e. acutely ill, geriatric patients, etc.)
  - Alcohol may exacerbate low blood pressure and urinary frequency
  - Modest increases in glucose, although not typically clinically significant, it may happen in our diabetes patients
  - Possible cause of weight loss

Metoprolol (Toprol XL, Lopressor)

- Class: Antihypertensive, beta-blocker
- Mechanism of Action: Blocks beta receptors leading to lower pulse/BP
- Common Uses: Treatment of hypertension and atrial fibrillation
- Memorable Side Effects: Low pulse, low BP, fatigue
- Clinical Pearls:
  - Common error in practice I've seen is confusion with metoprolol succinate (Toprol XL) versus metoprolol tartrate (Lopressor). Succinate is the "sustained" release formulation while tartrate is the immediate release formulation and usually dosed twice daily
  - Trick to remembering beta receptors: you have 1 heart and 2 lungs (beta-1 is primarily on the heart and beta-2 primarily in the lungs). You will see beta receptors again with respiratory medications. If beta-1 is stimulated, heart rate increases. If beta-1 is blocked, heart rate decreases
  - The selectivity of these drugs is really important; metoprolol is beta-1 selective, so in a patient with asthma, we would likely not see much of a problem however this selectivity may start to disappear as you push to doses higher
  - Pulse and blood pressure are going to be the two most important monitoring parameters you will want to follow
  - Often in practice, providers will place a hold order on beta-blockers if the pulse is too low. This is obviously done to reduce the risk of significant bradycardia; clinically, it may depend upon the situation, but in an ambulatory setting, you may see the order set to hold the beta blocker when pulse is less than 55 or 60.
- Monitoring: Pulse, blood pressure, EKG as clinically indicated (i.e. acute atrial fibrillation)

192

- Drug and Diet Considerations:
  - Ideally given with food, water (oral medication)

Metronidazole (Flagyl)
- Class: Antibiotic
- Mechanism of Action: Interferes with bacterial DNA and can inhibit protein synthesis
- Common Uses: Treatment of C. diff, H. pylori, anaerobic infections (gut infections), bacterial vaginosis
- Memorable Side Effects: GI side effects, metallic taste
- Clinical Pearls:
  - Can be utilized for anaerobic bacteria
  - Commonly used in combo in treatment of Helicobacter pylori which is a common cause of GI ulcers
  - IV and PO available
- Monitoring: LFTs, CBC as clinically indicated (long term therapy)
- Drug and Diet Considerations:
  - NO ALCOHOL with this medication – causes disulfiram reaction
  - Give with food to reduce GI upset

Micafungin (Mycamine)
- Class: Antifungal, echinocandin
- Mechanism of Action: Inhibition of 1,3 beta-D glucan synthase, a key enzyme involved in fungal cell wall synthesis
- Common Uses: Alternative to fluconazole if the patient has a resistant infection
- Memorable Side Effects: Low blood pressure, GI upset, diarrhea, edema, tachycardia, infusion reaction, electrolytes imbalances possible, but rare
- Clinical Pearls:
  - Typically better tolerated and lower risk than other IV antifungals, like azole antifungals and amphotericin B
- Monitoring: Liver function, renal function (as clinically indicated), CBC (as clinically indicated)
- Drug and Diet Considerations:
  - No major diet concerns
  - Monitor fluid and electrolyte status and alter dietary intake accordingly

Midazolam (Versed)
- Class: Benzodiazepine, sedative
- Mechanism of Action: Enhances activity of GABA, an inhibitory neurotransmitter that causes sedation
- Common Uses: Sedation/amnesia for procedures in a hospitalized patient and seizures
- Memorable Side Effects: Sedation, confusion, fall risk, dizziness, amnesia, respiratory depression
- Clinical Pearls:
  - Injectable/IV
  - Primary use is to cause sedation and amnesia in the hospital setting for various procedures/surgery

- o Monitoring of respirations will be important as cases of respiratory arrest have been reported
- o Can be used for surgery as well as seizure
- o Flumazenil is antidote in overdose
- Monitoring: Pulse, blood pressure, oxygen saturation
- Drug and Diet Considerations:
  - o Grapefruit juice can cause an increase in drug levels

Midodrine (Proamatine)

- Class: Alpha agonist
- Mechanism of Action: By stimulating alpha receptors, it causes vasoconstriction leading to an increase in blood pressure and reduction in the risk of orthostasis
- Common Uses: Treatment of orthostasis
- Memorable Side Effects: Hypertension, urinary retention
- Clinical Pearls:
  - o Use cautiously in patients with heart disease history
  - o Opposite of alpha blocker
    - ▪ May negatively impact urinary flow, causing BPH exacerbation
  - o Occasionally administered prior to dialysis sessions
  - o Boxed warning – should only be used in patients with significant hypotension that is interfering with normal function
- Monitoring: Blood pressure, pulse, renal function
- Drug and Diet Considerations:
  - o Increases in caffeine intake may exacerbate hypertensive effects
  - o May be given without regard to meals

Miglitol (Glyset)

- Class: Antidiabetic, alpha-glucosidase inhibitor
- Mechanism of Action: Prevents breakdown of complex sugars in the gut thus reducing blood sugar
- Common Uses: Treatment of type 2 diabetes
- Memorable Side Effects: Use is limited by significant GI side effects (diarrhea, pain and flatulence), increase in LFTs (rare)
- Clinical Pearls:
  - o Seldom used due to GI side effects and frequent dosing
  - o If patient has hypoglycemic episode, you MUST use simple sugars (i.e. glucose tablets) to treat it; complex sugars may not be broken down due to the drugs mechanism of action
  - o Hypoglycemia risk typically not an issue if used alone
- Monitoring: Blood sugar, HbA1c, LFTs as clinically indicated
- Drug and Diet Considerations:
  - o Must be administered with meals to be effective
  - o Targets post-prandial glucose lowering
  - o Implementation of a diabetic diet

Mineral Oil

- Class: Lubricant laxative
- Mechanism of Action: Softens and lubricates the intestine which helps constipation

194

- Common Uses: Treatment of constipation
- Memorable Side Effects: GI upset, diarrhea, oily stools, anal leakage and irritation
- Clinical Pearls:
  - Avoid use in geriatrics and those with swallowing disorders as it may increase the risk for aspiration pneumonitis
- Monitoring: Bowel movements, vitamin levels as clinically indicated (i.e. vitamin D)
- Drug and Diet Considerations:
  - Mineral oil may bind fat soluble vitamins A, D, E, K and contribute to deficiency when used long term
  - Avoid giving with food due to the risk of aspiration

Minocycline (Minocin)
- Class: Tetracycline, antibiotic
- Mechanism of Action: Inhibits bacterial protein synthesis
- Common Uses: Treatment of acne and skin infections
- Memorable Side Effects: GI side effects, photosensitivity (increased risk of sunburn), rash, dizziness
- Clinical Pearls:
  - Can cause birth defects (category D)
  - Can make patients more susceptible to sunburn
  - Possibility to cause tooth and skin discoloration when used long term use or for multiple courses
- Monitoring: LFTs, renal function, and CBC (only in cases with clinical concerns or in long term therapy)
- Drug and Diet Considerations:
  - Avoid taking calcium, iron, magnesium, zinc, and antacids at the same time as minocycline, absorption may be blocked, decreasing the amount of drug absorbed; separate by 2 hours
  - May give with meals if GI upset is a problem
  - Take with a full glass of water to avoid GI irritation

Minoxidil (Loniten)
- Class: Vasodilator, antihypertensive
- Mechanism of Action: Directly dilates arteries and arterioles (decreases BP)
- Common Uses: Treatment of hypertension and hair growth
- Memorable Side Effects: Low BP, EKG changes, hair growth, fluid retention and weight gain
- Clinical Pearls:
  - Boxed warning on the risk for pericardial effusion, angina exacerbation, and risk of cardiac tamponade
  - Fall/orthostatic blood pressure risk
  - May exacerbate heart failure
  - May be given to promote hair growth as a topical agent for alopecia
- Monitoring: Blood pressure, electrolytes, EKG, and fluid status
- Drug and Diet Considerations:
  - May be given without respect to food

Mirabegron (Myrbetriq)

- Class: Bladder beta agonist
- Mechanism of Action: Binds beta-3 receptors in the bladder which relaxes detrusor smooth muscle
- Common Uses: Treatment of overactive bladder
- Memorable Side Effects: Hypertension, tachycardia, dry mouth
- Clinical Pearls:
  - Does have selectivity for bladder beta receptors, but systemic side effects still possible (beta-1 agonist activity will increase blood pressure and pulse) especially at higher doses
- Monitoring: Blood pressure, pulse
- Drug and Diet Considerations:
  - May be administered with or without food, consistency is recommended

Mirtazapine (Remeron)

- Class: Antidepressant
- Mechanism of Action: Blocks alpha 2 which increases norepinephrine and serotonin; also antagonist at certain serotonin receptors and H1 receptors
- Common Uses: Treatment of depression, insomnia and anorexia
- Memorable Side Effects: Sedation, weight gain (can be good or bad), CNS effects, dry mouth, constipation
- Clinical Pearls:
  - Can be used to help with sleep as it tends to be more sedating at lower doses due to H1 blocking effects
  - Takes weeks to work for depression or anxiety, not beneficial on an as needed basis
  - Sedative properties may work in the short term (as needed)
- Monitoring: Weight, CBC (as clinically indicated), LFTs (as clinically indicated)
- Drug and Diet Considerations:
  - Weight gain can be a problem in younger patients, but can be a positive in frail, elderly

Misoprostol (Cytotec)

- Class: Prostaglandin
- Mechanism of Action: Inhibits gastric acid release by binding the prostaglandin receptor in parietal cells
- Common Uses: GI ulcer prevention and abortion
- Memorable Side Effects: Diarrhea, GI upset, cramping
- Clinical Pearls:
  - Boxed warning to avoid in females of child bearing age
  - PPIs generally preferred as they are more tolerable and do not have severe pregnancy risks like misoprostol
- Monitoring: Pregnancy testing
- Drug and Diet Considerations:
  - Give with food to minimize GI upset

Mitomycin (Mutamycin)

- Class: Oncology agent, antibiotic

- Mechanism of Action: Prevents DNA cross-linking which ultimately prevents proliferation and growth of cells
- Common Uses: Treatment of various GI cancers, pancreatic cancers and other metastatic cancers
- Memorable Side Effects: Nausea, vomiting, weight loss, myelosuppression, thrombocytopenia, hair loss, lung toxicity, heart failure
- Clinical Pearls:
  - Boxed warning for the risk of myelosuppression and hemolytic uremic syndrome
- Monitoring: CBC, renal function, pulmonary testing
- Drug and Diet Considerations:
  - Nausea and vomiting may increase the risk for weight loss and nutritional deficiencies
  - Monitor fluid status and replace if patient experiences vomiting/fluid loss

Moexipril (Univasc)

- Class: Antihypertensive, ACE inhibitor
- Mechanism of Action: Inhibits angiotensin converting enzyme which prevents the production of angiotensin 2 and leads to lower BP; Angiotensin 2 is a potent vasoconstrictor
- Common Uses: Treatment of hypertension, acute MI and heart failure
- Memorable Side Effects: Cough, kidney impairment, low blood pressure, hyperkalemia, angioedema
- Clinical Pearls:
  - ACE inhibitors are notoriously known for causing a dry chronic cough
  - Angiotensin Receptor Blockers (ARBs) are the cousins to the ACE inhibitors and are the first line substitute to a patient who has had a cough with an ACE inhibitor
  - ACE inhibitors can exacerbate kidney impairment as well as contribute to acute renal failure especially in patients who are already on other potential renal toxic medications (i.e. diuretics, NSAIDs etc.) even though in conditions like heart failure, diuretics and ACE inhibitors are often used together
  - ACE inhibitors can cause elevated potassium levels; if your patient has hyperkalemia, you must make sure the ACE inhibitor has been addressed
  - In some cases, patients of African descent may not respond to ACE inhibitors as well as other ethnicities
  - ACE inhibitors should not be used in combination with an ARB
  - ACE inhibitors (and ARBs) are frequently used in patients with hypertension and a history of diabetes, stroke, CAD, CKD, or CHF
  - Angioedema (swelling of the lips/airway) is classically caused by ACE inhibitors; it is an extremely rare, but very serious reaction requiring immediate discontinuation
- Monitoring: Renal function, potassium, blood pressure
- Drug and Diet Considerations:
  - Be cautious and monitor potassium closely in patients with high dietary intake of potassium as this could contribute to hyperkalemia in combination with this medication

197

- To maximize absorption, take an hour before eating

Mometasone (Asmanex)

- Class: Inhaled corticosteroid
- Mechanism of Action: Inhaled steroid that helps to reduce inflammation
- Common Uses: Treatment of asthma and COPD
- Memorable Side Effects: Pretty well tolerated, thrush, cough, rhinitis, systemic corticosteroid effects are possible, but not very likely, as absorption is low (see prednisone for adverse effects)
- Clinical Pearls:
    - Educate patients that it is not meant to provide emergency relief of symptoms
    - Rinse mouth after administration
- Monitoring: FEV1, peak-flow, growth in pediatric patients
- Drug and Diet Considerations:
    - Certain formulations main contain lactose which could cause a reaction in patients with milk protein allergy

Mometasone (Nasonex)

- Class: Nasal corticosteroid
- Mechanism of Action: Nasal steroid that helps reduce inflammation
- Common Uses: Relief of allergy symptoms
- Memorable Side Effects: Pretty well tolerated, nasal irritation, possible nose bleeds
- Clinical Pearls:
    - Gently shake the product for nasal inhalation and you may need to prime the nasal delivery device if it is the first time using it
    - Educate patients that it may not work right away, it may take a few hours or up to a day or two to start working (because of this, it may not be the best to use this as needed, but I've certainly seen it prescribed this way before)
    - It may only be necessary to use this medication seasonally based upon timing and duration of allergy symptoms
    - Be sure to educate patients to clean the tip of the nasal delivery device as it can get pretty nasty
- Monitoring: No lab work is necessary; minimal systemic absorption
- Drug and Diet Considerations:
    - No notable issues with diet

Mometasone and Formoterol (Dulera)

- Class: Inhaled corticosteroid and long acting beta-agonist
- Mechanism of Action: Provides anti-inflammatory effects through mometasone and formoterol stimulates beta-2 receptors leading to relaxation of smooth muscle and opening of airways
- Common Uses: Management of asthma and COPD
- Memorable Side Effects: Thrush, tachycardia, tremor, and anxiousness; rare effects include: reduced bone mineral density, HPA suppression hypokalemia, hyperglycemia
- Clinical Pearls:

- o Inhaled corticosteroids have a very low rate of systemic absorption, so issues such as reduced bone mineral density, hyperglycemia, and HPA suppression are unlikely to be clinically significant
- Monitoring: Frequency of use, FEV1, peak-flow, pulse, blood pressure, and potassium (usually only necessary in high dosages), glucose (rarely clinically significant
- Drug and Diet Considerations:
  - o Assess potassium intake and blood levels of potassium if the patient is using a beta agonist frequently or has a history of hypokalemia
  - o Be aware of caffeine intake in combination with a beta-agonist as it can have an additive effect on blood pressure and heart rate
  - o Monitor diabetes patients for elevations in blood sugar

Montelukast (Singulair)
- Class: Leukotriene receptor blocker
- Mechanism of Action: Blocks leukotriene receptors which can help reduce inflammation
- Common Uses: Treatment of asthma and allergic rhinitis
- Memorable Side Effects: Pretty well tolerated; psychiatric or unusual behavior changes are possible but rare
- Clinical Pearls:
  - o Usually dosed in the evening, however in patients with ONLY allergies, they may give it at the time of day that works the best
  - o Overall, usually well tolerated
  - o This medication is meant to control asthma, NOT provide acute relief with an exacerbation (albuterol is used for an asthma attack)
  - o Rare post-marketing case reports of neuropsychiatric problems (abnormal behavior, aggression, depression, etc.)
- Monitoring: No lab work is necessary; minimal systemic absorption
- Drug and Diet Considerations:
  - o No notable issues with diet

Morphine (MS Contin, Oramorph)
- Class: Opioid, analgesic
- Mechanism of Action: Binds opioid receptors inhibiting CNS pain pathways to provide pain relief
- Common Uses: Management of pain disorders, both chronic and acute
- Memorable Side Effects: Constipation, sedation, respiratory depression, CNS effects like confusion, delirium
- Clinical Pearls:
  - o Morphine is a scheduled 2 controlled substance; risk of addiction and dependence
  - o Very frequently used short term for pain and post-op procedures
  - o It is critical to educate/assess patients for constipation if they are taking frequent opioids like morphine
  - o Driving/working machinery is certainly risky when using opioids as they can cause significant sedation (usually patients get used to this side effect if they take the medication chronically)
  - o MS Contin is the brand name of the extended release morphine
  - o Naloxone is reversal agent for opioids

- o You should not see MS Contin used on an as needed basis as it is intended to have a slower/steady absorption over a longer period of time
- o Very high risk for significant error as different liquid concentrations are available – be careful!
- Monitoring: Bowel movements, pain management, risk for addiction
- Drug and Diet Considerations:
  - o Alcohol can exacerbate the CNS depressant effect from morphine
  - o Giving with food and water can reduce the risk of GI upset
  - o Encourage a constipation friendly diet including fiber, fluids and exercise as morphine can be very constipating

Moxifloxacin (Avelox)

- Class: Quinolone, antibiotic
- Mechanism of Action: Inhibits bacterial DNA synthesis
- Common Uses: Treatment of pneumonia and complicated skin infections
- Memorable Side Effects: GI side effects, QTc prolongation (rare)
- Clinical Pearls:
  - o Typically used only for pneumonia which is different from ciprofloxacin and levofloxacin
  - o Watch out for binding interactions that can decrease absorption, like co-administration with calcium or iron
  - o May increase QTc prolongation risk especially in patients already at risk (on antiarrhythmic medications or other meds that may prolong QTc interval)
  - o Spontaneous tendon rupture has been reported, but is extremely rare
- Monitoring: In the short term, lab monitoring is typically not necessary; in long term therapy, renal function, LFTs, CBC, and risk for hypoglycemia in diabetes may be assessed as clinically indicated
- Drug and Diet Considerations:
  - o Antacids, iron, calcium, zinc, magnesium, aluminum, and dairy products can interfere with the absorption of this drug; give 4 hours before or 8 hours after

Mycophenolate (Cellcept, MMF)

- Class: Immunosuppressant
- Mechanism of Action: Converted to mycophenolic acid, a prodrug, which inhibits inosine-5-monophosphate dehydrogenase, leading to a reduction in guanosine nucleotide availability in T and B lymphocytes which are important in a normally function immune system
- Common Uses: Organ rejection prevention
- Memorable Side Effects: GI upset, blood pressure changes, edema, insomnia, dizziness, risk for infections
- Clinical Pearls:
  - o Mycophenolate has different dosage forms that are not interchangeable for dosing
  - o Boxed warning that it should be used by an experienced clinician who specializes in areas where this medication might be used
  - o Additional boxed warnings for risk of serious infection and malignancy
  - o When you may want to reassess levels
    - ▪ Monitor adherence

- - - Changes in drug therapy and monitoring of drug interactions
    - Adjusting of dose
    - Signs of toxicity or rejection
- Monitoring: Drug levels, renal function, CBC, blood pressure, LFTs
- Drug and Diet Considerations:
  - Can be given with or without meals, consistency and monitoring of drug level is critical
  - Calcium carbonate supplements and other antacids may reduce drug concentrations

Nabumetone (Relafen)

- Class: NSAID, analgesic
- Mechanism of Action: Inhibits Cyclooxygenase-1 and 2 (COX-1 and COX-2); results in a reduction of prostaglandins which cause pain, fever and inflammation
- Common Uses: Reduction of pain, fever and inflammation
- Memorable Side Effects: GI ulcer, worsening kidney function, edema, hypertension, inhibits platelets (can exacerbate bleed risk)
- Clinical Pearls:
  - NSAIDs are one of the most common causes of GI bleeding; this risk increases in the elderly and those on medications that increase risk of bleeding (anticoagulants and antiplatelet medications)
  - Because of the side effects of GI upset/bleeding, NSAIDs should be taken with food
  - Due to effects on platelets, NSAIDs are typically held before/after surgery to reduce the risk of bleeding
  - NSAIDs can contribute to edema and exacerbate CHF (congestive heart failure); be on the lookout and have NSAIDs reassessed if you see a patient with a CHF exacerbation or a patient requiring increasing diuretics like furosemide
  - NSAIDs can cause worsening kidney function (creatinine should be monitored); this risk can be greatly increased in patients on ACE inhibitors or ARBs and/or diuretic type medications
  - Due to above reasons on kidney function, GI bleed risk, and CHF, NSAIDs are not the safest medication in the elderly; acetaminophen is generally preferred for generalized pain with a few exceptions
  - Although generally considered riskier in the elderly, a big advantage of NSAIDs over acetaminophen is that they can reduce inflammation
  - Pregnancy category C/D when >30 weeks gestation; NSAIDs are generally avoided in pregnancy and especially after 30 weeks gestation
- Monitoring: Renal function, hemoglobin, platelets (contained within CBC), blood pressure, signs of bruising or bleeding, weight (risk for edema)
- Drug and Diet Considerations:
  - Because of significant incidence of GI upset, it is recommended to give with food or milk
  - Dehydration coupled with nabumetone may increase the risk for acute renal failure
  - Excessive alcohol may increase GI bleed risk

- Vitamin E, Omega-3 fatty acids, gingko, garlic, ginseng, turmeric, and fish oil supplements have been purported to have antiplatelet type activity which in theory could increase the risk of bleed – clinical significance is questionable; the most common resolution is to discontinue the supplements if they are not necessary

Nadolol (Corgard)
- Class: Antihypertensive, non-selective beta-blocker
- Mechanism of Action: Blocks beta receptors leading to lower pulse/BP
- Common Uses: Treatment of hypertension, atrial fibrillation, migraines, tremor, variceal hemorrhage in patients with cirrhosis (prophylaxis)
- Memorable Side Effects: Low pulse, low BP, fatigue
- Clinical Pearls:
  - Trick to remembering beta receptors: you have 1 heart and 2 lungs (beta-1 is primarily on the heart and beta-2 primarily in the lungs) – non selective beta blockers can contribute to airway restriction (beta-2) as well as lower cardiac output (beta-1)
  - The selectivity of these drugs is really important. Nadolol is the classic example of a beta blocker that is not selective for beta-1 receptors. It also blocks beta-2 receptors which makes it more likely that it could potentially exacerbate respiratory conditions like asthma
  - Nadolol has a unique use of migraine prophylaxis as well as being used for portal hypertension in patients with cirrhosis, tremor, and possibly stress/anxiety type issues
  - Often in practice, providers will place a hold order on beta-blockers if the pulse is too low, this is done to reduce the risk of significant bradycardia
- Monitoring: Pulse, blood pressure, EKG as clinically indicated (i.e. acute atrial fibrillation)
- Drug and Diet Considerations:
  - Alcohol may have variable effects on drug concentrations
  - Can be given with or without food
  - May mask signs and symptoms of hypoglycemia

Nafcillin (Nafcil)
- Class: Antibiotic, penicillin
- Mechanism of Action: Inhibits bacterial cell wall formation
- Common Uses: Treatment of endocarditis, skin and soft tissue infections, meningitis and joint infections
- Memorable Side Effects: GI side effects most common, allergy, rash Clostridium difficile diarrhea
- Clinical Pearls:
  - Be sure to check allergies, don't use if allergic to penicillin, amoxicillin, etc.
  - Diarrhea and GI upset are going to be the major/common side effects with nafcillin, hopefully the patient can tolerate it and continue therapy
  - Monitor the response of the patient, hopefully they will begin feeling better by day 2 or 3 of treatment
  - Temperature would be an important symptom to monitor in patients who were significantly febrile

- o   Available as injection only
- Monitoring: Signs of infection improvement (i.e. fever and symptoms), rash, labwork is typically not necessary with short term use
- Drug and Diet Considerations:
  - o   GI upset and diarrhea is the most common adverse effect and could contribute to a short term reduction in caloric intake
  - o   Bland foods that reduce GI upset and diarrhea can be helpful
  - o   Maintain adequate hydration to avoid dehydration if diarrhea is a significant problem
  - o   Consult prescriber/pharmacist if adverse effects are severe for an alternative antibiotic

Naltrexone (Vivitrol, ReVia)

- Class: Opioid antagonist
- Mechanism of Action: Blocks mu receptors, not completely understood how, but it helps reduce reward sensation from drinking
- Common Uses: Opioid use disorder, alcohol used disorder, combined with bupropion as a weight loss medication
- Memorable Side Effects: Opioid withdrawal symptoms possible in patients currently taking opioids, insomnia, headache, GI upset, reduced appetite, elevated LFTs
- Clinical Pearls:
  - o   Be careful in patients who are also on opioids as this medication will precipitate opioid withdrawal
  - o   Injection site reactions like hematoma can happen with the injectable formulation
  - o   Use is not recommended with hepatic impairment
- Monitoring: LFTs
- Drug and Diet Considerations:
  - o   May be given with or without food
  - o   Dietary changes are possible with this medication; it may also be due to alcohol or opioid withdrawal as well

Naproxen (Naprosyn, Aleve)

- Class: NSAID, analgesic
- Mechanism of Action: Inhibits Cyclooxygenase-1 and 2 (COX-1 and COX-2); results in a reduction of prostaglandins which cause pain, fever and inflammation
- Common Uses: Reduction of pain, fever and inflammation
- Memorable Side Effects: GI ulcer, worsening kidney function, edema, hypertension, inhibits platelets (can exacerbate bleed risk)
- Clinical Pearls:
  - o   NSAIDs are one of the most common causes of GI bleeding; this risk increases in the elderly and those on medications that increase risk of bleeding (anticoagulants and antiplatelet medications)
  - o   Because of the side effects of GI upset/bleeding, NSAIDs should be taken with food
  - o   Due to effects on platelets, NSAIDs are typically held before/after surgery to reduce the risk of bleeding
  - o   NSAIDs can contribute to edema and exacerbate CHF (congestive heart failure); be on the lookout and have NSAIDs reassessed if you

see a patient with a CHF exacerbation or a patient requiring increasing diuretics like furosemide
  - o NSAIDs can cause worsening kidney function (creatinine should be monitored); this risk can be greatly increased in patients on ACE inhibitors or ARBs and/or diuretic type medications
  - o Due to above reasons on kidney function, GI bleed risk, and CHF, NSAIDs are not the safest medication in the elderly; acetaminophen is generally preferred for generalized pain with a few exceptions
  - o Although generally considered riskier in the elderly, a big advantage of NSAIDs over acetaminophen is that they can reduce inflammation
  - o Pregnancy category C/D when >30 weeks gestation; NSAIDs are generally avoided in pregnancy and especially after 30 weeks gestation
- Monitoring: Renal function, hemoglobin, platelets (contained within CBC), blood pressure, signs of bruising or bleeding, weight (risk for edema)
- Drug and Diet Considerations:
  - o Because of significant incidence of GI upset, it is recommended to give with food or milk
  - o Dehydration coupled with naproxen may increase the risk for acute renal failure
  - o Excessive alcohol may increase GI bleed risk
  - o Vitamin E, Omega-3 fatty acids, gingko, garlic, ginseng, turmeric, and fish oil supplements have been purported to have antiplatelet type activity which in theory could increase the risk of bleed – clinical significance is questionable; the most common resolution is to discontinue the supplements if they are not necessary

Naratriptan (Amerge)
- Class: Anti-migraine, triptan
- Mechanism of Action: Serotonin 5HT agonist, which causes vasoconstriction and reduction in inflammation associated with migraine
- Common Uses: Acute relief of migraine
- Memorable Side Effects: Dizziness, changes in CNS
- Clinical Pearls:
  - o Meant for acute relief of migraine, not prophylaxis
  - o Be sure to assess frequent use, and if using frequently, need to have control of migraines assessed and have controller medication added (valproic acid, propranolol, topiramate, etc.)
  - o Often used with NSAIDs, like naproxen, in migraine treatment
  - o Does have serotonin activity so it could potentially contribute o serotonin syndrome (higher risk in patients already on SSRIs, tramadol, etc.)
- Monitoring: Blood pressure, EKG when clinically indicated to assess risk for QTc prolongation
- Drug and Diet Considerations:
  - o Given as needed for migraine, so administration at any point is fine with regards to food

Nateglinide (Starlix)
- Class: Anti-diabetic agent, glinide

- Mechanism of Action: Stimulates pancreatic cells to release insulin by blocking ATP-dependent potassium channels, which depolarizes the cell membrane and increases calcium influx; calcium in the cell stimulates the release of insulin
- Common Uses: Treatment of diabetes
- Memorable Side Effects: Hypoglycemia, weight gain
- Clinical Pearls:
  - Via its mechanism of action, whenever you increase insulin, hypoglycemia is of highest concern
  - Be attentive to appetite changes or new diabetes medications and monitor for hypoglycemia
  - Elderly can be especially at risk for hypoglycemia
  - Frequent dosing can be difficult for treatment adherence
- Monitoring: HbA1c, blood glucose, risk for hypoglycemia
- Drug and Diet Considerations:
  - Be very cautious for the risk of hypoglycemia if there is a significant reduction in dietary intake (i.e. acute illness, nausea/vomiting)
  - Patient without caloric intake will likely have to hold this medication (i.e. before surgery, missed meals)
  - Possible increase in concentration from grapefruit juice
  - Needs to be administered up to 30 minutes before meals which can be difficult to manage if the patient has a variable meal schedule
  - Post-prandial glucose reduction

Nebivolol (Bystolic)

- Class: Antihypertensive, beta-blocker
- Mechanism of Action: Blocks beta receptors leading to lower pulse/BP
- Common Uses: Treatment of hypertension and atrial fibrillation
- Memorable Side Effects: Low pulse, low BP, fatigue
- Clinical Pearls:
  - Trick to remembering beta receptors: you have 1 heart and 2 lungs (beta-1 is primarily on the heart and beta-2 primarily in the lungs). If beta-1 is stimulated, heart rate increases; if beta-1 is blocked, heart rate decreases
  - Usually only dosed once daily which is a nice advantage over some other beta-blockers
  - Often in practice, providers will place a hold order on beta-blockers if the pulse is too low; this is done to reduce the risk of significant bradycardia
  - Clinically, it may depend upon the situation, but in an ambulatory setting, you may see the order set to hold the beta blocker when pulse is less than 55 or 60
- Monitoring: Blood pressure, pulse, EKG as clinically indicated
- Drug and Diet Considerations:
  - No notable diet concerns

Nefazodone (Serzone)

- Class: Antidepressant
- Mechanism of Action: Inhibits reuptake of serotonin and norepinephrine, but differs from SNRIs in that it has blocking activity on alpha 1 receptors

205

- Common Uses: Treatment of depression and insomnia
- Memorable Side Effects: Sedation, dizziness, orthostasis, dry mouth, GI upset, elevated LFTs
- Clinical Pearls:
  - Boxed warning on hepatotoxicity limits its use
  - Must educate patients on its sedative properties and risk of driving
  - Keep an eye out for postural hypotension (dizziness upon rising) especially in our elderly patients and those already on blood pressure lowering medications – if you remember from the mechanism of action above, it does have alpha blocking activity
- Monitoring: LFTs as clinically indicated, blood pressure
- Drug and Diet Considerations:
  - Give with a meal or small snack to reduce the risk for orthostasis, but this may also reduce drug absorption; recommend consistency and monitor for benefit and adverse effects
  - Alcohol can increase the CNS depressant effect

Niacin (Vitamin B3, Niaspan, Slo-Niacin)
- Class: Antilipemic
- Mechanism of Action: Converted to nicotinamide which can affect lipid metabolism
- Common Uses: Treatment of hyperlipidemia
- Memorable Side Effects: Flushing, GI, increase uric acid
- Clinical Pearls:
  - Flushing from niacin can be treated with aspirin
  - Slow release formulation may help minimize flushing
  - Can possibly exacerbate gout due to the increase of uric acid
  - Rare possibility of liver issues
  - Usual RDA for most adults is 14-16 mg/day
- Monitoring: Lipids, blood sugar (diabetes), uric acid (gout), LFTs
- Drug and Diet Considerations:
  - Give medication with food
  - Alcohol, spicy food and drinks can worsen flushing reaction
  - Possibly can increase blood sugars, but usually not clinically significant; if a patient had persistent high blood sugars, might be a good idea to avoid niacin
  - A cholesterol friendly diet should be implemented in combination with this medication

Nicotine Replacement Products
- Class: Nicotine replacement
- Mechanism of Action: Replacement of nicotine to reduce withdrawal symptoms and ease cravings
- Common Uses: Smoking cessation
- Memorable Side Effects: Headache, irritation at site of administration (i.e. skin, mouth), stimulant effects such as tachycardia, insomnia, elevated blood pressure; patches have a higher likelihood of causing abnormal dreams, GI upset
- Clinical Pearls:
  - Patches (Nicoderm CQ)

- - Takes up to an hour or so to get to adequate concentrations; not meant for acute cravings like the other nicotine replacement agents
    - Can be worn while sleeping, but may be at risk of insomnia, vivid dreams; start by removing at bedtime and apply a new patch in the morning
  - Smoking is generally discouraged while using nicotine replacement products so the patient doesn't double up on nicotine intake; if patients still feel the need to continue smoking, nicotine replacement product dose may not be high enough
  - Gum (Nicorette)
  - Inhaler (Nicotrol Inhaler)
  - Lozenge (Nicorette)
  - Nasal Spray (Nicotrol)
  - Vaping is not considered a nicotine replacement product for medical treatment, there is limited long term evidence about safety; unclear if same long term risks as smoking or not at this time
- Monitoring: Pulse and blood pressure (if excessive dose is suspected)
- Drug and Diet Considerations:
  - Foods and drinks that are acidic may reduce absorption of nicotine
  - Weight gain is often a complaint of patients who have tried to quit smoking in the past, this may occur as a patient reduces their nicotine intake and smoking amounts

Nifedipine (Procardia)

- Class: Antihypertensive, dihydropyridine calcium channel blocker
- Mechanism of Action: Blocks calcium ions from entering voltage smooth muscle, resulting in relaxation (vasodilation)
- Common Uses: Treatment of hypertension
- Memorable Side Effects: Low blood pressure, edema, constipation
- Clinical Pearls:
  - Very important distinction: you will not see nifedipine used in atrial fibrillation, because its activity is primarily on the vessels; this differs from non-dihydropyridine calcium channel blockers like verapamil and diltiazem that act on the heart AND blood vessels; this also means that pulse monitoring will not be necessary with nifedipine
  - The higher you push the dose on these medications, the more likely you will see the side effect of edema
  - Keep an eye out for new requirement of diuretic prescriptions to treat the edema caused by the calcium channel blockers
  - Educate our patients to get up slowly to minimize risk of orthostatic hypotension
  - Nifedipine has an extended release formulation available
- Monitoring: Blood pressure, weight (in association with edema risk)
- Drug and Diet Considerations:
  - May give with food if GI upset occurs
  - St. John's wort may reduce effectiveness
  - Standard calcium supplementation typically will not impact the effectiveness of nifedipine; excessive doses of calcium may have a higher likelihood of blunting the effects of nifedipine
  - Alcohol may increase drug concentrations

207

- o Avoid grapefruit and its juice as they can raise concentrations

Nitrofurantoin (Macrobid)
- Class: Antibiotic
- Mechanism of Action: Inhibits bacterial protein synthesis, metabolism, DNA, RNA, and cell wall synthesis
- Common Uses: Treatment of urinary tract infection
- Memorable Side Effects: GI, CNS (more likely in elderly), neuropathy(rare), pulmonary distress (rare)
- Clinical Pearls:
  - o Use is contraindicated in kidney disease, reassess use as the drug can accumulate and have reduced effects in the urinary tract
  - o May cause urine to be a brown/orange color, be sure to educate patients
  - o Rare adverse effect of respiratory issues
  - o Generally not first line in the elderly for UTIs
  - o Category B, potential option in pregnancy
- Monitoring: Lung function, CBC, LFTs, renal function as clinically indicated and more appropriate with long term use
- Drug and Diet Considerations:
  - o Taking with food can improve absorption and lower GI side effects risk
  - o Rarely may be associated with higher phosphate levels

Nitroglycerin (Nitrostat)
- Class: Antihypertensive, antianginal, nitrate
- Mechanism of Action: Metabolized into nitric oxide which leads to smooth muscle relaxation (vasodilation)
- Common Uses: Treatment of angina (chest pain)
- Memorable Side Effects: Low BP, headache
- Clinical Pearls:
  - o Sublingual used most commonly for acute relief of angina
  - o Make sure patients are well educated on emergency care when chest pain doesn't resolve with use
  - o Recommended to only use 3 tablets every 5 minutes, max of 3 tabs
  - o Also long acting products available, dosed daily (isosorbide mononitrate) or multiple times daily (isosorbide dinitrate)
  - o Patch formulation available as well for those that have trouble swallowing or tolerating the oral formulation
- Monitoring: Blood pressure, pulse
- Drug and Diet Considerations:
  - o Alcohol could exacerbate low blood pressure risk

Nitroglycerin Patch (Nitro-Dur)
- Class: Antihypertensive, antianginal, nitrate
- Mechanism of Action: Direct acting vasodilation by nitric oxide which causes smooth muscle relaxation and reduction in blood pressure
- Common Uses: Treatment of angina (chest pain)
- Memorable Side Effects: Low BP, headache, dizziness
- Clinical Pearls:

- o Tolerance can develop without a break in drug therapy during the day
- o An 8-12 hour off period is recommended to reduce the risk of tolerance
- o The patch is typically placed for 12 hours and then removed for 12 hours every day
- o Avoid combination with PDE-5 inhibitors, like sildenafil, for erectile dysfunction
- Monitoring: Blood pressure, pulse
- Drug and Diet Considerations:
  - o Alcohol could exacerbate low blood pressure risk

Nitroprusside (Nitropress)

- Class: Antihypertensive, vasodilator
- Mechanism of Action: Direct vasodilation on vessel smooth muscle
- Common Uses: Treatment of hypertensive crisis and heart failure
- Memorable Side Effects: Low blood pressure, changes in heart rate, dizziness, metabolic acidosis
- Clinical Pearls:
  - o Too much drug may lead to a drop in blood pressure
  - o Injection type reaction can happen resulting in pain, redness, rash and warmth
  - o Cyanide toxicity is a black box warning if used at too high of a dose or for too long
- Monitoring: Blood pressure, blood pH, cyanide levels as clinically indicated
- Drug and Diet Considerations:
  - o No notable concerns

Nizatidine (Axid)

- Class: H2 blocker
- Mechanism of Action: Blocks histamine 2 receptors which results in reduced gastric acid secretion and a higher pH in the stomach
- Common Uses: Treatment of GERD, heartburn and GI bleed
- Memorable Side Effects: Well tolerated overall, drowsiness, dry mouth
- Clinical Pearls:
  - o H2 blockers are cleared by the kidney, so they can accumulate/require dose adjustments in CKD
  - o Generally less effective at suppressing stomach acid than PPIs
  - o Available over the counter, inexpensive
  - o CNS effects are more common in elderly, higher doses, and in patients with kidney disease
  - o Generally used before PPIs if something more than Tums (calcium carbonate) is needed in pregnancy
- Monitoring: No routine lab work is typically necessary; LFTs, hemoglobin when clinically indicated
- Drug and Diet Considerations:
  - o Reduced stomach acid (high pH) may impair the absorption of iron supplements
  - o Associations with B12 deficiency in chronic users

Norepinephrine (Levophed)

- Class: Alpha and beta agonist
- Mechanism of Action: Stimulates alpha and beta receptors
- Common Uses: Treatment of shock (severe hypotension)
- Memorable Side Effects: Hypertension, arrhythmias, anxiety
- Clinical Pearls:
    - Clamps down on vessels causing an increase in BP
    - Chest pain possible due to reduced blood flow through the heart
    - Boxed warning for extravasation
- Monitoring: Blood pressure, pulse, cardiac output and PCWP as clinically indicated
- Drug and Diet Considerations:
    - No notable concerns

Nortriptyline (Pamelor)

- Class: TCA, antidepressant
- Mechanism of Action: Inhibits reuptake of serotonin and possibly norepinephrine
- Common Uses: Treatment of depression, neuropathy, pain syndromes, anxiety and PTSD
- Memorable Side Effects: Confusion, fall risk in elderly
- Clinical Pearls:
    - Highly anticholinergic (can't spit, see, pee, or sh*t and increases confusion/fall risk) which can be especially problematic in geriatric patients – avoid if possible
    - In addition, cognitive impairment is not good in the elderly due to possibility of preexisting dementia
    - TCAs may have some benefit in neuropathy, generally much cheaper than SNRIs which can be beneficial in neuropathy
    - Not a good first line choice for sleep or depression; other agents exist that are much safer
    - Considered a more tolerable choice than amitriptyline in the elderly
    - Look out for TCAs causing the prescribing cascade; addition of artificial tears for dry eyes, constipation medications, BPH medications like tamsulosin, dementia medications, or artificial saliva would be a red flag
- Monitoring: EKG, and possibly electrolytes, in at risk patients (especially in overdose), behavioral changes, weight, sodium (in patients with signs of hyponatremia),
- Drug and Diet Considerations:
    - Weight gain is possible and may be problematic
    - Slows the motility of the GI tract which could increase the risk for constipation, maintain adequate fluids and non-constipating diet
    - If GI upset occurs, no issues in giving the drug with food
    - Dry mouth may increase thirst and alter taste/pleasure of food
    - Poor intake may place the patient at higher risk for complications from electrolyte abnormalities (i.e. hyponatremia, hypokalemia, or hypomagnesemia)

Octreotide (Sandostatin)

- Class: Somatostatin analog

210

- Mechanism of Action: Somatostatin has multiple physiologic affects including reducing growth hormone and inhibiting gastrin, insulin, glucagon, and other chemomediator secretions
- Common Uses: Treatment of variceal bleeding, acromegaly and chemotherapy induced diarrhea
- Memorable Side Effects: GI upset, CNS changes like fatigue, headache, and dizziness, hypertension, bradycardia, hyperglycemia, alterations in thyroid function
- Clinical Pearls:
  - Laboratory monitoring may depend upon indication and length of use
- Monitoring: Thyroid function, B12, blood sugar, zinc, EKG, renal function/fluid status
- Drug and Diet Considerations:
  - B12 and zinc deficiency is possible
  - Monitor diabetes patients as blood sugar fluctuations may result from use
  - Give injection between meals to avoid alteration in fat absorption
  - If using for diarrhea, be aware of fluid and electrolyte status

Ofloxacin (Floxin)
- Class: Quinolone, antibiotic
- Mechanism of Action: Inhibits bacterial DNA synthesis
- Common Uses: Treatment of pneumonia, UTIs and complicated skin infections
- Memorable Side Effects: GI side effects, QTc prolongation (rare)
- Clinical Pearls:
  - Commonly used for both UTIs and Pneumonia
  - Watch out for binding interactions that can decrease absorption like co-administration with calcium or iron
  - May increase QTc prolongation risk especially in patients already at risk (on antiarrhythmic medications or other meds that may prolong QTc interval)
  - Spontaneous tendon rupture has been reported, but is extremely rare
  - May exacerbate myasthenia gravis
- Monitoring: In the short term, lab monitoring is typically not necessary; in long term therapy, renal function, CBC, and risk for hypoglycemia in diabetes may be assessed as clinically indicated
- Drug and Diet Considerations:
  - Antacids, iron, calcium, zinc, magnesium, aluminum, and dairy products can interfere with the absorption of this drug; administer oral ofloxacin 2 hours before or up to 6 hours after any of the above listed products

Olanzapine (Zyprexa)
- Class: Antipsychotic
- Mechanism of Action: Blocks dopamine receptors
- Common Uses: Treatment of schizophrenia, bipolar disorder and off-label for dementia-related behaviors like aggression, hallucinations and delusions
- Memorable Side Effects: Sedation, fall risk, orthostatic BP changes, EPS, metabolic syndrome

- Clinical Pearls:
  - Usually higher doses are required for younger patients with schizophrenia and/or bipolar disorder while lower doses can and should be used in the elderly
  - Remember with antipsychotic medications that they block dopamine and can exacerbate conditions where there is a shortage of dopamine like Parkinson's disorder (remember that we use dopamine to treat Parkinson's – i.e. carbidopa/levodopa or pramipexole)
  - Sedation, orthostatic hypotension, movement disorder side effects can all increase the risk of falls, especially in our elderly patients
  - NMS (neuroleptic malignant syndrome) is a very rare but very serious complication with antipsychotic medications; a few symptoms of NMS include: fever, hyperreflexia, confusion, delirium and tremor
  - Antipsychotics increase risk of metabolic syndrome (diabetes, elevated lipids, weight gain, etc.); it is important to periodically monitor for this, especially in younger patients with schizophrenia and/or bipolar disorder who may be likely to require long term use of higher doses; Olanzapine is one of the worst antipsychotics as far as this side effect goes
  - Anticholinergic effects are possible as well with antipsychotics, dry eyes, dry mouth, exacerbation of urinary retention (i.e. BPH), constipation (SLUD – can't salivate, lacrimate, urinate or defecate)
  - Antipsychotics can contribute to QTc prolongation, which can be especially problematic in patients who are already at risk (i.e. on antiarrhythmic medications)
- Monitoring: Weight, BMI, lipids, HbA1c, blood sugars, EKG as clinically appropriate, electrolytes (potassium and magnesium are important if the patient is at risk for QTc prolongation)
- Drug and Diet Considerations:
  - Increased appetite and risk for metabolic syndrome, olanzapine is one of the higher risk agents)
  - Increased blood sugars can result in our diabetes patients, monitor blood sugars closely with acute changes in the drug
  - Alcohol may exacerbate the CNS depressant effect
  - Can be administered with or without meals

Olmesartan (Benicar)
- Class: Antihypertensive, ARB
- Mechanism of Action: Block the angiotensin 2 receptor, which prevents vasoconstriction, aldosterone release, etc.
- Common Uses: Treatment of hypertension and heart failure
- Memorable Side Effects: Hyperkalemia, exacerbate/worsen kidney function, low blood pressure
- Clinical Pearls:
  - When you think of ARBs and ACE inhibitors, you can lump the side effects together as they are overall the same; one major exception to this rule is the side effect of cough
  - Kidney function changes and monitoring of potassium is critical when doses are changed or an ARB is initiated
  - Orthostatic BP and/or dizziness upon rising is important to ask patients about

- o Risk of kidney injury increases when patients are also on an NSAID and/or diuretic(s)
- o You shouldn't ever see an ACE inhibitor like lisinopril and an ARB used together
- o Hyperkalemia risk will increase when using potassium supplements, ACE inhibitors, or potassium sparing diuretics with ARBs
- Monitoring: Renal function, potassium, blood pressure
- Drug and Diet Considerations:
  - o Be cautious and monitor potassium closely in patients with high dietary intake of potassium as this could contribute to hyperkalemia in combination with this medication
  - o Administer with or without food

Olsalazine (Dipentum)

- Class: 5-Aminosalicylic acid derivative (5-ASA compound)
- Mechanism of Action: Not well understood, but likely reduces inflammation by impacting leukotrienes
- Common Uses: Treatment of inflammatory bowel disease (ulcerative colitis)
- Memorable Side Effects: GI upset, belching, diarrhea
- Clinical Pearls:
  - o Slow onset to beneficial effects
  - o Diarrhea adverse effect may exacerbate symptoms in some patients
- Monitoring: LFTs, CBC, and renal function as clinically indicated
- Drug and Diet Considerations:
  - o Give with food

Omeprazole (Prilosec)

- Class: PPI
- Mechanism of Action: Inhibits proton pumps in the stomach leading to a less acidic environment
- Common Uses: Treatment of GERD, ulcer and Barrett's esophagus
- Memorable Side Effects: Usually well tolerated; long term use possibly linked to increased fracture risk, reduced B12 levels, C. diff risk, and low magnesium
- Clinical Pearls:
  - o PPIs are the most potent acid blocker on the market
  - o PPIs are generally dosed 30 minutes or so before meals; this is a recommendation, not an absolute (example, if a patient likes to get up and eat right away upon rising, the medication will still likely be beneficial, but may not have a maximal effect)
  - o For some patients PPIs may not work very quickly, i.e. it might take a few days for maximal effect; this is a disadvantage compared to other acid blocking agents
  - o For the above reason, as needed (PRN) PPIs can possibly be effective, but are generally not recommended
  - o Use short term if possible due to increased risk of osteoporosis, low magnesium, and B12 deficiency if used long term
  - o Barrett's esophagus, high risk GI medications (i.e. NSAIDs, prednisone), or chronic GI bleed are a few examples where a patient may require indefinite therapy
  - o If GI bleed is problematic, monitoring hemoglobin and/or hemoccult might be appropriate to assess possible blood loss

- Monitoring: Magnesium and B12 in chronic use
- Drug and Diet Considerations:
    - When it is used chronically, it is a possible cause or contributing factor to B12 and magnesium deficiency
    - PPIs are typically best given at least 30-60 minutes before a meal
    - St. John's wort should be avoided as it can significantly reduce concentrations of the drug
    - Reduced stomach acid (high pH) may impair the absorption of iron supplements

Ondansetron (Zofran)

- Class: Antiemetic, serotonin receptor antagonist
- Mechanism of Action: Blocks serotonin at 5HT3 receptors; acts centrally in the chemoreceptor trigger zone
- Common Uses: Management of nausea/vomiting
- Memorable Side Effects: Constipation, sedation, QTc prolongation is a risk, but rare unless the patient is on other drugs that can contribute to QTc prolongation or has risk factors
- Clinical Pearls:
    - Frequently used in patients undergoing chemotherapy (nausea/vomiting common with chemo)
    - Can be used as needed or scheduled
    - Can cause QTc prolongation especially when used in combination with other QTc prolonging agents
    - Has serotonin activity, be on the lookout for other serotonergic medications (like SSRIs, tramadol, etc.)
- Monitoring: Assessment for QTc prolongation and associated risk factors such as EKG, magnesium, and potassium
- Drug and Diet Considerations:
    - If vomiting is problematic, there is an injectable and orally disintegrating tablet formulation
    - With or without food is acceptable

Oral Contraceptives (Combination Estrogen and Progestin)

- Class: Birth control, contraceptive, estrogen and progestin
- Mechanism of Action: Inhibits ovulation by changing gonadotropin, FSH, and luteinizing hormone release
- Common Uses: Contraception and acne treatment
- Memorable Side Effects: Abnormal vaginal bleeding, DVT, hypertension, nausea, weight changes
- Clinical Pearls:
    - Age and smoking can put patients at higher risk of clot
    - Can exacerbate hypertension
    - Adherence to regimen is very important to prevent unplanned pregnancy
    - Enzyme inducers like carbamazepine and phenytoin can possibly reduce effectiveness of birth control
    - List of brand names: Beyaz, Gianvi, Loryna, Nikki, Yaz, Amethyst, Aviane, Balcoltra, Falmina, Larissia, Lessina, Lutera, Orsythia, Sronyx, Blisovi, Junel, Larin, Loestrin, Melodetta, Microgestin, Minastrin, Taytulla, Apri, Cyred, Emoquette, Enxkyce, Juleber, Reclipsen, Ocella, Safyral, Tydemy, Yasmin, Zarah, Chateal,

Kurvelo, Levora, Marlissa, Portia, Cryselle, Elinest, Low-Ogestrel, Kelnor, Pirmella, Zovia, Balziva, Briellyn, Philith, Vyfemia, Brevicon, Necon, Nortrel, Wera, Alyacen, Cyclafen, Dasetta, Nortrel, Ortho-Novum, Mili, Femynor, MonoNessa, Ortho-Cyclen, Previfem, Sprintec, VyLibra, Cleo, Cyestra, Diane, Azurette, Beekyree, Kariva, Mircette, Pimtrea, Viorele, Volnea, Ortho-Tri-Cyclen Lo, Tri-Lo-Sprintec, Tri-Sprintec, TriNessa, Cyclafen, Dasetta

- Monitoring: Blood clot risk, blood pressure, weight
- Drug and Diet Considerations:
  - St. John's wort should be avoided as it can significantly reduce concentrations of the drug
  - Vitamin C and grapefruit juice may increase estrogen concentrations, monitor for estrogen side effects
  - Weight changes can present as an adverse effect, note the timing of initiation in correlation to any weight changes
  - Consistency in administration time is the most important factor, with or without food is acceptable
  - Give with food and/or consider a dose reduction in the estrogen if nausea is a problem
  - Possible alterations in potassium with some products

Oral Contraceptives (Progestin-only)

- Class: Birth control, contraceptive, progestin
- Mechanism of Action: Progestins block ovulation, helps reduce sperm delivery by thickening cervical mucous, alters FSH and LH, and alters ovum movement through the fallopian tubes
- Common Uses: Contraception, abnormal bleeding and endometriosis treatment
- Memorable Side Effects: Acne, mood swings, headache, GI upset, breast tenderness
- Clinical Pearls:
  - VERY sensitive to missed doses, even if a dose is missed by > 3 hours, use backup protection
  - Enzyme inducers like carbamazepine and phenytoin can possibly reduce effectiveness of birth control
  - List of brand names: Jolivette, Camila, Errin, Heather, Incassia, Jencycla, Nora-BE, Ortho Micronor, Sharobel, Slynd
- Monitoring: Blood clot risk, blood pressure, weight
- Drug and Diet Considerations:
  - St. John's wort should be avoided as it can significantly reduce concentrations of the drug
  - Weight changes can present as an adverse effect, note the timing of initiation in correlation to any weight changes
  - Consistency in administration time is the most important factor, with or without food is acceptable
  - Possible alterations in blood glucose and lipids

Orlistat (Xenical, Alli)

- Class: Weight loss agent, lipase inhibitor
- Mechanism of Action: Blocks the action of gut lipases which reduces absorption of ingested fats and ultimately lowers caloric intake

- Common Uses: Weight loss therapy
- Memorable Side Effects: Diarrhea, oily stools, fat soluble vitamin deficiencies
- Clinical Pearls:
  - Oily stool leakage can be very troublesome and embarrassing for patients
- Monitoring: Weight, dietary intake, LFTs and renal function as clinically indicated, blood sugar in diabetes patients
- Drug and Diet Considerations:
  - Given during a meal or within at least 1 hour of a meal
  - Separate timing of vitamin supplements, particularly fat soluble vitamins, by at least 2 hours
  - GI adverse effects will likely be worse with higher fat intake
  - If vitamin K intake is altered, it may affect INR in patients taking warfarin

Oseltamivir (Tamiflu)
- Class: Antiviral, neuraminidase inhibitor
- Mechanism of Action: Inhibits viral neuraminidase, preventing influenza virus from replicating
- Common Uses: Influenza treatment and prophylaxis
- Memorable Side Effects: GI, psych events like delirium (rare, more likely in pediatrics)
- Clinical Pearls:
  - Drug of choice for influenza prophylaxis or treatment
  - Prophylaxis is especially common for patients at high risk who've been exposed to infected individuals (immunosuppressed, elderly, or living in a healthcare institution)
  - Dose adjustments in patients with poor kidney function
  - GI upset is going to be the most common side effect
  - With or without food is ok, but likely better tolerated with food
  - Encourage influenza vaccination
- Monitoring: No routine lab work is necessary
- Drug and Diet Considerations:
  - Take with food if the patient encounters GI upset

Oxaliplatin (Eloxatin)
- Class: Oncology agent, platinum compound
- Mechanism of Action: Blocks DNA synthesis and alters the natural double helix of DNA to inhibit cell growth
- Common Uses: Treatment of numerous types of cancers
- Memorable Side Effects: Neuropathy, vomiting, nausea, fatigue, anemia, increased LFTs, myelosuppression, thrombocytopenia
- Clinical Pearls:
  - Boxed warning for anaphylaxis
  - Cold stimuli may exacerbate neuropathic pain
- Monitoring: CBC, renal function, electrolytes, LFTs
- Drug and Diet Considerations:
  - Weight loss and poor nutrition may result on account of nausea and vomiting adverse effects
  - Assess for the need of fluid and electrolyte replacement in patients with vomiting and/or diarrhea

Oxazepam (Serax)
- Class: Antianxiety, benzodiazepine
- Mechanism of Action: Enhances activity of GABA, an inhibitory neurotransmitter that causes sedation
- Common Uses: Treatment of anxiety, seizure and insomnia
- Memorable Side Effects: Sedation, confusion, fall risk, dizziness
- Clinical Pearls:
  - The best way I remember benzodiazepines is that they are very close to "alcohol in a pill"
  - Sedation, slurred speech, and trouble walking (ataxia) are all common with benzos/alcohol; they are also commonly used in alcohol withdrawal
  - Be cautious with patients on high doses of benzodiazepines to make sure they aren't abruptly stopped
  - Educate patients on driving/operating machinery; remember that benzodiazepines are often used for sleep as well as anxiety
  - Unlike SSRIs for anxiety, a great advantage of benzos is that they work quickly and can be used as needed
  - Fall risk in the elderly is a big downside to using these medications
  - Benzos are a controlled substance, they can cause addiction and dependence
  - Can be used for acute behavioral issues as well as seizure
  - Flumazenil is antidote in overdose
- Monitoring: Routine lab monitoring typically isn't necessary unless clinically indicated; respiratory rate in overdose risk
  - Alcohol intake can have additive side effects of sedation, confusion, slurred speech, and other CNS depressant effects
  - May give with or without food

Oxcarbazepine (Trileptal)
- Class: Antiepileptic
- Mechanism of Action: Multiple mechanisms suspected, but ultimately believed to alter sodium ion flow across cell membranes and decrease synaptic firing
- Common Uses: Treatment of seizures and trigeminal neuralgia
- Memorable Side Effects: Sedation, dizziness, rash, hyponatremia (SIADH), N/V
- Clinical Pearls:
  - Similar adverse effect profile to carbamazepine
  - Typically less risk for drug interactions compared to carbamazepine
- Monitoring: Sodium, CBC, LFTs
- Drug and Diet Considerations:
  - Alcohol may exacerbate CNS depressant effects
  - Vitamin D deficiency may be possible from oxcarbazepine

Oxybutynin (Ditropan, Oxytrol)
- Class: Bladder anticholinergic
- Mechanism of Action: Blocks muscarinic receptors in the bladder which increases urine volume in the bladder and potentially decreases frequency/urge
- Common Uses: Treatment of overactive bladder and bladder spasms

- Memorable Side Effects: Anticholinergic effects possible (dry mouth, dry eyes, urinary retention, constipation)
- Clinical Pearls:
    - Anticholinergic effects
    - Many patients don't benefit from this class of medication, be sure to assess if the medication is working for incontinence/frequency
    - Keep an eye out for patients on diuretics and if urinary frequency is the major issue, make sure that they are minimized if possible (not always possible to reduce diuretics with CHF history, etc.)
    - Urinary frequency can be especially problematic in patients who have an active social life as well as night when trying to sleep
    - Oxybutynin (Oxytrol) has a patch formulation available that is applied twice weekly
- Monitoring: Renal function as clinically indicated
- Drug and Diet Considerations:
    - Slows the motility of the GI tract which could increase the risk for constipation, maintain adequate fluids and non-constipating diet
    - If GI upset occurs, there are no issues in giving the drug with food
    - Dry mouth may increase thirst and alter taste/pleasure of food
    - Patch may be administered without regard to oral intake

Oxycodone (Oxycontin, Oxyfast, Oxy IR)

- Class: Opioid, analgesic
- Mechanism of Action: Binds opioid receptors inhibiting CNS pain pathways which provides pain relief
- Common Uses: Management of pain disorders, both chronic and acute
- Memorable Side Effects: Constipation, sedation, respiratory depression, CNS effects like confusion, delirium, etc.
- Clinical Pearls:
    - Oxycodone is a scheduled 2 controlled substance; risk of addiction and dependence
    - Very frequently used short term for pain and post-op procedures
    - It is critical to educate/assess patients for constipation if they are taking frequent opioids like oxycodone
    - Naloxone is reversal agent for opioids
    - Driving/working machinery is certainly risky when using opioids as they can cause significant sedation; usually patients get used to this side effect if they take the medication chronically
    - Hydrocodone and oxycodone are NOT interchangeable
    - Oxycontin is the brand name of the extended release oxycodone
    - You should not see Oxycontin (oxycodone ER) used on an as needed basis as it is intended to have a slower/steady absorption over a longer period of time
    - Oxycodone ER is usually dosed twice daily, occasionally patients may need three times daily if pain is increasing as drug is wearing off
    - If the immediate release formulation is used in an institutional setting, be sure that parameters, usually based upon pain scale, are set up; for example, if pain is 1-5 give 1 tablet and if pain is 6-10 give 2 tablets
- Monitoring: Bowel movements, pain management, risk for addiction
- Drug and Diet Considerations:
    - Alcohol can exacerbate the CNS depressant effect from oxycodone

- o Giving with food and water can reduce the risk of GI upset
- o Encourage a constipation friendly diet including fiber, fluids and exercise as hydrocodone can be very constipating

Oxycodone/APAP (Percocet)

- Class: Opioid, analgesic – also see acetaminophen
- Mechanism of Action: Binds opioid receptors, inhibiting CNS pain pathways which provides pain relief; acetaminophen is believed to inhibit prostaglandin production, but does not have anti-inflammatory effects like NSAIDs
- Common Uses: Management of pain disorders, both chronic and acute
- Memorable Side Effects: Constipation, sedation, respiratory depression, CNS effects like confusion, delirium, etc., liver toxicity (acetaminophen in large doses >4 grams/day)
- Clinical Pearls:
  - o Risk of acetaminophen overdose is certainly a possibility; need to educate patients that this contains acetaminophen as well as many common OTCs, cough and cold medicines, etc.
  - o Oxycodone is a scheduled 2 controlled substance; risk of addiction and dependence
  - o Very frequently used short term for pain and post-op procedures
  - o It is critical to educate/assess patients for constipation if they are taking frequent opioids like oxycodone
  - o Naloxone is reversal agent for opioids
  - o Driving/working machinery is certainly risky when using opioids as they can cause significant sedation; usually patients get used to this side effect if they take the medication chronically
  - o Hydrocodone and oxycodone are NOT interchangeable
  - o Oxycodone/acetaminophen is meant for acute pain relief and certainly can and is used on an as needed basis
  - o In an institutional setting, be sure that parameters, usually based upon pain scale, are set up; for example, if pain is 1-5 give 1 tablet and if pain is 6-10 give 2 tablets
- Monitoring: See individual agents
- Drug and Diet Considerations:
  - o See individual agents

Paclitaxel (Taxol)

- Class: Oncology agent, taxane
- Mechanism of Action: Stimulates tubulin dimers, interferes with G2 mitotic phase and prevents cell replication by inhibiting microtubule disassembly
- Common Uses: Treatment of numerous types of cancers
- Memorable Side Effects: Neuropathy, CNS toxicity, muscle soreness, stomatitis, nausea, vomiting, diarrhea, myelosuppression, hair loss, anaphylaxis, CV changes such as bradycardia or blood pressure changes with infusion
- Clinical Pearls:
  - o Peripheral neuropathy is one of the most common complications with this medication
  - o Pre-medicate with steroids, diphenhydramine, and an H2 blocker, like. famotidine, to reduce the risk of infusion reactions

- Monitoring: CBC, LFTs, renal function, electrolytes, EKG (as clinically indicated), vital signs with infusion
- Drug and Diet Considerations:
    - Weight loss and poor nutrition may result on account of nausea, vomiting, and stomatitis adverse effects
    - May cause taste alterations that can impact dietary preferences

Paliperidone (Invega, Trinza, Sustenna)

- Class: Antipsychotic
- Mechanism of Action: Blocks dopamine receptors
- Common Uses: Treatment of schizophrenia, bipolar disorder and off-label for dementia related behaviors like aggression, hallucinations and delusions
- Memorable Side Effects: Sedation, fall risk, orthostatic BP changes, EPS, metabolic syndrome
- Clinical Pearls:
    - Usually higher doses are required for younger patients with schizophrenia and/or bipolar disorder while lower doses can and should be used in the elderly
    - Remember with antipsychotic medications that they block dopamine and can exacerbate conditions where there is a shortage of dopamine like Parkinson's disorder (remember that we use dopamine to treat Parkinson's – i.e. carbidopa/levodopa or pramipexole)
    - Sedation, orthostatic hypotension, movement disorder side effects can all increase the risk of falls especially in our elderly patients
    - NMS (neuroleptic malignant syndrome) is a very rare, but serious complication with antipsychotic medications; a few symptoms of NMS include: fever, hyperreflexia, confusion, delirium and tremor
    - Antipsychotics increase risk of metabolic syndrome (diabetes, elevated lipids, weight gain, etc.); it is important to periodically monitor for this, especially in younger patients with schizophrenia and/or bipolar disorder who may be likely to require long term use of higher doses
    - Anticholinergic effects are possible as well with antipsychotics - dry eyes, dry mouth, exacerbation of urinary retention (i.e. BPH), constipation
    - Antipsychotics can contribute to QTC prolongation, which can be especially problematic in patients who are already at risk (i.e. on antiarrhythmic medications)
- Monitoring: Weight, lipids, HbA1c, blood sugars
- Drug and Diet Considerations:
    - Increased appetite and risk for metabolic syndrome
    - Increased blood sugars can happen in our diabetes patients, monitor blood sugars closely with acute changes in the drug
    - Can be administered with or without meals
    - Alcohol may exacerbate CNS depressant effect

Palonosetron (Aloxi)

- Class: Antiemetic, serotonin receptor antagonist
- Mechanism of Action: Blocks serotonin at 5HT3 receptors, acts centrally in the chemoreceptor trigger zone
- Common Uses: Prevention and treatment of nausea/vomiting

- Memorable Side Effects: Constipation, sedation, QTc prolongation is a risk (pretty rare unless the patient is on other drugs that can contribute to QTc prolongation or has risk factors)
- Clinical Pearls:
  - Frequently used in patients undergoing chemotherapy (nausea/vomiting common with chemo)
  - Can be used as needed or scheduled
  - Can cause QTc prolongation especially when used in combination with other QTc prolonging agents
  - Has serotonin activity, be on the lookout for other serotonergic medications (like SSRIs, tramadol, etc.)
  - IV only
- Monitoring: Assessment for QTc prolongation and associated risk factors such as EKG, magnesium, and potassium
- Drug and Diet Considerations:
  - Typically timed before chemotherapy

Pancrelipase (Creon, Pancreaze, Zenpep)

- Class: Enzyme replacement
- Mechanism of Action: Product that is derived from porcine pancreatic glands that contains enzymes such as lipase, amylase, and protease
- Common Uses: Treatment of pancreatic insufficiency
- Memorable Side Effects: GI upset, irritation to the oral cavity is more likely if chewing or opening capsule
- Clinical Pearls:
  - Porcine products may have purines within them which could exacerbate gout
  - Renal impairment could exacerbate uric acid level concerns in combination with the product
  - Hypersensitivity reaction is rare, but possible
  - Different products are not considered interchangeable
- Monitoring: Stool consistency, growth in pediatric patients, nutritional status
- Drug and Diet Considerations:
  - Alkaline food may exacerbate inactivation of the product (food should have a pH of <4.5 if the capsules are opened and sprinkled
  - Take with acidic food, such as applesauce with a pH < 4.5, if the capsules are opened and sprinkled
  - Take with food and encourage a healthy, balanced diet

Pantoprazole (Protonix)

- Class: PPI
- Mechanism of Action: Inhibits proton pumps in the stomach leading to a less acidic environment
- Common Uses: Treatment of GERD, ulcer and Barrett's esophagus
- Memorable Side Effects: Usually well tolerated; in long term use there is a possibility to increase fracture risk, decrease B12 levels, C. diff risk and low magnesium
- Clinical Pearls:
  - PPIs are the most potent acid blocker on the market

221

- o PPIs are generally dosed 30 minutes or so before meals; this is a recommendation, not an absolute (example if a patient likes to get up and eat right away upon rising, the medication will still likely be beneficial, but may not have a maximal effect)
  - o For some patients, PPIs may not work very quickly, and take a few days for maximal effect
  - o For the above reason, as needed PPIs can possibly be effective, but are generally not used
  - o Use short term if possible due to increased risk of osteoporosis, low magnesium, and B12 deficiency if used long term
  - o Barrett's esophagus, high risk GI medications (i.e. NSAIDs, prednisone), or chronic GI bleed may require indefinite therapy
  - o If GI bleed is problematic, monitoring hemoglobin and/or hemoccult might be appropriate to assess possible blood loss
- Monitoring: Magnesium and B12 levels with chronic use
- Drug and Diet Considerations:
  - o When it is used chronically, it is a possible cause or contributing factor to B12 and magnesium deficiency
  - o PPIs are typically best given at least 30-60 minutes before a meal
  - o Reduced stomach acid, high pH, may impair the absorption of iron supplements
  - o With the use of IV pantoprazole, zinc supplementation may be necessary

Pantothenic Acid (Vitamin B5)

- Class: Vitamin
- Mechanism of Action: Important cofactor for coenzyme A activity; coenzyme A is necessary for production and oxidation of fatty acids and actions in the Krebs Cycle
- Common Uses: Supplement in deficient diet
- Memorable Side Effects: Well tolerated, change in urine color
- Clinical Pearls:
  - o Target RDA is in the range of 5-7 mg/day for most adults, with pregnancy and breast-feeding typically requiring the upper end
  - o Water soluble
- Monitoring: Routine lab work is not necessary
- Drug and Diet Considerations:
  - o May be given with or without food
  - o No major drug interactions

Paroxetine (Paxil)

- Class: Antidepressant, SSRI
- Mechanism of Action: Selective serotonin reuptake inhibitor; increases serotonin in the brain
- Common Uses: Treatment of depression, anxiety and PTSD
- Memorable Side Effects: GI side effects (N/V/D), can cause sedation or activation depending upon the patient, changes in mental status, hyponatremia (rare)
- Clinical Pearls:
  - o SSRIs are generally considered first line medication to treat depression, they are generally well tolerated, and less risky than

other antidepressants in the situation of attempted suicide by overdose
- o Constipation may be a little more common with paroxetine versus other SSRIs
- o There is a boxed warning for an increased risk of suicidal thinking when first starting these medications
- o Paroxetine tends to be a little more sedating than other SSRIs like sertraline or fluoxetine
- o Although not terribly common, hyponatremia (low sodium) is a possible unique side effect with SSRIs and much more likely in patients already prone to hyponatremia; classic example would be patients who are taking diuretics, which can also lower sodium
- o Remember that these drugs are not an immediate fix! SSRI take weeks to months before a patient will start improving; however side effects will be apparent from the start of the medication, making it difficult to coach our patients to continue the medication in the first few weeks after starting it
- o SSRI are used in pregnancy, but the risk versus the benefits need to be assessed on a case by case basis (paroxetine is actually category D)
- o SSRIs can decrease libido
- Monitoring: EKG, potassium and magnesium if the patient is at risk for QTc prolongation; sodium level if the patient is displaying symptoms of hyponatremia
- Drug and Diet Considerations:
  - o Weight gain or weight loss can happen with SSRIs; monitor for changes over time once started, increased, reduced, or discontinued
  - o Constipation may be more common with paroxetine when compared to other SSRIs; consider constipation friendly diet in patients who have this complaint
  - o If the patient has a prolonged QT interval, out of range electrolytes like potassium and magnesium could increase the risk for Torsades de Pointes
  - o Low sodium can be a rare adverse effect
  - o Can be taken with or without food
  - o Alcohol can have additive, unpredictable effects when used with SSRIs
  - o St John's wort may have additive effects on any drug that has serotonergic type activity

Pegfilgrastim (Neulasta)
- Class: Colony Stimulating Factor (CSF)
- Mechanism of Action: Stimulates production of WBC's
- Common Uses: Prevention of neutropenia in chemo patients
- Memorable Side Effects: Ostealgia (bone pain), anaphylaxis (rare)
- Clinical Pearls:
  - o Helps patients continue on chemotherapy by increasing white blood cells and decreasing risk of infection
  - o Bone pain is common and you will often see use of NSAIDs and/or acetaminophen used to help treat this (remember that it stimulates bone marrow which resides inside the bones – source of pain)

223

- o CBC (white blood cell count is incredibly important to monitor for positive response)
- o Fever and signs of infection are also incredibly important to watch for in a patient on pegfilgrastim
- o Long acting version of filgrastim and it is dosed less frequently
- Monitoring: CBC, including white blood cell count and absolute neutrophil count
- Drug and Diet Considerations:
  - o No notable diet considerations

Penicillin (Pen-VK)

- Class: Antibiotic, penicillin
- Mechanism of Action: Inhibits bacterial cell wall formation
- Common Uses: Treatment of ear infection, sinusitis, strep throat and skin infections
- Memorable Side Effects: GI side effects most common, allergy, rash
- Clinical Pearls:
  - o Many patients have an allergy to penicillin; should not be used in patients with a severe allergy; if it is an intolerance like stomach upset, it may be prudent to try a "penicillin" type antibiotic again depending upon the patient's situation
  - o Diarrhea and GI upset are going to be the major/common side effects with penicillin; with mild GI upset and/or diarrhea, hopefully the patient can tolerate it and continue therapy
  - o Giving penicillin with food or a snack may help reduce GI upset
  - o We are going to want to monitor the response of the patient, hopefully they will begin improving by day 2 or 3 of treatment
  - o Temperature would be an important thing to monitor in patients who were significantly febrile
  - o Usually dosed multiple times throughout the day
- Monitoring: Signs of infection improvement (i.e. fever and symptoms), rash, lab work is typically not necessary with short term use
- Drug and Diet Considerations:
  - o Ideally take 1-2 hours before eating to maximize absorption
  - o Maintain adequate hydration to avoid dehydration if diarrhea is a significant problem
  - o Consult prescriber/pharmacist if adverse effects are severe for an alternative antibiotic

Pentamidine (Pentam, Nebupent)

- Class: Antiprotozoal agent, antifungal
- Mechanism of Action: Disrupts RNA/DNA, and protein synthesis by blocking phosphorylation
- Common Uses: Alternative to Bactrim in the treatment of PCP pneumonia
- Memorable Side Effects: Injection reaction, worsening renal function, QTc prolongation, hypotension, hypoglycemia, and blood dyscrasias (IV agent), respiratory problems such as coughing, dyspnea (nebulized formulation
- Clinical Pearls:
  - o Nebulized formulation is indicated in PCP prevention
  - o IV agent is indicated for treatment
- Monitoring: Renal function, electrolytes, CBC, EKG, blood pressure, LFTs, EKG as clinically indicated

- Drug and Diet Considerations:
  - Monitor blood sugars more closely upon initiation in those taking insulin products or sulfonylureas; or in those who have a history of hypoglycemia
  - Reduced appetite may occur with nebulized formulation

Pentoxifylline (Trental)
- Class: Blood viscosity reducer
- Mechanism of Action: Inhibits erythrocyte phosphodiesterase which increases erythrocyte cAMP action; ultimately leading to lower blood viscosity
- Common Uses: Treatment of intermittent claudication
- Memorable Side Effects: GI upset, mild increased bleed risk
- Clinical Pearls:
  - Can increase risk of bleed especially in those on antiplatelet medications/anticoagulants
- Monitoring: Blood pressure, CBC, renal function
- Drug and Diet Considerations:
  - Give with food
  - Vitamin E, Omega-3 fatty acids, gingko, garlic, ginseng, turmeric, and fish oil supplements have been purported to have antiplatelet type activity which in theory could increase the risk of bleed – clinical significance is questionable; the most common resolution is to discontinue the supplements if they are not necessary
  - Alcohol may have an additive antiplatelet type effect and increase the risk of GI bleed

Phenazopyridine (Pyridium)
- Class: Urinary analgesic
- Mechanism of Action: Local anesthetic action in the bladder/urinary tract
- Common Uses: Relief of painful urination (dysuria)
- Memorable Side Effects: GI, low risk of dizziness
- Clinical Pearls:
  - Very important to identify patients who are taking this and have them assessed for infection or something else going on
  - Often will see it used short term for painful urination associated with UTI
  - Not intended for long term use
  - Ensure adequate fluid intake if patient is having UTIs and/or using this medication frequently
  - Can accumulate in kidney disease
- Monitoring: No routine lab work is necessary
- Drug and Diet Considerations:
  - Give medication with food or right after eating to minimize GI upset risk

Phenelzine (Nardil)
- Class: Mono-amine oxidase inhibitor, antidepressant
- Mechanism of Action: Inhibits the action of monoamine oxidase which increases the CNS neurotransmitters serotonin, norepinephrine, and epinephrine

- Common Uses: Treatment of depression
- Memorable Side Effects: Nausea, dizziness, blood pressure fluctuations, hypertension (with tyramine), hypotension, tachycardia, unusual behavior, SIADH (hyponatremia), serotonin syndrome
- Clinical Pearls:
    o Boxed warning for an increased risk of suicidal thoughts in pediatric patients and young adults
    o Avoid use of other serotonergic agents (i.e. SSRIs)
    o Not a first line agent in depression due to adverse effect profile, diet interactions, and drug interactions
- Monitoring: Blood pressure, pulse, electrolytes (as clinically indicated), renal function, LFTs
- Drug and Diet Considerations:
    o Patch may be administered consistently without regard to meals while oral disintegrating table is typically given before breakfast
    o Alcohol should be avoided as it may increase risk for toxicity
    o MAOI/Tyramine interaction (less likely than traditional MAOIs)
        ▪ Foods high in tyramine: fermented, cured, aged foods such as cheese, smoked meats/fish, beer
        ▪ Reaction: tachycardia, N/V, headache
        ▪ Risk of reaction increases as the dose of the medication increases
    o Food and beverages with large amounts of caffeine, tyrosine, phenylalanine, dopamine, or tryptophan may also cause elevated blood pressure

Phenobarbital (Luminal)
- Class: Antiepileptic, barbiturate
- Mechanism of Action: Stimulates the GABA receptor, activation has CNS inhibitory effects, which decreases neuron activity
- Common Uses: Management of seizures
- Memorable Side Effects: CNS changes, sedation, ataxia, vitamin D deficiency, slurred speech, respiratory depression
- Clinical Pearls:
    o Enzyme inducer, reduces concentrations of many other drugs
    o Seldom used
    o 10-40 mcg/mL is the therapeutic range for adults
    o Increases fall risk, particularly in the elderly
    o Controlled substance, risk for dependence and abuse
- Monitoring: Drug levels, CBC and CMP as clinically indicated
- Drug and Diet Considerations:
    o Folic acid, vitamin B12, riboflavin, pyridoxine, and vitamin D may all be reduced; assess for signs of deficiency and if supplementation may be necessary
    o Alcohol may exacerbate the CNS depressant effect
    o Low protein diet may lengthen the duration of action

Phentermine (Fastin)
- Class: CNS stimulant, weight loss agent
- Mechanism of Action: Stimulates release of norepinephrine in the central nervous system which can cause a reduction in appetite
- Common Uses: Obesity treatment

- Memorable Side Effects: Anxiety, insomnia, poor appetite, weight loss, twitching, shakiness, hypertension, tachycardia, emotional lability
- Clinical Pearls:
    o Remembering that this medication ramps you up (stimulant) will help you remember its side effects (anxiety, insomnia, weight loss, poor appetite, increased BP, increased pulse, etc.)
    o Be cautious in adult patients who may already be at cardiovascular risk (hypertension, congenital defects, etc.)
    o It is a controlled substance with abuse potential
    o Avoid dosing late in the evening to avoid insomnia
- Monitoring: Blood pressure, pulse, weight, cardiac monitoring (in patients with preexisting cardiac condition or at risk for cardiac complications)
- Drug and Diet Considerations:
    o Typically give before meals to allow medication to be absorbed prior to beginning to eat (dosage form dependent)
    o Use caution with other foods/supplements that may have additive effects to heart rate, blood pressure, and insomnia (i.e. caffeine)
    o Diet, exercise, and behavioral weight loss counseling is important in combination with the use of this medication
    o Vitamin C may reduce concentrations of the drug by reducing absorption

Phenylephrine (Sudafed PE)
- Class: Decongestant
- Mechanism of Action: Stimulates alpha receptors causing vasoconstriction (beneficial in the respiratory tract)
- Common Uses: Nasal congestion
- Memorable Side Effects: hypertension, urinary retention (watch out for BPH patients), dry mouth, anxiety, insomnia
- Clinical Pearls:
    o Watch out for elderly/patients at high risk for cardiovascular problems as it can raise BP
    o Can exacerbate BPH
    o Can cause/worsen insomnia and/or anxiety
- Monitoring: Blood pressure and pulse as clinically indicated
- Drug and Diet Considerations:
    o Giving with or without food is acceptable
    o Dry mouth and stimulant-type effect can impact appetite
    o Small quantities of sodium may be contained within some products

Phenytoin, Fosphenytoin (Dilantin, Cerebyx)
- Class: Antiepileptic
- Mechanism of Action: Has effects on sodium movement across cells which stabilizes the cell membrane
- Common Uses: Management of seizures
- Memorable Side Effects: GI, CNS changes, ataxia, vitamin D deficiency, liver function changes (rare)
- Clinical Pearls:
    o If new meds are started, recommend looking up potential interactions; a few examples are, fluconazole, amiodarone, alcohol, cimetidine and fluvoxamine

227

- o Very sensitive to changes in dose, a small increase may lead to toxicity)
- o Usual phenytoin level is from 10-20, this can be misleading if patient has low albumin
- o Toxicity resembles alcohol toxicity in many ways including, ataxia (difficulty walking), confusion, GI side effects like nausea, slurred speech, etc.
- o Boxed warning for cardiovascular risks with fast infusion rates
- o Fosphenytoin can be more rapidly administered, has lower tissue injection complications, has a lower cardiac toxicity risk, and does not need an IV filter compared to phenytoin
- Monitoring: Drug levels, CBC, LFTs, EKG, and albumin (as clinically indicated),
- Drug and Diet Considerations:
  - o Folic acid, calcium, vitamin B12, riboflavin, pyridoxine, and vitamin D may all be reduced; assess for signs of deficiency and if supplementation may be necessary
  - o Alcohol may exacerbate the CNS depressant effect
  - o IV formulation contains phosphate

Pilocarpine (Salagen)
- Class: Cholinergic agonist
- Mechanism of Action: Agonist activity at cholinergic receptors which results in secretion from salivary glands
- Common Uses: Treatment of dry mouth
- Memorable Side Effects: Nausea, diarrhea, sweating, flushing, dizziness, weakness, urinary frequency
- Clinical Pearls:
  - o May exacerbate breathing issues (opposes anticholinergic effects)
  - o Use cautiously in patients with a history of renal stones
- Monitoring: No routine lab work
- Drug and Diet Considerations:
  - o If sweating occurs, may exacerbate risk for dehydration, assess fluid status
  - o May be given with or without food; avoid large fat intake with administration as it can reduce absorption

Pioglitazone (Actos)
- Class: Antidiabetic, TZD
- Mechanism of Action: Improves tissue sensitivity to insulin leading to a reduction in blood glucose
- Common Uses: Treatment of type 2 diabetes
- Memorable Side Effects: Edema, CHF exacerbation, possible elevations in LFT's (rare)
- Clinical Pearls:
  - o Usually dosed once daily which is nice
  - o If you see a patient on furosemide or other medications that might indicate CHF, pioglitazone is not a good choice as it can worsen edema and exacerbate CHF
  - o Monitor for low blood sugar risk, especially in patients on sulfonylureas (i.e. glipizide) or insulins

- o HbA1c will be important to monitor in any patient on diabetes medications
- o Goal is to keep HbA1c low and minimize risk of hypoglycemia; this will help decrease risk of diabetes complications like neuropathy, retinopathy, worsening kidney function, etc.
- Monitoring: Blood sugars, HbA1c, lipids, weight, BNP (as clinically indicated in patients at risk for heart failure), and LFTs as clinically indicated
- Drug and Diet Considerations:
  - o Can be taken with or without food
  - o Weight gain and edema can occur with this medication
  - o Appropriate diet education for patient with diabetes

Piperacillin/tazobactam (Zosyn)
- Class: Antibiotic, penicillin
- Mechanism of Action: Inhibits bacterial cell wall formation
- Common Uses: Treatment of moderate to severe nosocomial pneumonia
- Memorable Side Effects: GI side effects most common, allergy, rash
- Clinical Pearls:
  - o Commonly used for complex bacterial infections, provides broad bacterial coverage
  - o Has coverage against Pseudomonas, a common drug resistant hospital infection
  - o Similar to penicillin in chemical structure so have to look out for penicillin, amoxicillin, etc. allergy
- Monitoring: Renal function, CBC, electrolytes, signs of infection
- Drug and Diet Considerations:
  - o IV formulation only which may contain some amount of sodium – could negatively impact patients sensitive to sodium load (i.e. heart failure)

Piroxicam (Feldene)
- Class: NSAID, analgesic
- Mechanism of Action: Inhibits Cyclooxygenase-1 and 2 (COX-1 and COX-2); results in a reduction of prostaglandins which cause pain, fever and inflammation
- Common Uses: Reduction of pain, fever and inflammation
- Memorable Side Effects: GI ulcer, worsening kidney function, edema, hypertension, inhibits platelets (can exacerbate bleed risk)
- Clinical Pearls:
  - o NSAIDs are one of the most common causes of GI bleeding; this risk increases in the elderly and those on medications that increase risk of bleeding (anticoagulants and antiplatelet medications)
  - o Due to effects on platelets, NSAIDs are typically held before/after surgery to reduce the risk of bleeding
  - o NSAIDs can contribute to edema and exacerbate CHF (congestive heart failure); be on the lookout and have NSAIDs reassessed if you see a patient with a CHF exacerbation or a patient requiring increasing diuretics like furosemide
  - o NSAIDs can cause worsening kidney function (creatinine should be monitored); this risk can be greatly increased in patients on ACE inhibitors or ARBs and/or diuretic type medications

- - - Due to above reasons on kidney function, GI bleed risk, and CHF, NSAIDs are not the safest medication in the elderly, acetaminophen is generally preferred for generalized pain with a few exceptions
    - Although generally considered riskier in the elderly, a big advantage of NSAIDs over acetaminophen is that they can reduce inflammation
    - Pregnancy category C/D when >30 weeks gestation; NSAIDs are generally avoided in pregnancy and especially after 30 weeks gestation
- Monitoring: Renal function, hemoglobin, platelets (contained within CBC), blood pressure, signs of bruising or bleeding, weight (risk for edema)
- Drug and Diet Considerations:
    - Because of significant incidence of GI upset, it is recommended to give with food or milk
    - Dehydration may exacerbate the risk for acute renal failure
    - Excessive alcohol may increase GI bleed risk
    - Vitamin E, Omega-3 fatty acids, gingko, garlic, ginseng, turmeric, and fish oil supplements have been purported to have antiplatelet type activity which in theory could increase the risk of bleed – clinical significance is questionable; the most common resolution is to discontinue the supplements if they are not necessary

Pitavastatin (Livalo)

- Class. Statin, antilipemic
- Mechanism of Action: HMG Co-A reductase inhibitor,
- Common Uses: Reduction of cholesterol, particularly LDL
- Memorable Side Effects: Muscle aches, rhabdomyolysis (rare but serious)
- Clinical Pearls:
    - Statins, like pitavastatin, are one of the mainstays of therapy to reduce cholesterol, and more particularly LDL (bad cholesterol)
    - The most notable side effect with statins that you will likely hear patients complain about is myopathy (muscle aches/pain)
    - Usually muscle aches are all over which can help you differentiate from other pain conditions or pain/soreness from an injury or overuse
    - Contraindicated in pregnancy
    - Patients who do not tolerate pitavastatin may try another statin as long as adverse effects aren't too severe (i.e. rhabdomyolysis); if you notice that the patient had an allergy or intolerance, you need to clarify with the provider
    - CPK will be the primary lab to test for rhabdomyolysis, the breakdown of muscle; this elevation in CPK may eventually lead to kidney failure
    - Patients usually will present with myopathy when the medication is first started or increased, but be on the lookout for new medications that can interact with statins like CYP3A4 inhibitor drug interactions with medications like fluconazole or erythromycin (this will cause pitavastatin concentrations in the body to go up potentially leading to toxicity)
    - Gemfibrozil is a cholesterol medication that also interacts with pitavastatin; this drug interaction should be addressed with the primary provider

- o For many statins it is "recommended" to give them at night but pitavastatin may be given without respect to the time of day
- Monitoring: Lipids, LFTs, CPK if experiencing muscle pain (myopathy)
- Drug and Diet Considerations:
  - o Liver toxicity risk from excessive alcohol may be increased if used in combination with statins
  - o Low, often not clinically significant, risk of elevating blood sugars in patients with diabetes
  - o Can be taken with or without food
  - o Encourage a lipid lowering diet for any patient taking a cholesterol medication

Polycarbophil (FiberCon, Fiber-Caps, Fiber-Lax)
- Class: Bulk-forming laxative, fiber supplement
- Mechanism of Action: Fiber and fiber-like substances absorb water and keep it in the gut lumen which helps stimulate peristalsis and bowel movements; in patients with alternative diarrhea and constipation, it may help bulk up the stool and improve regularity
- Common Uses: Treatment of constipation or diarrhea
- Memorable Side Effects: Cramping, diarrhea, obstruction risk
- Clinical Pearls:
  - o May cause swallowing issues in at risk patients (elderly, Parkinson's, swallowing disorders, etc.) particularly if not taken with adequate fluids
- Monitoring: No routine monitoring is necessary
- Drug and Diet Considerations:
  - o Encourage adequate fluid intake, at least 8 ounces of water, at time of administration and continued intake throughout the day
  - o Calcium may be an ingredient in some formulations

Polyethylene Glycol (Miralax)
- Class: Osmotic laxative
- Mechanism of Action: It works by pulling water into the gut which promotes motility and bowel movements
- Common Uses: Treatment of constipation and bowel prep prior to colonoscopy
- Memorable Side Effects: Diarrhea, abdominal cramps, GI upset
- Clinical Pearls:
  - o Rare electrolyte imbalances have occurred with higher doses and long term use being the most likely culprits
  - o Renal impairment may increase the risk of rare electrolyte complications
  - o Over-the-counter availability
  - o Ensure that patients are educated to consult a healthcare professional if use is needed for longer than 1-2 weeks
- Monitoring: Bowel movements, electrolytes and renal function as clinically indicated
- Drug and Diet Considerations:
  - o Mix in 4-8 ounces of water, juice, coffee, tea, or soda until dissolved

- o Assess fluid and electrolyte status in patients who may be taking this medication on a chronic basis; electrolyte depletion is more likely in patients with low dietary intake

Potassium chloride (Klor-Con)
- Class: Potassium supplement
- Mechanism of Action: Replaces body's potassium
- Common Uses: Potassium replacement
- Memorable Side Effects: GI side effects (oral), hyperkalemia
- Clinical Pearls:
  - o High risk electrolyte as hyperkalemia can cause cardiac arrhythmias
  - o Often, supplementation is necessary in patients who are on diuretics, like furosemide; however, potassium sparing diuretics, like triamterene or spironolactone, can increase potassium levels and do not require potassium supplementation
  - o With the wax-matrix formulation of potassium, patients may find the outer coating remaining in their stool; the drug is designed to leak out of the matrix shell, educate patients that this is normal and that they are getting their potassium
  - o Normal potassium level: 3.5-5.1 mEq/L but may vary slightly depending upon lab
  - o By adding ACE inhibitors, ARBs, or potassium sparing diuretics to the patients' medication regimen, we may be able to get away with less potassium supplement
  - o Sodium polystyrene sulfonate is used to treat hyperkalemia
- Monitoring: Electrolytes, renal function, EKG as clinically indicated (i.e. high or low potassium levels)
- Drug and Diet Considerations:
  - o GI upset is the most common adverse effect and it is best to take with food and a glass of water

Potassium Citrate (Urocit-K)
- Class: Bicarbonate agent, alkalizing agent
- Mechanism of Action: Causes crystallization of salts such as calcium oxalate, calcium phosphate, and uric acid which can raise urinary pH
- Common Uses: Treatment of kidney stones
- Memorable Side Effects: GI side effects (oral), hyperkalemia,
- Clinical Pearls:
  - o Be cautious in patients with poor kidney function, potassium may be more likely to accumulate and cause hyperkalemia
- Monitoring: Electrolytes, renal function, EKG as clinically indicated (i.e. high or low potassium levels), CBC, urine pH
- Drug and Diet Considerations:
  - o Take with food
  - o Hydration/fluid intake is important to emphasize
  - o Most patients will benefit from limiting salt

Potassium Phosphate (K-Phos)
- Class: Potassium supplement, electrolyte replacement
- Mechanism of Action: IV agent provides replenishment of potassium and phosphate; oral agent can help acidify the urine
- Common Uses: Urine acidification and electrolyte replacement

- Memorable Side Effects: GI side effects (oral), hyperkalemia, symptoms associated with electrolyte abnormalities such as arrhythmias, weakness, and CNS changes
- Clinical Pearls:
    ○ Oral agent is most often used for urine acidification which can help prevent kidney stones
    ○ May be used to help manage UTIs in patients taking methenamine
- Monitoring: Electrolytes, renal function, EKG as clinically indicated (i.e. high or low potassium levels)
- Drug and Diet Considerations:
    ○ Calcium supplements and antacids may decrease oral phosphate absorption
    ○ Foods containing oxalate can increase the risk of calcium oxalate stones which is what we try to mitigate with urine acidification; foods such as nuts, berries, tomatoes, beans, chocolate, beer, coffee, dark green vegetables have high oxalate content and should be avoided

Potassium phosphate and sodium phosphate (Neutral Phos, K-Phos Neutral, Phos-NaK)
- Class: Phosphorus supplement
- Mechanism of Action: Supplements dietary phosphorus
- Common Uses: Phosphate replacement and urinary acidification
- Memorable Side Effects: Diarrhea, hyperkalemia, hypernatremia, hyperphosphatemia
- Clinical Pearls:
    ○ Renal impairment will increase risk for electrolyte abnormalities
- Monitoring: Renal function, electrolytes
- Drug and Diet Considerations:
    ○ Typically given with meals, may help reduce diarrhea risk, and at bedtime
    ○ Give with 8 ounces of water
    ○ Iron, magnesium, and calcium supplements may reduce absorption

Pramipexole (Mirapex)
- Class: Anti-Parkinson's agent, dopamine agonist
- Mechanism of Action: Stimulates dopamine receptors
- Common Uses: Treatment of restless leg syndrome and Parkinson's disorder
- Memorable Side Effects: Orthostasis, edema, OCD symptoms (very rare)
- Clinical Pearls:
    ○ Indicated for Parkinson's but more commonly drug of choice for RLS
    ○ Often patients struggle with RLS at night, this is likely the indication if you see it dosed once daily at nighttime
    ○ Keep an eye out for orthostasis, especially in the elderly and patients who are already taking numerous antihypertensives
    ○ Make sure the diagnosis is clear and the medication actually helps the patient
- Monitoring: Blood pressure, pulse (as clinically indicated)
- Drug and Diet Considerations:

- o Can be given with food if nausea occurs
- o Rare associations with impulsive behaviors which could include but is not limited to binge eating
- o Any drug with dopamine type activity can cause nausea and vomiting
- o Alcohol may have additive CNS adverse effects like sedation

Prasugrel (Effient)
- Class: Antiplatelet, thienopyridine
- Mechanism of Action: Blocks ADP receptors, leading to inhibition of platelets
- Common Uses: MI and stroke prevention
- Memorable Side Effects: Bleeding (GI, nose bleeds, etc.)
- Clinical Pearls:
  - o Prasugrel is often used after a heart attack (MI) with aspirin to prevent further heart attacks; how long a patient should remain on this medication can vary depending upon cardiac and/or stroke risk – length of therapy should be addressed by the primary provider and in many situations may be 12 months, but can be longer or indefinite depending upon risk factors
  - o Boxed warning to avoid in patients over the age of 75 due to an increased risk for intracranial bleeding
  - o Prasugrel may be a substitute if a patient cannot take or tolerate aspirin to help prevent stroke or heart attack
  - o Due to its ability to inhibit platelets, the major complication is bleeding; assess patients for bruising, blood in the stool, any abnormal sign of bleeding, etc.
  - o Thrombotic thrombocytopenic purpura (rare)
  - o Avoids the CYP2C19 metabolic pathway which is different from clopidogrel
- Monitoring: CBC with platelets
- Drug and Diet Considerations:
  - o Generally avoid supplements that may be associated with antiplatelet activity such as ginseng, garlic, glucosamine, vitamin E, etc. or at a minimum, monitor for bruising and bleed risk
  - o Can be administered with or without food

Pravastatin (Pravachol)
- Class: Antilipemic, statin
- Mechanism of Action: HMG Co-A reductase inhibitor, eventually decreasing LDL
- Common Uses: Reduction of cholesterol, particularly LDL
- Memorable Side Effects: Muscle aches, rhabdomyolysis (rare but serious)
- Clinical Pearls:
  - o Statins like pravastatin are one of the mainstays of therapy to reduce cholesterol, and more particularly LDL (bad cholesterol)
  - o The most notable side effect with statins that you will likely hear patients complain about is myopathy (muscle aches/pain)
  - o Usually muscle aches are all over which can help you differentiate from other pain conditions or pain/soreness from an injury or overuse
  - o Contraindicated in pregnancy

- - o Patients who do not tolerate pravastatin, may try another statin as long as adverse effects aren't too severe (i.e. rhabdomyolysis); if you notice that the patient had an allergy or intolerance, you need to clarify with the provider
    - o CPK will be the primary lab to test for rhabdomyolysis -- breakdown of muscle; this elevation in CPK may eventually lead to kidney failure
    - o Pravastatin tends to have less drug interactions than other statins (atorvastatin, simvastatin, etc.) with CYP3A4 inhibitors like fluconazole or erythromycin
    - o For many, but not all, statins it is "recommended" to give them at night; this is not an absolute, but the drugs ideally work best when given at night
    - o Pravastatin is used less frequently because it doesn't reduce LDL as much as newer statins like atorvastatin, simvastatin, and rosuvastatin
- Monitoring: Lipids, LFTs, CPK if experiencing muscle pain (myopathy)
- Drug and Diet Considerations:
  - o Liver toxicity risk from excessive alcohol may be increased if used in combination with statins
  - o Low, but usually not clinically significant, risk of elevating blood sugars in patients with diabetes
  - o Can be taken with or without food
  - o Encourage a lipid lowering diet for any patient taking a cholesterol medication

Prazosin (Minipress)
- Class: Alpha blocker, antihypertensive
- Mechanism of Action: Blocks alpha receptors causing smooth muscle relaxation, vasodilation and opening of the ureter
- Common Uses: Treatment of BPH, urinary obstruction, hypertension and nightmares
- Memorable Side Effects: Low BP, dizziness
- Clinical Pearls:
  - o Non-selective alpha blocker, so it can be used for both hypertension and BPH
  - o High risk for syncope and low blood pressure especially in geriatric patients
  - o In the case of worsening urinary retention due to BPH and initiation of these agents, be sure to assess if your patient is on anticholinergic medications (diphenhydramine, TCAs, etc.)
  - o Usually dosed at night to minimize the risk of orthostasis
  - o Risk of floppy iris syndrome for those undergoing eye surgery
- Monitoring: Blood pressure
- Drug and Diet Considerations:
  - o Administer with or without food

Prednisone (Deltasone)
- Class: Corticosteroid
- Mechanism of Action: Suppresses leukocytes and ultimately reduces inflammation, also suppresses adrenal function and the immune system

235

- Common Uses: Treatment of many acute inflammatory states including, dermatitis, arthritis flare, Crohn's, pneumonia, and asthma exacerbation
- Memorable Side Effects: GI side effects, insomnia, hyperglycemia, long term use; suppress immune system, increase osteoporosis risk as well as cause adrenal insufficiency
- Clinical Pearls:
    o Be sure to take steroids with food as they can be pretty hard on the stomach
    o In patients with diabetes, educate them that a fluctuation in blood sugar may occur when starting, changing doses, or discontinuing this medication due to the adverse effect of hyperglycemia
    o Long term corticosteroid use can lead to increased risk Cushing's (moon face), diabetes, and osteoporosis; make sure long term use is assessed frequently to minimize duration of use and dose of steroids
    o In patients on long term use, they should be assessed if vitamin D and/or calcium and bisphosphonates should be added to reduce osteoporosis risk
    o Insomnia is common in the short term, but may resolve with chronic use
    o Short "bursts" (3 days to 1-2 weeks) are often used to relieve acute inflammatory states causing patient distress (asthma, rheumatoid arthritis, etc.)
    o Corticosteroids (especially long term and higher doses) can also suppress the immune system
- Monitoring: Blood sugar (in diabetes patients), blood pressure, bone mineral density (longer term use), HPA suppression, weight, development (pediatric patients)
- Drug and Diet Considerations:
    o Give with food as it can cause GI upset
    o In patients with diabetes, educate them that a fluctuation in blood sugars may occur when starting, changing doses, or discontinuing this medication due to the adverse effect of hyperglycemia
    o May reduce effectiveness of calcitriol (active vitamin D)
    o Long term use may increase the need for certain nutrients and vitamins such as folic acid, calcium, phosphorus, vitamin C, and vitamin D
    o May increase appetite and weight gain
    o Potassium and sodium may be elevated due to corticosteroids

Pregabalin (Lyrica)

- Class: Antiepileptic, analgesic
- Mechanism of Action: Inhibits excitatory neurotransmitters by binding voltage gated calcium channels in the CNS
- Common Uses: Treatment of neuropathy, fibromyalgia and seizures
- Memorable Side Effects: Edema, sedation, dizziness, confusion
- Clinical Pearls:
    o Think similar side effect/treatment profile as gabapentin; it's more expensive, but may be more effective when higher doses are needed
    o Generally classified as an anti-seizure medication, but often used for neuropathy
    o Keep an eye out for patients with kidney disease who may be experiencing side effects, this drug can accumulate in patients with poor renal function

- o Watch out for dizziness and sedation in our elderly patients as this can potentially contribute to fall risk
- o Weight gain in the form of edema may potentially happen with pregabalin; be on the lookout for patients with a history of CHF and edema issues, as well as those who may already be receiving diuretics like furosemide
- Monitoring: Seizures (if being used for seizures), weight/edema
- Drug and Diet Considerations:
  - o Can be taken with or without food
  - o Alcohol may have additive CNS depressant effects

Primidone (Mysoline)
- Class: Antiepileptic, barbiturate
- Mechanism of Action: Suppresses neuron activity and excitability
- Common Uses: Treatment of tremor and seizures
- Memorable Side Effects: CNS changes, ataxia, sedation, vitamin D deficiency
- Clinical Pearls:
  - o Converted to phenobarbital
  - o If concerned about toxicity, check primidone and phenobarbital levels
  - o Levels aren't routinely checked for tremor if patient is not having signs of toxicity
  - o While initially developed as a seizure medication, it is more frequently used for tremor
  - o Numerous drug interactions
- Monitoring: Drug levels, CBC and CMP as clinically indicated
- Drug and Diet Considerations:
  - o Folic acid, vitamin B12, riboflavin, pyridoxine, and vitamin D may all be reduced, assess for signs of deficiency and if supplementation may be necessary
  - o Alcohol may exacerbate the CNS depressant effect
  - o Low protein diet may lengthen the duration of action

Probenecid (Benemid)
- Class: Anti-gout, uricosuric
- Mechanism of Action: Inhibits reabsorption of uric acid in the kidney which facilitates removal of uric acid in the body through the kidney
- Common Uses: Treatment of gout and hyperuricemia
- Memorable Side Effects: GI upset, flushing, dizziness
- Clinical Pearls:
  - o Can increase the concentrations of beta-lactam antibiotics
  - o For this drug to be effective, the patient needs decent kidney function (creatinine clearance <30 mL/min; possibly less than 50 mL/min)
  - o Hemolytic anemia is a rare adverse effect that may be more likely in patients with G6PD deficiency
- Monitoring: Uric acid, CBC, renal function
- Drug and Diet Considerations:
  - o Give with food to reduce GI upset
  - o Plenty of fluids may help flush uric acid out through the kidneys; encourage adequate hydration

237

Prochlorperazine (Compazine)

- Class: Antiemetic, dopamine blocker, anticholinergic
- Mechanism of Action: Blocks dopamine receptors as well as H1 receptors
- Common Uses: Treatment of nausea/vomiting and migraine headaches
- Memorable Side Effects: Sedation, fall risk, orthostatic BP changes, EPS, metabolic syndrome (typically not an issue with short term use)
- Clinical Pearls:
  - While prochlorperazine is classically considered an antipsychotic (blocks dopamine), it is most often used for its antiemetic effect
  - Prochlorperazine also has anticholinergic effects, which leads to its sedative type effects, and also its ability to be used for allergy symptoms
  - If prochlorperazine is used on a regular basis, we need to monitor for development of tardive dyskinesia; this is normally not an issue when promethazine is used short term and as needed for nausea/vomiting
  - Elderly may be more susceptible to adverse effects
- Monitoring: EKG, and possibly electrolytes, in at risk patients (especially in overdose)
- Drug and Diet Considerations:
  - Slows the motility of the GI tract which could increase the risk for constipation, maintain adequate fluids and non-constipating diet
  - May give with food
  - Dry mouth may increase thirst and alter taste/pleasure of food
  - CNS depressant activity which could be exacerbated by alcohol
  - Recommended to increase riboflavin intake

Promethazine (Phenergan)

- Class: Antiemetic, dopamine blocker, antihistamine
- Mechanism of Action: Blocks dopamine receptors as well as H1 receptors
- Common Uses: Treatment of nausea/vomiting and motion sickness
- Memorable Side Effects: Sedation, fall risk, orthostatic BP changes, EPS, metabolic syndrome
- Clinical Pearls:
  - While promethazine is classically considered an antipsychotic (blocks dopamine), it is most often used for its antiemetic effect
  - Promethazine also has antihistamine effects, which leads to its sedative type effects, and also its ability to be used for allergy type symptoms
  - If promethazine is used on a regular basis, we need to monitor for development of tardive dyskinesia; this is normally not an issue when promethazine is used short term and as needed for nausea/vomiting
  - When using injectable forms, which can obviously be beneficial for nausea and vomiting to avoid the oral route, the preferred route of administration is intramuscular (into deep muscle)
  - Sedation, orthostatic hypotension, movement disorder side effects can all increase the risk of falls especially in our elderly patients
- Monitoring: EKG, and possibly electrolytes, in at risk patients (especially in overdose)
- Drug and Diet Considerations:

- o Slows the motility of the GI tract which could increase the risk for constipation, maintain adequate fluids and non-constipating diet
- o If GI upset occurs, no issues in giving the drug with food
- o Dry mouth may increase thirst and alter taste/pleasure of food
- o CNS depressant activity which could be exacerbated by alcohol

Propofol (Diprivan)

- Class: Anesthetic
- Mechanism of Action: Possible agonist activity on GABA and blockade of NMDA
- Common Uses: Anesthesia in intubated/ICU type patients
- Memorable Side Effects: Hypotension, respiratory apnea, elevated triglycerides, respiratory acidosis
- Clinical Pearls:
  - o Rare risk for anaphylaxis
  - o Can be riskier in patients who already have lower blood pressure
  - o Very fast onset, less than 1 minute
- Monitoring: Blood pressure, triglycerides (as clinically indicated), arterial blood gases as clinically indicated, potassium, LFTs, renal function, and CPK as clinically indicated, zinc
- Drug and Diet Considerations:
  - o Infusion contains lipids, explains the possibility for elevated triglycerides
  - o Propofol-related infusion syndrome may cause low pH (acidosis), hyperkalemia, and elevated lipids which can lead to rhabdomyolysis and renal failure
  - o May lower zinc levels
  - o Alcohol can exacerbate CNS depressant effects

Propranolol (Inderal LA)

- Class: Antihypertensive, beta-blocker
- Mechanism of Action: Blocks beta receptors leading to lower pulse/BP
- Common Uses: Treatment of hypertension, atrial fibrillation, migraines, tremor and prophylaxis of variceal hemorrhage in patients with cirrhosis
- Memorable Side Effects: Low pulse, low BP, fatigue
- Clinical Pearls:
  - o Trick to remembering beta receptors: you have 1 heart and 2 lungs (beta-1 is primarily on the heart and beta-2 primarily in the lungs) – non selective beta blockers can contribute to airway restriction (beta-2) as well as lower cardiac output (beta-1)
  - o The selectivity of these drugs is really important. Propranolol is the classic example of a beta blocker that is not selective for beta-1 receptors. It also blocks beta-2 receptors which makes it more likely that it could potentially exacerbate respiratory conditions like asthma
  - o Propranolol has a unique use of migraine prophylaxis as well as being used for portal hypertension in patients with cirrhosis, tremor, and possibly stress/anxiety type issues
  - o Often in practice, providers will place a hold order on beta-blockers if the pulse is too low, and this is done to reduce the risk of significant bradycardia

- Monitoring: Pulse, blood pressure, EKG as clinically indicated (i.e. acute atrial fibrillation)
- Drug and Diet Considerations:
  - Recommended to take immediate release tablets without food
  - Alcohol may have variable effects on drug concentrations
  - May mask signs and symptoms of hypoglycemia
  - Consistency is important with administration as diet changes can alter absorption, particularly with the extended release formulation
  - High protein foods may increase the amount absorbed

Propylthiouracil (PTU)
- Class: Antithyroid
- Mechanism of Action: Inhibits thyroid synthesis by interfering with oxidation of iodine; this is done via inhibition of the peroxidase enzyme
- Common Uses: Treatment of hyperthyroidism
- Memorable Side Effects: GI upset, hepatitis, agranulocytosis, anemia, lupus reaction
- Clinical Pearls:
  - Boxed warning on liver failure makes this a second line medication versus methimazole
  - Pay attention to symptoms of hyperthyroid and hypothyroid as these may indicate under-dosing or overdosing
  - Three times daily dosing is a disadvantage compared to once daily methimazole
  - Typically, it will take a little while for the drug to work
- Monitoring: Thyroid function (TSH, T4, T3), LFTs, CBC
  - Under-dosing may result in weight loss
  - Overdosing of medication may result in weight gain
  - May give with or without food, but consistency is recommended

Pseudoephedrine (Sudafed)
- Class: Decongestant
- Mechanism of Action: Stimulates alpha receptors causing vasoconstriction (beneficial in the respiratory tract)
- Common Uses: Relief from nasal congestion
- Memorable Side Effects: Hypertension, urinary retention (watch out for BPH patients), dry mouth, anxiety
- Clinical Pearls:
  - Watch out for elderly/high risk patients for cardiovascular problems as it can raise BP
  - Can exacerbate BPH
  - Can cause/worsen insomnia and/or anxiety
  - Due to methamphetamine abuse, use is restricted in the U.S; all products containing pseudoephedrine are kept behind the counter and require a signature to purchase
- Monitoring: Blood pressure and pulse as clinically indicated
- Drug and Diet Considerations:
  - Give with food if the patient has GI upset when taking it
  - Dry mouth and stimulant-type effect can impact appetite
  - Small quantities of sodium may be contained within some products

Psyllium (Metamucil, Fiber-Therapy, Evac)

- Class: Bulk-forming laxative, fiber supplement
- Mechanism of Action: Fiber and fiber like substances absorb water and keep it in the gut lumen which helps stimulate peristalsis and bowel movements
- Common Uses: Treatment of constipation
- Memorable Side Effects: Cramping, diarrhea, obstruction risk
- Clinical Pearls:
  - If inadvertently inhaled, it may cause a hypersensitivity- type reaction (rare)
- Monitoring: No routine monitoring is necessary
- Drug and Diet Considerations:
  - Encourage adequate fluid intake at time of administration and all throughout the day
  - Review specific product as there may be additional ingredients/electrolytes, although typically not clinically significant

Pyridoxine (Vitamin B6)

- Class: Vitamin
- Mechanism of Action: Gets converted to pyridoxal and is an important cofactor in metabolizing carbohydrates, proteins, and fats
- Common Uses: Nausea and vomiting in pregnancy, pyridoxine deficiency and prevention of neurologic toxicity form isoniazid
- Memorable Side Effects: Usually well tolerated, nausea, CNS changes or acidosis risk (typically only with excessively high dosages)
- Clinical Pearls:
  - Target RDA is in the range of 1.5-2 mg/day for most adults depending upon the population (pregnancy and breast-feeding typically requires the upper end)
  - Water soluble
  - Potential signs of pyridoxine deficiency include weakness, neuropathy, fatigue, cutaneous reactions and CNS changes
- Monitoring: >50ng/mL is typically acceptable but is not routinely monitored
- Drug and Diet Considerations:
  - Oral absorption is acceptable
  - True replacement may be up to 600 mg per day in severe cases while dosing for isoniazid neuropathy prevention and nausea and vomiting in pregnancy are much lower (i.e. 25-100 mg/day)
  - May lower drug concentrations of phenytoin and barbiturates

Quetiapine (Seroquel)

- Class: Antipsychotic
- Mechanism of Action: Blocks dopamine receptors
- Common Uses: Treatment of schizophrenia, bipolar disorder and off-label for dementia-related behaviors like aggression, hallucinations and delusions
- Memorable Side Effects: Sedation, fall risk, orthostatic BP changes, EPS, metabolic syndrome
- Clinical Pearls:

241

- o Usually higher doses are required for younger patients with schizophrenia and/or bipolar disorder while lower doses can and should be used in the elderly
- o Remember with antipsychotic medications that they block dopamine and can exacerbate conditions where there is a shortage of dopamine like Parkinson's disorder (remember that we use dopamine to treat Parkinson's – i.e. carbidopa/levodopa or pramipexole)
- o Sedation, orthostatic hypotension, movement disorder side effects can all increase the risk of falls especially in our elderly patients
- o NMS (neuroleptic malignant syndrome) is a very rare but very serious complication with antipsychotic medications; a few symptoms of NMS include: fever, hyperreflexia, confusion, delirium and tremor
- o Antipsychotics increase risk of metabolic syndrome (diabetes, elevated lipids, weight gain, etc.); it is important to periodically monitor for this, especially in younger patients with schizophrenia and/or bipolar disorder who may be likely to require long term use of higher doses
- o Anticholinergic effects are possible as well with antipsychotics, dry eyes, dry mouth, exacerbation of urinary retention (i.e. BPH), constipation (SLUD – can't salivate, lacrimate, urinate or defecate)
- o Antipsychotics can contribute to QTc prolongation, which can be especially problematic in patients who are already at risk (i.e. on antiarrhythmic medications)
- Monitoring: Weight, lipids, HbA1c, blood sugars
- Drug and Diet Considerations:
  - o Increased appetite and risk for metabolic syndrome; this can occur, but less common with quetiapine, compared to other antipsychotics, like olanzapine
  - o Increased blood sugars can happen in our diabetes patients, monitor blood sugars closely with acute changes in the drug
  - o Can be administered with or without meals
  - o Alcohol may exacerbate CNS depressant effect
  - o St John's wort may reduce the effectiveness of quetiapine
  - o High-fat, large meal may increase drug concentrations

Quinapril (Accupril)

- Class: Antihypertensive, ACE inhibitor
- Mechanism of Action: Inhibits t angiotensin converting enzyme which prevents the production of angiotensin 2; angiotensin 2 is a potent vasoconstrictor, less angiotensin 2 equates to less vasoconstriction, and lower blood pressure
- Common Uses: Treatment of hypertension, acute MI and heart failure
- Common Side Effects: Cough, kidney impairment, low blood pressure, and hyperkalemia
- Clinical Pearls:
  - o ACE inhibitors are notoriously known for causing a dry chronic cough
  - o Angiotensin Receptor Blockers (ARBs) are the cousins to the ACE inhibitors, and are the first line substitute to a patient who has had a cough with an ACE inhibitor
  - o ACE inhibitors can exacerbate kidney impairment as well as contribute to acute renal failure especially in patients who are

already on other potential renal toxic medications (i.e. diuretics, NSAIDs, etc.) even though in conditions like heart failure, diuretics and ACE inhibitors are often used together
  - ○ ACE inhibitors are a classic cause of elevated potassium levels; if your patient has hyperkalemia, you must make sure the ACE inhibitor has been addressed
  - ○ In some cases, patients of African descent may not respond to ACE inhibitors as well as other ethnicities
  - ○ A common mistake I've seen clinicians make is using an ACE inhibitor with and ARB; this is generally not recommended
  - ○ ACE inhibitors (and ARBs) are frequently used in patients with hypertension and a history of diabetes, stroke, CAD, CKD, and CHF
  - ○ Angioedema (swelling of the lips/airway) is classically caused by ACE inhibitors, it is an extremely rare, but very serious adverse reaction requiring immediate discontinuation
- Monitoring: Renal function, potassium, blood pressure
- Drug and Diet Considerations:
  - ○ Be cautious and monitor potassium closely in patients with high dietary intake of potassium as this could contribute to hyperkalemia in combination with this medication
  - ○ Administer with or without food

Quinine (Qualaquin)

- Class: Malaria agent
- Mechanism of Action: Integrates into parasitic DNA which blocks the processes of replication and transcription
- Common Uses: Treatment of malaria and leg cramps
- Memorable Side Effects: GI upset, thrombocytopenia, arrhythmia, hypersensitivity reactions, ocular toxicity, QT prolongation, anemia
- Clinical Pearls:
  - ○ While rarely used for leg cramps, there is a boxed warning from the FDA to avoid this medication for the use of leg cramps as there are potential severe adverse effects like arrhythmia and thrombocytopenia
- Monitoring: LFTs, CBC, eye exams, blood sugar
- Drug and Diet Considerations:
  - ○ Give with food to reduce GI upset
  - ○ May exacerbate hypoglycemia risk in diabetes patients

Rabeprazole (Aciphex)

- Class: PPI
- Mechanism of Action: Inhibits proton pumps in the stomach leading to a less acidic environment
- Common Uses: Treatment of GERD, ulcer and Barrett's esophagus
- Memorable Side Effects: Usually well tolerated; when used long term there is a possibility to increase fracture risk, decrease B12 levels, C. diff risk, low magnesium
- Clinical Pearls:
  - ○ PPIs are the most potent acid blocker on the market

- o PPIs are generally dosed 30 minutes or so before meals, this is a recommendation, not an absolute (example if a patient likes to get up and eat right away upon rising, the medication will still likely be beneficial, but may not have a maximal effect)
        - o For some patients, PPIs may not work very quickly and may take a few days for maximal effect
        - o For the above reason, as needed (PRN) PPIs may be effective, but are generally not recommended
        - o Use short term if possible due to increased risk of osteoporosis, low magnesium, and B12 deficiency if used long term
        - o Most common primary outcome of PPI would be to improve symptoms likely heartburn and stomach from GERD, stomach ulcer, or other related condition
        - o Barrett's esophagus, high risk GI medications (i.e. NSAIDs, prednisone), or chronic GI bleed may require indefinite therapy
        - o If GI bleed is problematic, monitoring hemoglobin and/or hemoccult might be appropriate to assess possible blood loss
- Monitoring: Magnesium (chronic use), B12
- Drug and Diet Considerations:
    - o When used chronically, it is a possible cause or contributing factor to B12 and magnesium deficiency
    - o PPIs are typically best given at least 30-60 minutes before a meal
        - ▪ If this drug is used in the treatment of duodenal ulcers or Helicobacter pylori, it is ok to administer with meals
    - o Reduced stomach acid (high pH) may impair the absorption of iron supplements

Raloxifene (Evista)
- Class: Antineoplastic, anti-osteoporosis agent, selective estrogen receptor modulator
- Mechanism of Action: Stimulates estrogen receptors selectively in bone tissue leading to an increase in bone strength, also acts as an estrogen antagonist in other pathways
- Common Uses: Treatment of osteoporosis and breast cancer risk reduction
- Memorable Side Effects: Menopausal-type symptoms such as hot flashes, DVT/PE risk (boxed warning), stroke (boxed warning), elevated triglycerides
- Clinical Pearls:
    - o This medication makes a lot of sense in patients at risk for breast cancer and who have osteoporosis
    - o Avoid use in patients with a history of blood clots
- Monitoring: Bone mineral density, calcium, vitamin D levels, lipids
- Drug and Diet Considerations:
    - o Administer with or without food
    - o Ensure the patient has adequate vitamin D and calcium intake of at least 1,200 mg per day of calcium and 1,000 units in females with osteoporosis

Raltegravir (Isentress)
- Class: Integrase inhibitor, antiretroviral
- Mechanism of Action: Inhibits the viral enzyme integrase by binding enzyme cations and preventing viral DNA integration into the host genome
- Common Uses: HIV treatment

244

- Memorable Side Effects: Usually well tolerated, elevated LFTs, skin reaction risk/SJS (rare, but possible), CNS changes, GI adverse effects, CPK increase/myopathy
- Clinical Pearls:
  - Generally preferred now in place of protease inhibitors as they have less drug interactions and seem to be better tolerated
  - Typically included in healthcare associated post-exposure prophylaxis (PEP) regimens
- Monitoring: CBC, LFTs, HIV levels, CD4 count, Hepatitis B testing prior to initiation, CPK as clinically indicated
- Drug and Diet Considerations:
  - May be given without regard to food
  - There may be a modest increase of blood glucose, monitor in patients with diabetes and adjust diet accordingly
  - Supplements that have antacid activity like calcium carbonate and magnesium products may block absorption, separate by a minimum of 2 hours

Ramelteon (Rozerem)
- Class: Hypnotic, melatonin agonist
- Mechanism of Action: Stimulates the MT1 (Melatonin-1) and MT2 receptors to help induce sleep
- Common Uses: Treatment of insomnia
- Memorable Side Effects: Sedation, confusion, dizziness, GI upset, or change in behavior
- Clinical Pearls:
  - Typically ONLY used for insomnia (not anxiety or seizures)
  - The best way I remember benzodiazepines is that they are very close to "alcohol in a pill"
  - Sedation, confusion, slurred speech, trouble walking (ataxia), etc. are all common with benzos/alcohol
  - Be cautious with patients on higher doses of benzodiazepines to make sure they aren't abruptly stopped
  - Educate patients on driving/operating machinery risks
  - Fall risk in the elderly is a big downside to using these medications
  - Benzos are a controlled substance, they can cause addiction and dependence
  - Flumazenil is antidote in overdose
- Monitoring: Routine lab monitoring typically isn't necessary unless clinically indicated
- Drug and Diet Considerations:
  - Alcohol intake can have additive side effects of sedation, confusion, slurred speech, and other CNS depressant effects
  - Give on an empty stomach, typically at bedtime, because food, particularly fatty foods, may delay the onset of action

Ramipril (Altace)
- Class: Antihypertensive, ACE inhibitor
- Mechanism of Action: Inhibits the angiotensin converting enzyme which prevents the production of angiotensin 2; angiotensin 2 is a potent

vasoconstrictor, less angiotensin 2 equates to less vasoconstriction, and lower blood pressure
- Common Uses: Treatment of hypertension, acute MI and heart failure
- Common Side Effects: Cough, kidney impairment, low blood pressure, and hyperkalemia
- Clinical Pearls:
  - ACE inhibitors are notoriously known for causing a dry chronic cough
  - Angiotensin Receptor Blockers (ARBs) are the cousins to the ACE inhibitors, and are the first line substitute to a patient who has had a cough with an ACE inhibitor
  - ACE inhibitors can exacerbate kidney impairment as well as contribute to acute renal failure especially in patients who are already on other potential renal toxic medications (i.e. diuretics, NSAIDs, etc.) even though in conditions like heart failure, diuretics and ACE inhibitors are often used together
  - ACE inhibitors are a classic cause of elevated potassium levels; if your patient has hyperkalemia, you must make sure the ACE inhibitor has been addressed
  - In some cases, patients of African descent may not respond to ACE inhibitors as well as other ethnicities
  - A common mistake I've seen clinicians make is using an ACE inhibitor with and ARB; this is generally not recommended
  - ACE inhibitors (or ARBs) are frequently used in patients with hypertension and a history of diabetes, stroke, CAD, CKD, and CHF
  - Angioedema (swelling of the lips/airway) is classically caused by ACE inhibitors, it is an extremely rare, but very serious adverse reaction requiring immediate discontinuation
- Monitoring: Renal function, potassium, blood pressure
- Drug and Diet Considerations:
  - Be cautious and monitor potassium closely in patients with high dietary intake of potassium as this could contribute to hyperkalemia in combination with this medication
  - Administer with or without food

Ranitidine (Zantac)

- Class: Histamine-2 blocker
- Mechanism of Action: Blocks histamine 2 receptors which results in reduced gastric acid secretion and a higher pH in the stomach
- Common Uses: Treatment of GERD, heartburn and GI bleed
- Memorable Side Effects: Well tolerated overall, watch out for CNS changes in elderly
- Clinical Pearls:
  - ***Withdrawn from the US market in 2020 due to the risk of carcinogen substances***
  - H2 blockers are cleared by the kidney, so they can accumulate/require dose adjustments in CKD
  - Generally less effective at suppressing stomach acid than PPIs
  - Many alternative and inexpensive H2 blockers are available over the counter
  - CNS effects more common in elderly, on higher doses, and in patients with kidney disease

246

- o Generally used before PPIs if something more than Tums (calcium carbonate) is needed in pregnancy
- Monitoring: No routine lab work is typically necessary; LFTs, hemoglobin when clinically indicated
- Drug and Diet Considerations:
  - o Generally given with meals or at bedtime, can be taken with or without food
  - o Reduced stomach acid (high pH) may impair the absorption of iron supplements
  - o It has mild anticholinergic side effects so dry mouth could potentially alter taste and desire to eat
  - o Associations with B12 deficiency in chronic users

Repaglinide (Prandin)

- Class: Anti-diabetic agent, glinide
- Mechanism of Action: Stimulates pancreatic cells to release insulin by blocking ATP-dependent potassium channels which depolarizes the cell membrane and increases calcium influx; calcium in the cell stimulates the release of insulin
- Common Uses: Treatment of diabetes
- Memorable Side Effects: Hypoglycemia, weight gain
- Clinical Pearls:
  - o Due to increased insulin, hypoglycemia is of highest concern
  - o Be attentive to appetite changes or new diabetes medications and monitor for hypoglycemia
  - o Elderly can be especially at risk for hypoglycemia
  - o Frequent dosing can be difficult for patients to adhere to
- Monitoring: HbA1c, blood glucose, risk for hypoglycemia
- Drug and Diet Considerations:
  - o Be very cautious for the risk of hypoglycemia if there is a significant reduction in dietary intake (i.e. acute illness, nausea/vomiting)
  - o Patient without caloric intake will likely have to hold this medication (i.e. before surgery, missed meals)
  - o Possible increase in concentration from grapefruit juice
  - o Needs to be administered up to 30 minutes before meals which can be difficult to manage if the patient has a variable meal schedule
  - o Post-prandial glucose reduction

Revefenacin (Yuperlri)

- Class: Inhaled anticholinergic
- Mechanism of Action: Inhaled anticholinergic can open up airways and decrease secretions
- Common Uses: Treatment of COPD
- Memorable Side Effects: Dry mouth, cough, irritation to the lungs; usually well tolerated due to minimal systemic absorption
- Clinical Pearls:
  - o Revefenacin is primarily used for COPD, and because it has anticholinergic activity, it can help dry up the airways as well as open them up to allow for better breathing in patients who have thick mucus/sputum
  - o It is long acting and meant to be used as a controller medication

- o It is not meant to be a rescue inhalation product and will not provide acute relief from respiratory distress
- o Often by using this medication in COPD, our goal is likely to improve respiratory status, but also to reduce the amount of as needed albuterol and/or albuterol/ipratropium (Duoneb or Combivent)
- o Systemic anticholinergic effects are usually not a concern as systemic absorption is low
- o Nebulized formulation
- Monitoring: FEV1, peak flow
- Drug and Diet Considerations:
  - o Inhaled, local medication
  - o Dry mouth may impact dietary/fluid intake

Riboflavin (Vitamin B2)

- Class: Vitamin
- Mechanism of Action: Essential for flavoprotein enzyme function as well as necessary for the body to properly utilize pyridoxine
- Common Uses: Supplement and migraine prevention
- Memorable Side Effects: Well tolerated, change in urine color
- Clinical Pearls:
  - o Target RDA is in the range of 1.1 - 1.6 mg/day for most adults depending upon the population, pregnancy and breast-feeding typically require the upper end
  - o Water soluble
- Monitoring: Routine lab work is not necessary
- Drug and Diet Considerations:
  - o Generally given with food
  - o No major drug interactions

Rifampin (Rifadin)

- Class: Antibiotic
- Mechanism of Action: Inhibits bacterial RNA synthesis
- Common Uses: Treatment of TB and augmentation in MRSA/osteomyelitis
- Memorable Side Effects: increased LFTs , GI, rash
- Clinical Pearls:
  - o Enzyme inducer notorious for many drug interactions including, warfarin (causes lower INR when initiated), birth control, many HIV medications, some statins, and many more
  - o MRSA activity
- Monitoring: LFTs, CBC, renal function, risk for drug interactions
- Drug and Diet Considerations:
  - o Recommended to be given on an empty stomach with water to increase absorption
  - o GI upset, nausea, and anorexia are possible

Rifaximin (Xifaxan)

- Class: Antibiotic, rifamycin
- Mechanism of Action: Inhibits bacterial RNA synthesis which ultimately leads to death of ammonia producing bacteria
- Common Uses: Treatment of hepatic encephalopathy

- Memorable Side Effects: GI upset, rash, fatigue, dizziness, edema
- Clinical Pearls:
  - Dosed multiple times per day
  - Poor systemic absorption, incidence of systemic side effects is fairly low
  - Prevents bacteria from producing byproducts that increase the amount of ammonia
  - Very expensive at this time
- Monitoring: Ammonia levels in hepatic encephalopathy
- Drug and Diet Considerations:
  - Can be given with or without food
  - GI upset, nausea, and anorexia are possible, monitor dietary intake when initiating

Rilpivirine (Edurant)
- Class: Antiretroviral, non-nucleoside reverse transcriptase inhibitor
- Mechanism of Action: Bind to a hydrophobic site of the HIV reverse transcriptase and inactivate it, they do not require active conversion to triphosphate forms like the NRTIs
- Common Uses: HIV treatment
- Memorable Side Effects: Hallucinations, psychiatric changes, abnormal dreams, hepatotoxicity, rash, lowers seizure threshold
- Clinical Pearls:
  - Rash will usually occur within the first few days/weeks of starting the medication
  - May contribute to QTc prolongation risks
  - Resistance risk may be high especially if this medication is used alone
  - PPIs and H2 blockers may significantly impair the activity of the drug; recommended to avoid concomitant use if possible
- Monitoring: LFTs, cholesterol, HIV parameters
- Drug and Diet Considerations:
  - Give with meals
  - Cushing's-type appearance, including obesity and buffalo hump complications, may happen as a result of this medication
  - Recognize the risk for hypercholesterolemia and consider a lipid friendly diet and/or removing the agent
  - Antacids may reduce absorption, separate doses by at least 2 hours before or 4-6 hours after
  - Grapefruit and grapefruit juice may increase concentrations

Risedronate (Actonel)
- Class: Bisphosphonate
- Mechanism of Action: Inhibits osteoclasts (osteoclasts break down bone)
- Common Uses: Treatment of osteoporosis
- Memorable Side Effects: Esophageal ulceration (administration procedure important to decrease this risk), GI side effects in general
- Clinical Pearls:

- o Timing of administration is critical! Take on an empty stomach, usually right away in the morning with 6-8 ounces of plain water, 30 minutes prior to any food or drink (that isn't plain water)
- o Have patient remain sitting or standing upright for 30 minutes; this is to reduce the risk of esophageal irritation/ulceration
- o Absorption will be limited and drug will not be effective if taken with food or other medications
- o After 5 years of bisphosphonate use, some lower risk patients may be able to have the medication reassessed for ongoing need and possibly discontinued
- o Osteonecrosis (destruction or dying) of bone of the jaw is extremely rare, however, patient may be at increased risk if recently had an invasive dental procedure
- o Be cautious with oral bisphosphonates in patients who already have esophageal or GI related concerns, like a GI bleed or ulcer history
- o Always important to assure adequate vitamin D and calcium intake
- Monitoring: Bone mineral density, calcium, vitamin D levels
- Drug and Diet Considerations:
  - o Ensure the patient has adequate vitamin D and calcium intake, at least 1,200 mg per day of calcium and 1,000 units of vitamin D in females with osteoporosis
  - o Esophagitis and GI upset is possible which could cause changes in appetite and weight loss
  - o The drug must be taken in the morning prior to breakfast with 6-8 ounces of plain water and nothing else
  - o Wait at least 30 minutes prior to eating anything and remain upright
  - o If taken with food, juice, or other medications, the absorption, and effectiveness, will be reduced

Risperidone (Risperdal)

- Class: Antipsychotic
- Mechanism of Action: Blocks dopamine receptors
- Common Uses: Treatment of schizophrenia, bipolar disorder and off-label for dementia-related behaviors like aggression, hallucinations and delusions
- Memorable Side Effects: Sedation, fall risk, orthostatic BP changes, EPS, metabolic syndrome
- Clinical Pearls:
  - o Usually higher doses are required for younger patients with schizophrenia and/or bipolar disorder while lower doses can and should be used in the elderly
  - o Remember with antipsychotic medications that they block dopamine and can exacerbate conditions where there is a shortage of dopamine like Parkinson's disorder (remember that we use dopamine to treat Parkinson's – i.e. carbidopa/levodopa or pramipexole)
  - o Sedation, orthostatic hypotension and movement disorder side effects can all increase the risk of falls especially in our elderly patients
  - o NMS (neuroleptic malignant syndrome) is a very rare but very serious complication with antipsychotic medications; a few symptoms of NMS include: fever, hyperreflexia, confusion, delirium and tremor

- o   Antipsychotics increase the risk of metabolic syndrome (diabetes, elevated lipids, weight gain, etc.); it is important to periodically monitor for this, especially in younger patients with schizophrenia and/or bipolar disorder who may be likely to require long term use of higher doses
  - o   Anticholinergic effects are possible as well with antipsychotics, dry eyes, dry mouth, exacerbation of urinary retention (i.e. BPH), constipation (SLUD – can't salivate, lacrimate, urinate or defecate)
  - o   Antipsychotics can contribute to QTC prolongation, which can be especially problematic in patients who are already at risk (i.e. on antiarrhythmic medications)
- Monitoring: Weight, lipids, HbA1c, blood sugars
- Drug and Diet Considerations:
  - o   Increased appetite and risk for metabolic syndrome
  - o   Increased blood sugars can happen in our diabetes patients, monitor blood sugars closely with acute changes in the drug
  - o   Can be administered with or without meals
  - o   Alcohol may exacerbate CNS depressant effect
  - o   Oral solution can be mixed with water, orange juice, milk, or coffee

Ritonavir (Norvir)
- Class: Pharmacokinetic booster, protease inhibitor, antiretroviral
- Mechanism of Action: Boosts the concentration of other protease inhibitors which ultimately helps it to bind to the site where protein cleavage occurs and prevents protease from releasing essential proteins
- Common Uses: HIV treatment
- Memorable Side Effects: Buffalo hump, fat redistribution, metabolic effects like increased cholesterol and hyperglycemia, hepatotoxicity, skin reaction, nausea, vomiting, diarrhea
- Clinical Pearls:
  - o   Metabolic risks are a significant downside to long term use in younger populations
  - o   Boxed warning for numerous drug interactions through CYP3A4
- Monitoring: Lipids, glucose, HIV parameters (i.e. viral load and CD4 count), LFTs
- Drug and Diet Considerations:
  - o   Monitor hyperglycemia risk, may need to adjust diet accordingly
  - o   Lipid-lowering diet could help reduce the adverse effect of hypercholesterolemia
  - o   Take with food

Rivaroxaban (Xarelto)
- Class: Anticoagulant
- Mechanism of Action: Inhibits clotting factor 10A
- Common Uses: Prevention of stroke in patients with atrial fibrillation, DVT/PE prophylaxis or treatment
- Memorable Side Effects: Bleeding
- Clinical Pearls:
  - o   Is gaining popularity against warfarin
  - o   Less risk of drug interaction and patients do NOT need to do routine INRs

251

- o With bleed risk being the major side effect, hemoglobin (CBC) is important to monitor
- o Major use of this medication is to prevent or treat blood clots (DVT, PE, Stroke)
- o Expense is the major downside of rivaroxaban versus warfarin
- Monitoring: CBC, renal function
- Drug and Diet Considerations:
  - o Administer with or without food, typically given with the evening meal
  - o Vitamin E, Omega-3 fatty acids, gingko, garlic, ginseng, turmeric, and fish oil supplements have been purported to have antiplatelet type activity which in theory could increase the risk of bleed – clinical significance is questionable; the most common resolution is to discontinue the supplements if they are not necessary
  - o Alcohol may have an additive antiplatelet type effect and increase the risk of GI bleed
  - o St John's wort should not be taken with this medication as it can reduce drug concentrations

Rivastigmine (Exelon)
- Class: Dementia agent, acetylcholinesterase inhibitor
- Mechanism of Action: Inhibits acetylcholinesterase which increases acetylcholine in the CNS
- Common Uses: Management of Alzheimer's dementia
- Memorable Side Effects: GI (N/V/D), weight loss, insomnia, dizziness, bradycardia
- Clinical Pearls:
  - o One of the more common drug causes of weight loss in the elderly
  - o Will NOT reverse dementia symptoms, but may help with some symptom improvement
  - o Dementia medications in general can contribute to behavioral changes (good or bad)
  - o Patch formulation may have a lower risk of GI adverse effects
- Monitoring: Weight, GI adverse effects, pulse
- Drug and Diet Considerations:
  - o Significant cause of weight loss and poor appetite
  - o Assess for GI upset and loose stools
  - o Give oral formulation with food
  - o Patch may be administered at any time of the day, just be consistent

Rizatriptan (Maxalt)
- Class: Anti-migraine, triptan
- Mechanism of Action: Serotonin 5HT agonist, which causes vasoconstriction and reduction of inflammation associated with migraine
- Common Uses: Acute relief of migraine
- Memorable Side Effects: Dizziness, changes in CNS
- Clinical Pearls:
  - o Meant for acute relief of migraine, not prophylaxis
  - o Be sure to assess use, frequent use may indicate that a controller medication, like valproic acid, propranolol or topiramate, may need to be added to help prevent migraines
  - o Often used with NSAIDs, like naproxen, in migraine treatment

- o Does have serotonin activity so could potentially contribute to serotonin syndrome (higher risk in patients already on SSRIs, tramadol, etc.)
- Monitoring: Blood pressure, EKG when clinically indicated to assess risk for QTc prolongation
- Drug and Diet Considerations:
  - o Given as needed for migraine, so administration at any point is fine with regards to food
  - o Food may delay the onset

Ropinirole (Requip)
- Class: Anti-Parkinson's, dopamine agonist
- Mechanism of Action: Stimulates dopamine receptors
- Common Uses: Treatment of RLS and Parkinson's disorder
- Memorable Side Effects: Orthostasis, edema, OCD symptoms (very rare)
- Clinical Pearls:
  - o Indicated for Parkinson's but very commonly drug of choice for RLS
  - o Often patients struggle with RLS at night, so if you see it dosed once daily at night, this is likely the indication
  - o Keep an eye out for orthostasis, especially in the elderly and patients who may also be receiving numerous antihypertensives already
  - o Make sure the diagnosis is clear and the medication actually helps the patient; often this is inappropriately added for cramps or spasms
- Monitoring: Blood pressure
- Drug and Diet Considerations:
  - o Can be given with food if nausea occurs
  - o Rare associations with impulsive behaviors which could include, but is not limited to, binge eating
  - o Any drug with dopamine activity can cause nausea and vomiting
  - o Alcohol may have additive CNS adverse effects like sedation
  - o Smoking tobacco may reduce concentrations of ropinirole

Rosuvastatin (Crestor)
- Class: Antilipemic, statin
- Mechanism of Action: HMG Co-A reductase inhibitor, eventually leads to decreased LDL
- Common Uses: Reduction of cholesterol, particularly LDL
- Memorable Side Effects: Muscle aches, rhabdomyolysis (rare but serious)
- Clinical Pearls:
  - o Statins, like rosuvastatin, are one of the mainstays of therapy to reduce cholesterol, and more particularly LDL (bad cholesterol)
  - o The most notable side effect with statins that you will likely hear patients complain about is myopathy (muscle aches/pain)
  - o Usually muscle aches are all over which can help you differentiate from other pain conditions or pain/soreness from an injury or overuse
  - o Contraindicated in pregnancy
  - o Patients who do not tolerate rosuvastatin may try another statin, as long as adverse effects aren't too severe (i.e. rhabdomyolysis); if

you notice that the patient had an allergy or intolerance, you need to clarify with the provider
- o CPK will be the primary lab to test for rhabdomyolysis, the breakdown of muscle
- o For most statins it is "recommended" to give them at night; this is not an absolute, but the drugs ideally work the best when given at night; rosuvastatin is an exception to this rule
- Monitoring: Lipids, LFTs, CPK if experiencing muscle pain (myopathy)
- Drug and Diet Considerations:
    - o Liver toxicity risk from excessive alcohol may be increased if used in combination with statins
    - o Low, often not clinically significant, risk of elevating blood sugars in patients with diabetes
    - o Grapefruit juice can significantly increase the concentrations of rosuvastatin, avoid using grapefruit juice
    - o Can be taken with or without food
    - o Encourage a lipid lowering diet for any patient taking a cholesterol medication

Sacubitril and Valsartan (Entresto)

- Class: Heart failure agent, angiotensin receptor blocker (valsartan) and Neprilysin inhibitor (sacubitril)
- Mechanism of Action: See valsartan; sacubitril inhibits neprilysin which lead to an increase in vasodilation with an increase in sodium excretion
- Common Uses: Reduced ejection fraction heart failure
- Memorable Side Effects: Hypotension, hyperkalemia, serum creatinine elevations, dizziness, angioedema
- Clinical Pearls:
    - o Contraindicated in pregnancy
    - o Must not take with an ACE inhibitor and should have at least a 36 hour washout period
- Monitoring: Renal function, potassium, blood pressure
- Drug and Diet Considerations:
    - o May be given without respect to food
    - o Excessive dietary or supplemental potassium intake may exacerbate hyperkalemic effect

Salmeterol (Serevent)

- Class: Long acting beta-agonist
- Mechanism of Action: Stimulates beta-2 receptors leading to relaxation of smooth muscle and opening of airways
- Common Uses: Asthma prophylaxis and COPD treatment
- Memorable Side Effects: Tachycardia, tremor, anxiousness, hypokalemia (rare), hyperglycemia (rare)
- Clinical Pearls:
    - o Increased risk of asthma death in patients who take long acting beta agonists as monotherapy
- Monitoring: Frequency of use, FEV1, peak-flow, pulse, blood pressure, and potassium (usually only necessary in high dosages), glucose (rarely clinically significant
- Drug and Diet Considerations:

- o Assess potassium intake and blood levels of potassium if the patient is using a beta agonist frequently or has a history of hypokalemia
- o Be aware of caffeine intake in combination with a beta-agonist as it can have an additive effect on blood pressure and heart rate
- o Monitor diabetes patients for elevations in blood sugar

Salsalate (Disalcid)
- Class: Salicylate
- Mechanism of Action: Inhibits prostaglandin production which provides anti-inflammatory effects
- Common Uses: Arthritis, pain relief
- Memorable Side Effects: GI ulcer, worsening kidney function, edema, hypertension, inhibits platelets (can exacerbate bleed risk)
- Clinical Pearls:
  - o Essentially has a similar effect profile to NSAIDs
  - o Boxed warning on GI ulceration
  - o Boxed warning on association with cardiovascular events
- Monitoring: Renal function, hemoglobin, platelets (contained within CBC), blood pressure
- Drug and Diet Considerations:
  - o Because of significant incidence of GI upset, it is generally given with food or milk
  - o Dehydration coupled with salsalate may increase the risk for acute renal failure
  - o Excessive alcohol may increase GI bleed risk
  - o Vitamin E, Omega-3 fatty acids, gingko, garlic, ginseng, turmeric, and fish oil supplements have been purported to have antiplatelet type activity which in theory could increase the risk of bleed – clinical significance is questionable; the most common resolution is to discontinue the supplements if they are not necessary

Saquinavir (Invirase)
- Class: Protease inhibitor, antiretroviral
- Mechanism of Action: Binds to site where protein cleavage occurs and prevents protease from releasing essential proteins
- Common Uses: HIV treatment
- Memorable Side Effects: Buffalo hump, fat redistribution, metabolic effects like increased cholesterol and hyperglycemia, hepatotoxicity, skin reaction, nausea, vomiting, diarrhea, QTc prolongation, photosensitivity
- Clinical Pearls:
  - o Metabolic risks are a significant downside to long term use in younger populations
  - o Given in combination with ritonavir
- Monitoring: Lipids, glucose, HIV parameters (i.e. viral load and CD4 count), QTc as clinically indicated, electrolytes (magnesium and potassium)
- Drug and Diet Considerations:
  - o Product may contain lactose
  - o Monitor hyperglycemia risk and may need to adjust diet accordingly
  - o Lipid-lowering diet could help reduce the adverse effect of hypercholesterolemia

255

- o Ideal to give with a meal as food, fat in particular, will improve bioavailability

Saxagliptin (Onglyza)
- Class: Antidiabetic, DDP-4 inhibitor
- Mechanism of Action: Inhibits DPP-4 which increases incretin levels, incretin increases insulin and decreases glucagon in the body and also might help patients' stomachs "feel full"
- Common Uses: Treatment of type 2 diabetes
- Memorable Side Effects: Hypoglycemia if taken in combination with insulin or sulfonylurea, edema, pancreatitis concerns exist, but are rare
- Clinical Pearls:
  - o Usually well tolerated, once daily dosing is nice for a diabetes medication
  - o Generally avoided in heart failure where other options exist
- Monitoring: Blood sugar, HbA1c, and renal function as clinically indicated
- Drug and Diet Considerations:
  - o Administer with or without food
  - o Implementation of a diabetic diet
  - o Grapefruit juice may increase concentrations

Scopolamine (Transderm Scop)
- Class: Anticholinergic
- Mechanism of Action: Blocks acetylcholine receptors (anticholinergic), which relaxes parasympathetic smooth muscle, dries secretions and can provide motion sickness and nausea and vomiting relief
- Common Uses: Prophylaxis of motion sickness and nausea and vomiting from anesthesia
- Memorable Side Effects: Anticholinergic (can't spit, see, pee, or sh*t and increases confusion/fall risk) which can be especially problematic in geriatric patients – avoid if possible
- Clinical Pearls:
  - o Patch formulation
  - o Meant for prevention and is not immediately beneficial with a 6-8 hour onset of action
- Monitoring: No routine lab work is recommended
- Drug and Diet Considerations:
  - o Alcohol can exacerbate the CNS depressant effect
  - o The side effect of dry mouth could affect eating habits
  - o Timing in relation to food is not necessary given the use of the topical patch

Selegiline (Eldepryl, Emsam)
- Class: MAOI – type B, anti-Parkinson's agent
- Mechanism of Action: Inhibits the action of monoamine oxidase type B; helps to preserve dopamine
- Common Uses: Treatment of Parkinson's disease and a transdermal option for major depressive disorder
- Memorable Side Effects: Nausea, dizziness, blood pressure fluctuations, rash (localized with the patch only), dyskinesia, hallucinations, unusual behavior
- Clinical Pearls:

- o Patch formulation is only indicated for depression while oral formulations are indicated in Parkinson's
- o Increased risk of suicidal thoughts with the patch formulation
- o Avoid transdermal selegiline in patients under 12 years old
- o Serotonin syndrome is possible, but less likely than traditional MAO – type A inhibitors
- Monitoring: Blood pressure
- Drug and Diet Considerations:
  - o Patch may be administered consistently without regard to meals while oral disintegrating table is typically given before breakfast
  - o Alcohol should be avoided as it may increase risk for toxicity
  - o MAOI/Tyramine interaction is less likely than with traditional MAOIs
    - Avoid foods high in tyramine: fermented, cured, aged foods such as cheese, smoked meats/fish, beer
    - Reaction: tachycardia, N/V, headache
    - Risk of reaction increases as the dose of the medication increases

Semaglutide (Ozempic, Rybelsus)
- Class: Antidiabetic, GLP-1 agonist
- Mechanism of Action: Glucagon-like peptide 1 agonists enhance glucose dependent insulin secretion, slows gastric emptying, and reduces post prandial glucagon to reduce blood sugars
- Common Uses: Treatment of type 2 diabetes
- Memorable Side Effects: Nausea, vomiting, diarrhea, hypoglycemia if taken in combination with insulin or sulfonylurea, pancreatitis concerns exist, but are rare
- Clinical Pearls:
  - o Injection is dosed once weekly
  - o Oral dosage form is available, dosed once daily
  - o Boxed warning to avoid medication in certain types of thyroid tumors
  - o Promotes fullness, weight loss can be a beneficial effect
  - o Typically better in HbA1c reduction than most oral diabetes medications
- Monitoring: Blood sugar, HbA1c, renal function as clinically indicated
- Drug and Diet Considerations:
  - o Oral medication should be given with water 30-60 minutes prior to other food, beverage, or oral medications
  - o Injection can be administered without regard to meals
  - o Reduces appetite which can be helpful in obese type 2 diabetes patients
  - o Implementation of a diabetic diet

Sennosides (Senokot)
- Class: Stimulant laxative
- Mechanism of Action: Stimulates GI movement by irritating GI smooth muscle
- Common Uses: Treatment of constipation
- Memorable Side Effects: Abdominal pain
- Clinical Pearls:

- o Used to promote bowel movement
- o Often used in treatment/prevention of opioid induced constipation
- o Can be used as needed
- Monitoring: Bowel movements
- Drug and Diet Considerations:
  - o Implement constipation friendly diet

Sertraline (Zoloft)

- Class: Antidepressant, SSRI
- Mechanism of Action: Selective serotonin reuptake inhibitor; increases serotonin in the brain
- Common Uses: Treatment of depression, anxiety and PTSD
- Memorable Side Effects: GI side effects (N/V/D), can cause sedation or activation depending upon the patient, changes in mental status, hyponatremia (rare)
- Clinical Pearls:
  - o SSRIs are generally considered the first line medication to treat depression, they are generally well tolerated, and less risky than other antidepressants in the situation of attempted suicide through overdose
  - o Stomach/GI complaints like stomach upset and/or diarrhea are probably the most common adverse effects; sertraline is highest risk for causing diarrhea of all the SSRIs
  - o Boxed warning for an increased risk of suicidal thinking when first starting these medications
  - o Although not terribly common, hyponatremia (low sodium) is a possible unique side effect with SSRIs and much more likely in patients already prone to hyponatremia; classic example would be patients who are taking diuretics, which can also lower sodium
  - o SSRIs take weeks, sometimes months, before a patient will start improving; however, side effects will be apparent from the start of the medication, making it difficult to coach our patients to continue the medication in the first few weeks after starting it
  - o SSRIs are used in pregnancy, but the risk versus the benefits need to be assessed on a case by case basis
  - o SSRIs can decrease libido
- Monitoring: EKG, potassium and magnesium if the patient is at risk for QTc prolongation; sodium level if the patient is displaying symptoms of hyponatremia
- Drug and Diet Considerations:
  - o Weight gain or weight loss can happen with SSRIs, monitor for changes over time once started, increased, reduced, or discontinued
  - o Diarrhea is most common with sertraline compared to other SSRIs
  - o Low sodium can be a rare adverse effect
  - o Can be taken with or without food
  - o Alcohol has additive, unpredictable effects when used with SSRIs
  - o Grapefruit juice may increase concentrations
  - o St John's wort has additive effects on any drug that has serotonergic type activity

Sevelamer (Renagel, Renvela)

- Class: Phosphate binder

258

- Mechanism of Action: Binds with dietary phosphate in the gut and gets excreted in the feces
- Common Uses: Treatment of hyperphosphatemia associated with chronic kidney disease
- Memorable Side Effects: Nausea, vomiting, diarrhea, metabolic acidosis
- Clinical Pearls:
  - Used if elevated calcium level is a problem with calcium acetate
  - Administer with meals
  - GI side effects
  - May bind certain drugs like quinolone antibiotics, immunosuppressive drugs, and thyroid medications
- Monitoring: Phosphorus, calcium, parathyroid hormone (PTH), renal function, monitor for certain vitamin deficiencies as noted below
- Drug and Diet Considerations:
  - Patients on this medication need to have adequate education about appropriate use in the need to lower their phosphorus levels
  - The drug is ineffective if it is not given with food
  - Vitamins like A, D, E, K, and folic acid may have reduced absorption

Sildenafil (Viagra)
- Class: PDE-5 inhibitor
- Mechanism of Action: Inhibits phosphodiesterase Type 5 which enhances the release of nitric oxide which is necessary for erection
- Common Uses: Erectile dysfunction, pulmonary arterial hypertension
- Memorable Side Effects: Low blood pressure, vision color changes (seeing blue tinges in vision), flushing
- Clinical Pearls:
  - Originally developed as a blood pressure medication; caution patients about risk of low blood pressure
  - Drug interaction with systemic nitrate/nitroglycerin products; advise patients about potential interaction and elevated risk of low blood pressure
  - Be sure to assess if other medications may be contributing to sexual dysfunction, antidepressants like SSRIs are a classic example)
- Monitoring: Blood pressure
- Drug and Diet Considerations:
  - Can be given with or without food
  - Grapefruit juice can increase concentrations

Silodosin (Rapaflo)
- Class: Alpha blocker
- Mechanism of Action: Blocks alpha receptors causing smooth muscle relaxation and opening of the ureter
- Common Uses: Treatment of BPH and urinary obstruction
- Memorable Side Effects: Low BP, dizziness
- Clinical Pearls:
  - Usually dosed at night to try to avoid/minimize orthostasis risk
  - More selective for the prostate than other alpha blockers, (i.e. terazosin or doxazosin) so less risk of lowering blood pressure

259

- o Anticholinergics and pseudoephedrine can worsen BPH causing the initiation or increase of alpha blockers
- o May also be used to help patients pass a ureteral stone, it relaxes the smooth muscle and opens up the ureter to ease flow
- o Potential floppy iris syndrome risk in patients undergoing certain eye procedures like cataract surgery
- Monitoring: Blood pressure, PSA as clinically indicated
- Drug and Diet Considerations:
  - o Give with food
  - o Grapefruit juice may increase concentrations

Simethicone (Gas-X, Mi-Acid, Gas Relief)

- Class: Anti-gas/flatulence agent
- Mechanism of Action: Reduces surface tension of air bubbles which lowers gas bubble formation in the gut
- Common Uses: Relief from bloating, excessive flatulence and pain from GI gas buildup
- Memorable Side Effects: Typically well tolerated
- Clinical Pearls:
  - o Some formulations may contain benzyl alcohol
- Monitoring: No routine monitoring is necessary
- Drug and Diet Considerations:
  - o Avoid drinks, particularly carbonated beverages, that may exacerbate gas
  - o Gas forming foods may worsen condition (i.e. beans, lentils, some green vegetables, lactose, fructose); often offending foods can be patient specific

Simvastatin (Zocor)

- Class: Antilipemic, statin
- Mechanism of Action: Inhibits HMG Co-A reductase to eventually decrease LDL
- Common Uses: Reduction of cholesterol, particularly LDL
- Memorable Side Effects: Muscle aches, rhabdomyolysis (rare but serious)
- Clinical Pearls:
  - o Statins, like simvastatin, are one of the mainstays of therapy to reduce cholesterol, and more particularly LDL (bad cholesterol)
  - o The most notable side effect with statins that you will likely hear patients complain about is myopathy (muscle aches/pain)
  - o Usually muscle aches are all over which can help you differentiate from other pain conditions or pain/soreness from an injury or overuse
  - o Contraindicated in pregnancy
  - o Patients who do not tolerate simvastatin, may try another statin as long as adverse effects aren't too severe (i.e. rhabdomyolysis); if you notice that the patient had an allergy or intolerance, you need to clarify with the provider
  - o CPK will be the primary lab to test for rhabdomyolysis, breakdown of muscle; this elevation in CPK may eventually lead to kidney failure
  - o Patients usually will present with myopathy when the medication is first started or increased, but be on the lookout for new medications

that can interact with some statins like CYP3A4 inhibitor drug interactions with medications like fluconazole or erythromycin (this will cause drug concentrations in the body to go up, potentially leading to toxicity)
- o Amiodarone, amlodipine and diltiazem are a few other common drug interactions with simvastatin, doses should be reduced or monitored for risk of toxicity
- o Gemfibrozil is a cholesterol medication that also interacts with simvastatin, this drug interaction should be addressed with the primary provider
- o Simvastatin will have maximal effects when given at night
- Monitoring: Lipids, LFTs, CPK if experiencing muscle pain (myopathy)
- Drug and Diet Considerations:
  - o Liver toxicity risk from excessive alcohol may be increased if used in combination with statins
  - o Low, often not clinically significant, risk of elevating blood sugars in patients with diabetes
  - o Grapefruit juice can significantly increase the concentrations of simvastatin, avoid using grapefruit juice
  - o Can be taken with or without food
  - o St. John's wort can lower concentrations of simvastatin
  - o Encourage a lipid lowering diet for any patient taking a cholesterol medication

Sitagliptin (Januvia)
- Class: Antidiabetic, DDP-4 inhibitor
- Mechanism of Action: Inhibits DPP-4 which increases incretin levels, incretin increases insulin and decreases glucagon in the body and also might help patients' stomachs "feel full"
- Common Uses: Treatment of type 2 diabetes
- Memorable Side Effects: GI (usually well tolerated), pancreatitis and cardiovascular concerns exist, but are rare
- Clinical Pearls:
  - o Usually fairly well tolerated, once daily dosing is nice for a diabetes medication
  - o Watch out for dose adjustment and accumulation in CKD
  - o Janumet is a one pill option for patients taking both sitagliptin and metformin
- Monitoring: Blood sugar, HbA1c, and renal function as clinically indicated
- Drug and Diet Considerations:
  - o Administer with or without food
  - o Implementation of a diabetic diet

Sodium Bicarbonate (Alka-Seltzer, Neut)
- Class: Antacid, alkalinizing agent
- Mechanism of Action: Bicarbonate will neutralize acid in the gut and also help raise pH in the blood stream
- Common Uses: Treatment of heartburn, stomach upset, metabolic acidosis; also added to acidic IV solutions as an alkalizing agent to raise pH and minimize patient discomfort at infusion site
- Memorable Side Effects: Hypernatremia, alkalosis, edema

- Clinical Pearls:
  - Alka-Seltzer is a brand name that has numerous products with multiple combinations of different medications
- Monitoring: Sodium, renal function, ABGs (as clinically indicated)
- Drug and Diet Considerations:
  - Be aware of dietary sodium load in combination with this medication, particularly in higher risk patients. (i.e. heart failure)

Sodium phosphate (Fleets enema)
- Class: Osmotic laxative
- Mechanism of Action: It works by pulling water into the gut which promotes motility and bowel movements
- Common Uses: Treatment of constipation
- Memorable Side Effects: Diarrhea, abdominal cramps, GI upset, hyperphosphatemia, hypokalemia
- Clinical Pearls:
  - Rare electrolyte imbalances have occurred with higher doses and long term use being the most likely culprits
  - Acute phosphate nephropathy can be one of those complications
  - Renal impairment may increase the risk of rare electrolyte complications
  - Over-the-counter availability
- Monitoring: Bowel movements, electrolytes and renal function as clinically indicated
- Drug and Diet Considerations:
  - Rare reports of significant electrolyte abnormalities can occur; particularly with sodium, phosphate, calcium, or potassium with poor renal function increasing this risk for abnormalities
  - Fluid loss may occur, assess fluid status

Sodium Polystyrene Sulfonate (SPS, Kayexalate)
- Class: Potassium binder
- Mechanism of Action: Reduces potassium levels by pulling potassium into the gut and not allowing it to be reabsorbed
- Common Uses: Treatment of hyperkalemia
- Memorable Side Effects: GI upset, changes in stool consistency, intestinal necrosis, hypokalemia, hypocalcemia, hypomagnesemia, elevated sodium,
- Clinical Pearls:
  - Generally not a first line agent for hyperkalemia
  - Not intended to reduce potassium levels in an emergency, life-threatening situation
  - Avoid in patients who have low gut motility or obstruction
  - May bind other drugs like thyroid medications
- Monitoring: EKG, electrolytes
- Drug and Diet Considerations:
  - Avoid excess potassium in the diet of a patient taking this medication

Sofosbuvir/velpatasvir (Epclusa)
- Class: Hepatitis C antiviral, polymerase inhibitor

- Mechanism of Action: Velpatasvir inhibits NS5A, which is a viral phosphoprotein necessary for replication, assembly, and viral secretion; sofosbuvir is incorporated into the RNA chain which ends the chain and leads to stoppage of the replication processes
- Common Uses: Treatment of hepatitis C
- Memorable Side Effects: Fatigue, headache, increase in LFTs
- Clinical Pearls:
  - Potential association with new onset diabetes
  - Boxed warning for risk of hepatitis B reactivation
  - Very high cure rates (~95%)
  - Duration of treatment ranges from 8 to 24 weeks, but typically 12 weeks
- Monitoring: CBC, liver function, renal function, INR, cardiac monitoring if using it with amiodarone
- Drug and Diet Considerations:
  - May be given with or without food
  - May alter blood sugars, monitor in patients with diabetes
  - Calcium supplements and antacids may reduce the absorption, separate by at least 4 hours

Solifenacin (Vesicare)
- Class: Bladder anticholinergic
- Mechanism of Action: Blocks muscarinic receptors in the bladder which increases urine volume in the bladder and potentially decreases frequency/urge
- Common Uses: Treatment of overactive bladder and bladder spasms
- Memorable Side Effects: Anticholinergic effects possible (i.e. dry mouth, dry eyes, urinary retention, constipation)
- Clinical Pearls:
  - Anticholinergic effects
  - Solifenacin is less likely to cause anticholinergic effects than older bladder agents like oxybutynin as it is more selective for the bladder
  - Long acting product available, nice for once daily dosing
  - Be sure to assess if the medication is working for incontinence/frequency
  - Keep an eye out for patients on diuretics; if frequency is the major issue, make sure that diuretics are at the minimum effective dose (not always possible to reduce diuretics with CHF history.)
  - Frequency can be especially problematic in patients who have an active social life as well as at night when trying to sleep
- Monitoring: LFTs as clinically indicated
- Drug and Diet Considerations:
  - Slows the motility of the GI tract which could increase the risk for constipation, maintain adequate fluids and non-constipating diet
  - If GI upset occurs, there are no issues in giving the drug with food
  - Dry mouth may increase thirst and alter taste/pleasure of food
  - Grapefruit juice may increase concentrations

Sotalol (Betapace)
- Class: Non-selective beta-blocker, Class 2 and 3 antiarrhythmic
- Mechanism of Action: Non-selective beta blockade leads to decreased AV node conduction, reduced heart rate, and lengthened sinus cycle

- Common Uses: Treatment of atrial fibrillation
- Memorable Side Effects: Low pulse, low BP, fatigue, arrhythmias, dyspnea
- Clinical Pearls:
    - Trick to remembering beta receptors: you have 1 heart and 2 lungs (beta-1 is primarily on the heart and beta-2 primarily in the lungs) – non selective beta blockers can contribute to airway restriction (beta-2) as well as lower cardiac output (beta-1)
    - Boxed warning for potential to produce life-threatening arrhythmias
    - Sotalol is an example of a beta blocker that is not selective for beta-1 receptors. It also blocks beta-2 receptors which makes it more likely that it could potentially exacerbate respiratory conditions like asthma
- Monitoring: Pulse, blood pressure, EKG, renal function, and electrolytes
- Drug and Diet Considerations:
    - Ideally give oral medication with food and water
    - Concentrations may be reduced if taken with food, consistency with or without food in administration is recommended

Spironolactone (Aldactone)
- Class: Antihypertensive, potassium sparing diuretic, aldosterone antagonist
- Mechanism of Action: Aldosterone antagonist that increases water and sodium excretion but spares potassium
- Common Uses: Treatment of heart failure and cirrhosis with ascites
- Memorable Side Effects: Hyperkalemia, gynecomastia, low BP, hyponatremia, dehydration
- Clinical Pearls:
    - Much like all diuretics, in relation to the effects on the kidney, the risk of overdiuresis (promoting too much fluid loss) is worsening kidney function by inadequate flow through the kidney
    - The development of gynecomastia and breast tenderness can be very troubling for male patients on spironolactone
    - We can often reduce the potassium supplementation burden, especially in patients on high doses of KCl supplements, by using potassium sparing diuretics
- Monitoring: Renal function, potassium, blood pressure
- Drug and Diet Considerations:
    - Be cautious and monitor potassium closely in patients with high dietary intake of potassium as this could contribute to hyperkalemia in combination with this medication
    - Consistent administration is recommended, but can be given with or without food

Sucralfate (Carafate)
- Class: Stomach protectant
- Mechanism of Action: Creates a film type barrier that coats the stomach and protects it from stomach acid
- Common Uses: Treatment of stomach ulcer and GI upset
- Memorable Side Effects: Constipation
- Clinical Pearls:
    - Frequent dosing bothersome for some patients (usually TID or QID)

- o Binding interactions possible, particularly with levothyroxine and warfarin, administer other medications 2 hours before giving sucralfate
- Monitoring: No routine lab monitoring
- Drug and Diet Considerations:
  - o Given on an empty stomach
  - o Aluminum levels may be increased with sucralfate and should be monitored in patients with reduced renal function
  - o May reduce fat soluble vitamin absorption (A, D, E, K)
  - o Phosphate absorption may be reduced
  - o Oral suspension contains sugar and should be monitored in diabetes

Sulfasalazine (Azulfidine)

- Class: 5-Aminosalicylic acid derivative (5-ASA compound), DMARD
- Mechanism of Action: Reduces inflammation by blocking cyclooxygenase and reducing prostaglandin production
- Common Uses: Treatment of inflammatory bowel disease, rheumatoid arthritis, psoriasis and psoriatic arthritis
- Memorable Side Effects: GI upset, rash, abnormal LFTs, folic acid deficiency, hematologic effects
- Clinical Pearls:
  - o Slow onset to beneficial effects
  - o Multiple daily doses required
  - o Be aware of patients who may have a sulfa allergy as there may be cross-reactivity risks
  - o Patients with G6PD deficiency may be at higher, dose dependent risk for hemolytic anemia
- Monitoring: LFTs, CBC, folic acid
- Drug and Diet Considerations:
  - o Give with food to reduce GI upset risk
  - o Folic acid supplementation may be necessary
  - o May impact appetite, be sure to monitor weight and nutritional status
  - o Crystalluria is possible, adequate hydration can help reduce this risk

Sulindac (Clinoril)

- Class: NSAID, analgesic
- Mechanism of Action: Inhibits Cyclooxygenase-1 and 2 (COX-1 and COX-2); resulting in a reduction of prostaglandins which cause pain, fever and inflammation
- Common Uses: Reduction of pain, fever and inflammation
- Memorable Side Effects: GI ulcer, worsening kidney function, edema, hypertension, inhibits platelets (can exacerbate bleed risk)
- Clinical Pearls:
  - o NSAIDs are one of the most common causes of GI bleeding; this risk increases in the elderly and those on medications that increase risk of bleeding (anticoagulants and antiplatelet medications)
  - o Due to effects on platelets, NSAIDs are typically held before/after surgery to reduce the risk of bleeding
  - o NSAIDs can contribute to edema and exacerbate CHF (congestive heart failure); be on the lookout and have NSAIDs reassessed if you

see a patient with a CHF exacerbation or a patient requiring increasing diuretics, like furosemide
- o NSAIDs can cause worsening kidney function (creatinine should be monitored); this risk can be greatly increased in patients on ACE inhibitors or ARBs and/or diuretic type medications
- o Due to above reasons on kidney function, GI bleed risk, and CHF, NSAIDs are not the safest medication in the elderly; acetaminophen is generally preferred for generalized pain with a few exceptions
- o Although generally considered riskier in the elderly, a big advantage of NSAIDs over acetaminophen is that they can reduce inflammation
- o Pregnancy category C/D when >30 weeks gestation; NSAIDs are generally avoided in pregnancy and especially after 30 weeks gestation
- Monitoring: Renal function, hemoglobin, platelets (contained within CBC), blood pressure, signs of bruising or bleeding, weight (risk for edema)
- Drug and Diet Considerations:
  - o Because of significant incidence of GI upset, it is recommended to give with food or milk
  - o Dehydration may exacerbate the risk for acute renal failure
  - o Excessive alcohol may increase GI bleed risk
  - o Vitamin E, Omega-3 fatty acids, gingko, garlic, ginseng, turmeric, and fish oil supplements have been purported to have antiplatelet type activity which in theory could increase the risk of bleed – clinical significance is questionable; the most common resolution is to discontinue the supplements if they are not necessary

Sumatriptan (Imitrex)

- Class: Anti-migraine, triptan
- Mechanism of Action: Serotonin 5HT agonist which causes vasoconstriction and reduction of inflammation associated with migraine
- Common Uses: Acute relief of migraine
- Memorable Side Effects: Dizziness, changes in CNS
- Clinical Pearls:
  - o Meant for acute relief of migraine, not prophylaxis
  - o Comes in multiple formulations such as oral tablet, injection and nasal spray as some may struggle with oral intake due nausea when they have a migraine
  - o Be sure to asses use, frequent use may indicate that a controller medication, like valproic acid, propranolol or topiramate, may need to be added to help prevent migraines
  - o Often used with NSAIDs, like naproxen, in migraine treatment
  - o Does have serotonin activity so could potentially contribute to serotonin syndrome (higher risk in patients already on SSRIs, tramadol etc.)
- Monitoring: Blood pressure, EKG when clinically indicated to assess risk for QTc prolongation
- Drug and Diet Considerations:
  - o Given as needed for migraine, so administration at any point is fine with regards to food

Tacrolimus (Prograf, Astagraf XL)

- Class: Immunosuppressant, calcineurin inhibitor
- Mechanism of Action: Blocks T-cell activation by binding the FKBP-12 protein as part of the process to inhibit calcineurin activity
- Common Uses: Organ rejection prevention
- Memorable Side Effects: Hypertension, immunosuppression, elevated lipids, hyperglycemia, hyperkalemia, GI upset, neurotoxicity
- Clinical Pearls:
  - Numerous drug interactions through CYP3A4 that can alter concentrations
  - Dosage forms have varying bioavailability, any changes should prompt close monitoring of levels
  - Astagraf XL has a boxed warning for malignancy and mortality in liver transplantation
  - QTc prolongation risk has been reported
  - Reassess drug levels to monitor adherence, when there is a change in drug therapy or new drug interactions that may alter concentrations
    - Adjusting of dose
    - Signs of toxicity or rejection
- Monitoring: Drug levels, blood sugars in diabetes patients, electrolytes, renal function, CBC, blood pressure, LFTs
- Drug and Diet Considerations:
  - Consistency of administration is critical, but can be given with or without meals
  - Grapefruit juice can raise concentrations, avoid its use
  - Be aware of blood glucose, lipid effects, and elevations of potassium in relation to diet and the use of this medication
  - Alcohol may alter the pharmacokinetics, so it is recommended to avoid use altogether

Tadalafil (Cialis)

- Class: PDE-5 inhibitor
- Mechanism of Action: Inhibits phosphodiesterase type 5 to release nitric oxide which is necessary for erection
- Common Uses: Treatment of erectile dysfunction, pulmonary arterial hypertension and BPH
- Memorable Side Effects: Low blood pressure, vision color changes (seeing blue tinges in vision), flushing
- Clinical Pearls:
  - Originally developed as a blood pressure medication; caution patients at risk of low blood pressure
  - Drug interaction with systemic nitrate/nitroglycerin products; it is important to advise patients about potential interaction and elevated risk of low blood pressure
  - Be sure to assess if other medications may be contributing to sexual dysfunction, antidepressants like SSRIs are a classic example
- Monitoring: Blood pressure
- Drug and Diet Considerations:
  - Can be given with or without food
  - Grapefruit juice can increase concentrations

Tamoxifen (Nolvadex)

- Class: Antineoplastic, selective estrogen receptor modulator
- Mechanism of Action: Binds estrogen receptors in cancerous cells which prevents tumor growth by blocking DNA synthesis
- Common Uses: Breast cancer treatment
- Memorable Side Effects: Menopausal-type symptoms such as hot flashes, DVT/PE risk (boxed warning), stroke (boxed warning), elevated triglycerides, hypertension, edema, GI upset
- Clinical Pearls:
  - Tamoxifen is a prodrug activated by CYP2D6, therefore, inhibitors like paroxetine, bupropion, and fluoxetine can reduce efficacy
- Monitoring: Bone mineral density, calcium, vitamin D levels, lipids, CBC, LFTs and pregnancy testing, when appropriate
- Drug and Diet Considerations:
  - Administer with or without food
  - Grapefruit juice may increase concentrations

Tamsulosin (Flomax)

- Class: Alpha blocker
- Mechanism of Action: Blocks alpha receptors causing smooth muscle relaxation and opening of the ureter
- Common Uses: Treatment of BPH and urinary obstruction
- Memorable Side Effects: Low BP, dizziness
- Clinical Pearls:
  - Usually dosed at night to try to avoid/minimize orthostasis risk
  - More selective for the prostate than other alpha blockers, like terazosin and doxazosin, so less risk of lowering blood pressure
  - Anticholinergics and pseudoephedrine can worsen BPH causing the initiation or increase of alpha blockers like tamsulosin
  - May also be used to help patients pass a ureteral stone by relaxing the smooth muscle to open up the ureter and ease flow
- Monitoring: Blood pressure
- Drug and Diet Considerations:
  - Give 30 minutes after eating

Telmisartan (Micardis)

- Class: Antihypertensive, ARB
- Mechanism of Action: Blocks the angiotensin 2 (vasoconstrictor) receptor which ends up preventing vasoconstriction and aldosterone release to ultimately lower blood pressure
- Common Uses: Treatment of hypertension and heart failure
- Memorable Side Effects: Hyperkalemia, exacerbate/worsen kidney function, low blood pressure
- Clinical Pearls:
  - When you think of ARBs and ACE inhibitors, you can lump the side effects together as they are overall the same
  - One major exception to the above rule is the side effect of cough; patients who encounter this adverse effect from an ACE inhibitor may use an ARB as an alternative antihypertensive

- o Kidney function changes and monitoring of potassium is critical when doses are changed or an ARB is initiated
- o This worsening kidney function risk increases in patients who may be taking NSAIDs and/or diuretics
- o As with any medication used to treat hypertension, we need to educate our patients to rise slowly when getting up to minimize risk of orthostatic (sometimes called postural) hypotension
- Monitoring: Renal function, potassium, blood pressure
- Drug and Diet Considerations:
  - o Be cautious and monitor potassium closely in patients with high dietary intake of potassium as this could contribute to hyperkalemia in combination with this medication
  - o Administer with or without food

Temazepam (Restoril)
- Class: Benzodiazepine
- Mechanism of Action: Enhances activity of GABA (an inhibitory neurotransmitter that causes sedation)
- Common Uses: Treatment of insomnia
- Memorable Side Effects: Sedation, confusion, fall risk, dizziness,
- Clinical Pearls:
  - o Typically ONLY used for insomnia, not anxiety or seizures
  - o The best way I remember benzodiazepines is that they are very close to "alcohol in a pill"
  - o Sedation, confusion, slurred speech, trouble walking (ataxia), etc. are all common with benzos/alcohol
  - o Be cautious with patients on higher doses of benzodiazepines to make sure they aren't abruptly stopped
  - o Educate patients on driving/operating machinery risks
  - o Fall risk in the elderly is a big downside to using these medications
  - o Benzos are a controlled substance, they can cause addiction and dependence
  - o Flumazenil is antidote in overdose
- Monitoring: Routine lab monitoring typically isn't necessary unless clinically indicated
- Drug and Diet Considerations:
  - o Alcohol intake can have additive side effects of sedation, confusion, slurred speech, and other CNS depressant effects

Tenofovir alafenamide (Vemlidy, TAF)
- Class: Antiretroviral, nucleotide reverse transcriptase inhibitor (NRTI)
- Mechanism of Action: Phosphorylated to tenofovir diphosphate which blocks the action of viral DNA polymerase which prevents viral replication
- Common Uses: Treatment of HIV and hepatitis B
- Memorable Side Effects: Lactic acidosis/fatty liver warning, osteoporosis, GI adverse effects, elevation in cholesterol, fatigue, neuropathy, darkening of skin, renal toxicity
- Clinical Pearls:
  - o In combination products such as Stribild
  - o Boxed warning on risk of hepatitis B exacerbations

- o Reduced risk of renal and bone toxicity compared to tenofovir disoproxil fumarate
- Monitoring: Liver function, HIV viral load, CD4 count, renal function, hepatitis B testing prior to initiation, phosphorous
- Drug and Diet Considerations:
  - o May be given with or without meals
  - o Monitor cholesterol and implement cholesterol lowering diet in patients who may have elevated levels due to the adverse effects of the drug
  - o Assess dietary calcium and vitamin D intake, inadequate intake may place the patient at higher risk for reduced bone mineral density with this medication (less risk than tenofovir disoproxil fumarate)

Tenofovir disoproxil fumarate (Viread, TDF)
- Class: Antiretroviral, nucleotide reverse transcriptase inhibitor (NRTI)
- Mechanism of Action: Phosphorylated to tenofovir diphosphate which blocks the action of viral DNA polymerase which prevents viral replication
- Common Uses: Treatment of HIV and hepatitis B
- Memorable Side Effects: Lactic acidosis/fatty liver warning, osteoporosis, GI adverse effects, elevated cholesterol, fatigue, neuropathy, darkening of skin, renal toxicity
- Clinical Pearls:
  - o In combination products such as Atripla
  - o Rare reports of pancreatitis
  - o Boxed warning on risk of hepatitis B exacerbations
  - o Increased risk for renal toxicity when used in combination with NSAIDs
- Monitoring: Liver function, HIV viral load, CD4 count, renal function, hepatitis B testing prior to initiation
- Drug and Diet Considerations:
  - o Tablets may be given with or without meals, powder to be given with food
  - o Monitor cholesterol and implement cholesterol lowering diet in patients who may have elevated levels due to the adverse effects of the drug
  - o Assess dietary calcium and vitamin D intake, inadequate intake may place the patient at higher risk for reduced bone mineral density with this medication

Terazosin (Hytrin)
- Class: Antihypertensive, alpha blocker
- Mechanism of Action: Blocks alpha receptors causing smooth muscle relaxation, vasodilation, and opening of the ureter
- Common Uses: Treatment of BPH, urinary obstruction and hypertension
- Memorable Side Effects: Low BP, dizziness
- Clinical Pearls:
  - o Non-selective alpha blocker, so can be used for both hypertension and BPH
  - o Risk of orthostasis higher with a non-selective alpha blocker like terazosin

- o In the case of worsening urinary retention due to BPH and initiation of these agents, be sure to assess if your patient is on anticholinergic medications (diphenhydramine, TCA's, etc.)
  - o Usually dosed at night to minimize the risk of orthostasis
- Monitoring: Blood pressure
- Drug and Diet Considerations:
  - o Administer with or without food

Terbinafine (Lamisil)
- Class: Antifungal
- Mechanism of Action: Inhibits squalene epoxidase which is an important enzyme in the production of sterol in fungi; ergosterol, a necessary component of the fungal cell membrane is not formed by this inhibition
- Common Uses: Treatment of onychomycosis and severe cases of athlete's foot
- Memorable Side Effects: GI upset, elevated LFTs
- Clinical Pearls: Avoid use in patient with significant liver disease
- Monitoring: LFTs, CBC
- Drug and Diet Considerations:
  - o Can be given with or without food
  - o Alcohol may exacerbate the risk for liver complications, generally avoid
  - o Alterations in taste have been reported

Teriparatide (Forteo)
- Class: Parathyroid analog
- Mechanism of Action: Teriparatide has anabolic effects and works on building bone by stimulating osteoblasts
- Common Uses: Treatment of osteoporosis
- Memorable Side Effects: Risk of osteosarcoma (boxed warning), hypercalcemia, dizziness, GI upset, injection reaction, low blood pressure
- Clinical Pearls:
  - o Injection given once daily
  - o ONLY use for 2 years due to the risk for osteosarcoma
- Monitoring: Bone mineral density, calcium, vitamin D levels, blood pressure
- Drug and Diet Considerations:
  - o Ensure the patient has adequate vitamin D and calcium intake, at least 1,200 mg per day of calcium and 1,000 units of vitamin D in females with osteoporosis
  - o Give with or without food (injection)

Testosterone (Androgel, Androderm)
- Class: Androgen
- Mechanism of Action: Testosterone hormone responsible for development of male sex organs and muscle growth
- Common Uses: Treatment of testosterone deficiency and metastatic breast cancer
- Memorable Side Effects: Gynecomastia, hypertension, acne, mood changes
- Clinical Pearls:
  - o Drug of abuse in sports to increase muscle mass and boost performance

271

- o Schedule 3 controlled substance due to the risk of abuse
- o Testosterone can "amp" you up; think of "Roid Rage" – increased BP, irritability, mood swings, anger, etc.
- o Risk of DVT is possible, but rare
- o Increase in PSA and possible impotence especially with prolonged use
- Monitoring: Blood pressure, LFTs, lipids, electrolytes, blood sugar in patients with diabetes, bone mineral density, hemoglobin and hematocrit
- Drug and Diet Considerations:
  - o Numerous drug formulations (IM, nasal, buccal, subQ, topical); oral capsule can have lower absorption with fatty foods

Tetracycline (Sumycin)

- Class: Tetracycline, antibiotic
- Mechanism of Action: Inhibits bacterial protein synthesis
- Common Uses: Treatment of acne, skin infections and Helicobacter pylori
- Memorable Side Effects: GI side effects, photosensitivity (increased risk of sunburn), rash
- Clinical Pearls:
  - o Can cause birth defects (category D)
  - o Can make patients more susceptible to sunburn
  - o Long term use or multiple courses may cause tooth and skin discoloration
- Monitoring: LFTs, renal function, and CBC (only in cases with clinical concerns or in long term therapy)
- Drug and Diet Considerations:
  - o Avoid timing calcium, iron, magnesium, zinc, and antacids at the same time as tetracycline; take these medications at least 2 hours before or 4-6 hours after tetracycline to ensure adequate absorption
  - o Take with a full glass of water to avoid GI irritation
  - o Take on an empty stomach

Theophylline (Theochron, Elixophyllin, Theo-24)

- Class: PDE inhibitor
- Mechanism of Action: Inhibition of phosphodiesterase enzymes causes smooth muscle relaxation and bronchodilation
- Common Uses: Treatment of asthma and COPD
- Memorable Side Effects: Insomnia, anxiety, tachycardia, GI upset, tremor
- Clinical Pearls:
  - o Rarely used due to significant systemic adverse effects compared to newer inhaled medications
  - o Significant drug interactions exist
  - o Elderly are at higher risk for toxicity and complications
- Monitoring: Drug levels, heart rate, respirations
- Drug and Diet Considerations:
  - o Alcohol may increase drug concentrations
  - o Caffeine may exacerbate systemic effects such as tachycardia
  - o Monitor dietary changes as a high protein diet may reduce drug levels and a high carbohydrate diet may increase drug levels

Thiamine (Vitamin B1)
- Class: Vitamin
- Mechanism of Action: Important cofactor in metabolizing carbohydrates
- Common Uses: Supplementation in thiamine deficiency, Wernicke encephalopathy and alcohol use disorder
- Memorable Side Effects: Usually well tolerated, sweating, flushing type reaction with injection, stomach upset with oral replacement
- Clinical Pearls:
  - Being a cofactor in carbohydrate metabolism, as carbohydrate intake increases, the patient may require more thiamine
  - Target RDA is in the range of 1-1.5 mg for most adults depending upon the population, pregnancy and breast-feeding typically require the upper end
  - Water soluble
- Monitoring: Normal levels of thiamine range between 1.1 – 1.6 mg/dL
- Drug and Diet Considerations:
  - Patients with alcohol use disorder may be at risk for thiamine deficiency
  - Oral absorption is acceptable

Ticagrelor (Brilinta)
- Class: Antiplatelet, thienopyridine
- Mechanism of Action: Blocks ADP receptors which leads to inhibition of platelets
- Common Uses: MI and stroke prevention
- Memorable Side Effects: Bleeding (GI, nose bleeds, etc.)
- Clinical Pearls:
  - Due to its ability to inhibit platelets, the major complication is bleeding; assess patients for bruising, blood in the stool or any abnormal sign of bleeding
  - Can increase uric acid
  - Boxed warning for reduced effectiveness when patients are using aspirin doses greater than 100 mg
  - Metabolized via CYP3A4, this is a major pathway and presents with drug interaction risks
- Monitoring: CBC with platelets
- Drug and Diet Considerations:
  - Grapefruit juice may increase effects
  - Generally avoid supplements that may be associated with antiplatelet activity such as ginseng, garlic, glucosamine, vitamin E, etc. or at a minimum, monitor for bruising and bleed risk
  - Can be administered with or without food

Tiotropium (Spiriva)
- Class: Inhaled anticholinergic
- Mechanism of Action: Inhaled anticholinergic can open up airways and decrease secretions
- Common Uses: Treatment of COPD
- Memorable Side Effects: Dry mouth, cough, irritation to the lungs, usually well tolerated due to limited systemic absorption

- Clinical Pearls:
    - Tiotropium is primarily used for COPD, and because it has anticholinergic activity, it can help dry up the airways as well as open them up to allow for better breathing in patients who have thick mucus/sputum
    - It is long acting and meant to be used as a controller medication
    - It is not meant to be a rescue inhalation product as it will not provide acute relief from respiratory distress
    - Often by using this medication in COPD, our goal is likely to improve respiratory status, but also to reduce the amount of as needed albuterol and/or albuterol/ipratropium (Duoneb or Combivent)
    - Tiotropium comes with a special delivery device and capsules; to prepare the device for use, the capsules are inserted into the device and punctured for the contents to be inhaled by the patient
    - With the delivery device, it is imperative to assess if patients are able to adequately coordinate how to use the device, as well as if they are able to inhale quickly and forcefully enough to get the drug into their lungs
    - Systemic anticholinergic effects are usually not a concern as systemic absorption is low
- Monitoring: FEV1, peak flow
- Drug and Diet Considerations:
    - Inhaled, local medication, no notable drug/diet considerations
    - Dry mouth may impact dietary/fluid intake

Tiotropium and Oladaterol (Stiolto)

- Class: Inhaled anticholinergic and long acting beta-agonist
- Mechanism of Action: Provides anti-cholinergic effects and stimulates beta-2 receptors leading to relaxation of smooth muscle and opening of airways
- Common Uses: Treatment of COPD
- Memorable Side Effects: Tachycardia, tremor, anxiousness, hypokalemia (rare), hyperglycemia (rare), dry mouth
- Clinical Pearls:
    - See tiotropium (Spiriva) for further information on this medication
- Monitoring: Frequency of use, FEV1, peak-flow, pulse, blood pressure, and potassium (usually only necessary in high dosages), blood glucose (rarely clinically significant)
- Drug and Diet Considerations:
    - Assess potassium intake and blood levels of potassium if the patient is using a beta agonist frequently or has a history of hypokalemia
    - Be aware of caffeine intake in combination with a beta-agonist as it can have an additive effect on blood pressure and heart rate
    - Monitor diabetes patients for elevations in blood sugar
    - See tiotropium (Spiriva) for further information on this medication

Tobramycin

- Class: Aminoglycoside, antibiotic
- Mechanism of Action: Blocks bacterial protein synthesis
- Common Uses: Treatment of infections from gram negative bacteria such as, UTI's, sepsis and skin infections

274

- Memorable Side Effects: CNS changes, diarrhea, kidney impairment, changes in hearing
- Clinical Pearls:
  - Classic nephrotoxic drug so kidney function monitoring is critical
  - Monitoring of drug levels are also important
  - Usual trough target is less than 2mcg/mL
  - Ototoxicity (ear) is more likely with prolonged use
  - Peak sample usually drawn 30 minutes after infusion is complete and trough right before the next dose
- Monitoring: Renal function, drug levels, hearing test in patients on long-term therapy, electrolytes
- Drug and Diet Considerations:
  - Dehydration may exacerbate the risk of renal impairment caused by gentamicin
  - Supplementation of certain electrolytes might be considered if clinically indicated (potassium, magnesium, or calcium)
  - Monitor for anorexia risk with long term use

Tolterodine (Detrol LA, Detrol)
- Class: Bladder anticholinergic
- Mechanism of Action: Blocks muscarinic receptors in the bladder which increases urine volume in the bladder and potentially decreases frequency/urge
- Common Uses: Treatment of overactive bladder and bladder spasms
- Memorable Side Effects: Anticholinergic effects possible (i.e. dry mouth, dry eyes, urinary retention, constipation)
- Clinical Pearls:
  - Tolterodine is less likely to cause anticholinergic effects than older bladder agents like oxybutynin as it is more selective for the bladder
  - Long acting product available which is nice for once daily dosing
  - Be sure to assess if the medication is working for incontinence/frequency
  - Keep an eye out for patients on diuretics, if frequency is the major issue, make sure that diuretics are at the minimum effective dose (not always possible to reduce diuretics with CHF history, etc.)
  - Frequency can be especially problematic in patients who have an active social life as well as night when trying to sleep
- Monitoring: Renal function as clinically indicated
- Drug and Diet Considerations:
  - Slows the motility of the GI tract which could increase the risk for constipation, maintain adequate fluids and non-constipating diet
  - If GI upset occurs, there are no issues in giving the drug with food
  - Dry mouth may increase thirst and alter taste/pleasure of food

Topiramate (Topamax)
- Class: Antiepileptic
- Mechanism of Action: Not well understood; possible effects on sodium channels as well as GABA receptors
- Common Uses: Treatment of seizures and migraine prophylaxis
- Memorable Side Effects: Cognitive impairment, sedation
- Clinical Pearls:

- Cognitive slowing is probably the most concerning adverse effect for patients
- With the indication of migraines being a common issue with women of child-bearing age, be sure to remember that topiramate can reduce the effects of estrogen containing birth control
- Used for migraine prophylaxis, NOT acute relief
- With any medication being used to treat seizures, it is very important to not abruptly stop a medication unless there is a very good reason, such as a serious side effect
- Weight loss could potentially be a beneficial adverse effect in an overweight seizure or migraine patient
- Monitoring: Electrolytes (including bicarbonate), pH (risk for acidosis), weight
- Drug and Diet Considerations:
  - Can be given with or without food
  - Alcohol can have additive CNS depressant effects
  - High-fat, high protein, low-carb (ketogenic) diets may increase the risk for acidosis and/or renal stones
  - Adequate hydration can help reduce the risk of renal stones

Topotecan (Hycamtin)
- Class: Oncology agent, topoisomerase 1 inhibitor
- Mechanism of Action: Inhibits topoisomerase 1 which blocks the formation of the DNA strand
- Common Uses: Treatment of cervical, ovarian, and certain lung cancers, off-label for numerous types of other cancers
- Memorable Side Effects: Myelosuppression, nausea, vomiting, diarrhea, hair loss, anemia, thrombocytopenia
- Clinical Pearls:
  - Boxed warning for the risk of myelosuppression
- Monitoring: CBC, renal function, electrolytes, LFTs
- Drug and Diet Considerations:
  - Diarrhea can cause substantial fluid loss and electrolyte deficiencies, monitor and replace as appropriate
  - Weight loss and poor nutrition may result on account of nausea and vomiting adverse effects

Torsemide (Demedex)
- Class: Loop diuretic
- Mechanism of Action: Inhibits sodium and chloride reabsorption in the ascending "Loop" of Henle in the kidney
- Common Use: Treatment of edema, hypertension and heart failure
- Memorable Side Effects: Frequent urination, electrolyte depletion, low blood pressure, dehydration and renal impairment
- Clinical Pearls:
  - While furosemide can cause significant reductions in magnesium, calcium, and sodium, potassium is one of the most important electrolytes to monitor and often patients require potassium supplementation; this can sometimes be offset by potassium sparing diuretics, like spironolactone, ARBs, like losartan, and ACE inhibitors, like lisinopril (all potentially increase potassium)
  - Frequent urination can be significantly upsetting to patients and can greatly impact their wellbeing, including upsetting their sleep; make

sure these loop diuretics are not being given too close to bedtime if possible
- o Whenever you see a new Rx for a loop diuretic, be sure to look at the other medications the patient is taking to make sure that the edema is not a side effect; classic causes of edema include calcium channel blockers, pioglitazone, pregabalin, and NSAIDs.
- o Loops deplete volume in the body, so patients run the risk of not having adequate perfusion through the kidney; elevations in creatinine from baseline can help us monitor for this risk
- o Kidney function and electrolytes are going to be the primary labs to monitor
- o Urinary output and monitoring of weights can be very important patient factors to monitor and help assess the efficacy of how well the loop diuretic (or any diuretic) is working
- Monitoring: Renal function, electrolytes, weights, blood pressure, and hearing (when used at high doses)
- Drug and Diet Considerations:
  - o Potassium supplementation is usually required as torsemide can cause significant hypokalemia
  - o Monitor for dehydration warning signs
  - o With or without food is acceptable

Tramadol (Ultram)
- Class: Opioid, analgesic
- Mechanism of Action: Binds opioid receptors inhibiting CNS pain pathways which provides pain relief
- Common Uses: Management of pain disorders, both chronic and acute
- Memorable Side Effects: Constipation, sedation, respiratory depression, increases seizures risk, CNS effects like confusion, delirium
- Clinical Pearls:
  - o Has opioid like effects, so this medication is going to be a potential risk for abuse, drug diversion, addiction and dependence
  - o Tramadol is notoriously known for lowering seizure threshold (increasing risk of seizure); if you see a patient who has a seizure diagnosis or is on seizure medications, be sure that the risk versus benefit of tramadol is addressed
  - o Confusion, GI upset, constipation, lethargy can be problematic especially in our elderly population; there is a lower recommended maximum dose in the elderly – 300 mg versus 400 mg daily
  - o Naloxone is reversal agent for opioids
  - o Can be used on an as needed basis as this medication works fairly quickly
  - o It is not as highly controlled by the DEA as other medications in the opioid class (i.e. fentanyl, oxycodone, morphine) – It is a schedule 4 controlled substance where other opioids are schedule 2 controlled substances
  - o Can be given in combination with non-opioid analgesics like acetaminophen
  - o Tramadol can increase the risk of serotonin syndrome, and this is especially true at higher doses and patients who are already receiving other medications that can increase serotonin (i.e. SSRIs or SNRIs)

277

- Monitoring: Bowel movements, pain management, risk for addiction, blood pressure as clinically indicated
- Drug and Diet Considerations:
  - Alcohol can exacerbate the CNS depressant effect from tramadol
  - Giving with food and water can reduce the risk of GI upset
  - Encourage a constipation friendly diet including fiber, fluids, and exercise as tramadol can be very constipating

Tranylcypromine (Parnate)

- Class: Mono-amine oxidase inhibitor, antidepressant
- Mechanism of Action: Inhibits the action of monoamine oxidase which increases the CNS neurotransmitters serotonin, norepinephrine, and epinephrine
- Common Uses: Treatment of depression
- Memorable Side Effects: Nausea, dizziness, blood pressure fluctuations, hypertension (with tyramine), hypotension, tachycardia, unusual behavior, SIADH (hyponatremia), serotonin syndrome
- Clinical Pearls:
  - Boxed warning for increased risk of suicidal thoughts in pediatric patients and young adults
  - Avoid use of other serotonergic agents (i.e. SSRIs)
  - Not a first line agent in depression due to adverse effect profile, diet interactions, and drug interactions
- Monitoring: Blood pressure, pulse, electrolytes (as clinically indicated), renal function, LFTs
- Drug and Diet Considerations:
  - Patch may be administered consistently without regard to meals while oral disintegrating tablet is typically given before breakfast
  - Alcohol should be avoided as it may increase risk for toxicity
  - MAOI/Tyramine interaction (less likely than traditional MAOIs)
    - Avoid foods high in tyramine: fermented, cured, aged foods such as cheese, smoked meats/fish, beer
    - Reaction: tachycardia, N/V, headache
    - Risk of reaction increases as the dose of the medication increases
  - Food and beverages with significant amounts of caffeine, tyrosine, phenylalanine, dopamine, or tryptophan may also cause elevated blood pressure

Travoprost (Travatan)

- Class: Prostaglandin
- Mechanism of Action: Prostaglandin F2 alpha analog which decreases intraocular pressure
- Common Uses: Treatment of glaucoma
- Memorable Side Effects: Change in eye color, eye irritation
- Clinical Pearls:
  - Change in eye color to brown may be permanent
  - Many glaucoma patients will be on multiple eye drops; at least 5 minutes is the appropriate amount of time to wait between drops
- Monitoring: Eye exams, intraocular pressure
- Drug and Diet Considerations:
  - No notable concerns

Trazodone (Desyrel)

- Class: Antidepressant
- Mechanism of Action: Inhibits reuptake of serotonin, but differs from SSRIs in that it has blocking activity on H1 and alpha 1 receptors, H1 blocking activity gives this medication its sedative properties
- Common Uses: Treatment of insomnia and depression
- Memorable Side Effects: Sedation, dizziness, orthostasis
- Clinical Pearls:
  - While it is usually classified as an antidepressant, trazodone at lower doses is most frequently used for insomnia
  - Usually the antidepressant benefits of trazodone are seen at higher doses
  - Must educate patients on its sedative properties and risk of driving, etc.
  - Trazodone can be used "prn" or as needed for sleep, but you should never see it used as needed for depression as it usually takes significant time (like SSRIs) for the antidepressant effect to begin
  - Keep an eye out for postural hypotension (dizziness upon rising) especially in our elderly patients and those already on blood pressure lowering medications; remember from the mechanism of action above, it does have alpha blocking activity
  - Trazodone can contribute to dry mouth, be on the lookout for patients who complain about this or are using saliva substitute medications, like Biotene
- Monitoring: Blood pressure, LFTs as clinically indicated
- Drug and Diet Considerations:
  - Give with a meal or small snack to reduce the risk for orthostasis
  - Alcohol can increase the CNS depressant effect

Triamcinolone (Kenalog)

- Class: Topical corticosteroid
- Mechanism of Action: Suppresses mediators of inflammation (histamine, kinins, prostaglandins, etc.) resulting in less inflammation/redness
- Common Uses: Treatment of dermatitis
- Memorable Side Effects: Local irritation; increased risk of adrenal suppression, HPA-axis suppression with prolonged use and/or application to large areas
- Clinical Pearls:
  - If patients don't see improvement in condition in 1-2 weeks, be sure they know to get reassessed
  - Long term use, especially if large amounts are applied, can lead to significant systemic absorption and can suppress the HPA axis
  - Long term use is probably more concerning in young children
  - Systemic problems not likely if used short term
- Monitoring: If excessive use, monitor HPA suppression risk
- Drug and Diet Considerations:
  - No notable diet issues as this is a topical agent

Triamterene/hydrochlorothiazide (Dyazide)

- Class: Triamterene – potassium sparing diuretic; HCTZ – See Hydrochlorothiazide
- Mechanism of Action: Triamterene is a potassium sparing diuretic that blocks sodium channels in the kidney; hydrochlorothiazide is a thiazide diuretic
- Common Uses: Treatment of hypertension and edema
- Memorable Side Effects: Triamterene (hyperkalemia), HCTZ (hypokalemia), dehydration (rising creatinine and BUN), low blood pressure, orthostasis risk, electrolyte imbalances
- Clinical Pearls:
    - Much like all diuretics, in relation to the effects on the kidney, the risk of overdiuresis is worsening kidney function
    - We can often reduce the potassium supplementation burden, especially patients on high doses of KCl supplements, by using potassium sparing diuretics
    - Triamterene, while generally lumped into the group of potassium sparing diuretics because it causes elevations in potassium, does have a slightly different mechanism of action; it acts on sodium channels in the late distal convoluted tubule and unlike spironolactone, it does not compete with aldosterone
    - Patients often forget they are actually on two medications when they are used in combination in one pill
    - See HCTZ (hydrochlorothiazide) alone for its clinical pearls
- Monitoring: Electrolytes, renal function, blood pressure, weight
- Drug and Diet Considerations:
    - Can be given with food to minimize risk for GI upset
    - Potassium levels can go up on account of triamterene and down on account of hydrochlorothiazide, monitor dietary potassium intake and blood levels
    - Risk for weight loss (primarily through diuresis)
    - See hydrochlorothiazide

Triazolam (Halcion)

- Class: Benzodiazepine
- Mechanism of Action: Enhances activity of GABA, an inhibitory neurotransmitter that causes sedation
- Common Uses: Treatment of insomnia
- Memorable Side Effects: Sedation, confusion, fall risk, dizziness
- Clinical Pearls:
    - Typically ONLY used for insomnia (not anxiety or seizures)
    - The best way I remember benzodiazepines is that they are very close to "alcohol in a pill"
    - Sedation, confusion, slurred speech, trouble walking (ataxia), etc. are all common with benzos/alcohol
    - Be cautious with patients on higher doses of benzodiazepines to make sure they aren't abruptly stopped
    - Educate patients on driving/operating machinery risks
    - Fall risk in the elderly is a big downside to using these medications
    - Benzos are a controlled substance, they can cause addiction and dependence
    - Flumazenil is antidote in overdose

- Monitoring: Routine lab monitoring typically isn't necessary unless clinically indicated
- Drug and Diet Considerations:
    - Alcohol intake can have additive side effects of sedation, confusion, slurred speech, and other CNS depressant effects
    - Grapefruit juice can increase concentrations
    - Give on an empty stomach, typically at bedtime as it is only used for insomnia

Trihexyphenidyl (Artane)
- Class: Anticholinergic, anti-Parkinson's agent
- Mechanism of Action: Blocks muscarinic (anticholinergic) receptors and also has antihistamine effects
- Common Uses: Management of EPS associated with antipsychotic medications, Parkinsonism
- Memorable Side Effects: Anticholinergic, sedation
- Clinical Pearls:
    - Highly anticholinergic so lookout for dry eyes, dry mouth, constipation, urinary retention and confusion/fall risk
    - Rarely used for Parkinson's because of the anticholinergic impacts in the elderly
    - Most common clinical use is for extrapyramidal disorders (movement side effects with antipsychotics)
- Monitoring: Pulse
- Drug and Diet Considerations:
    - Slows the motility of the GI tract which could increase the risk for constipation, maintain adequate fluids and non-constipating diet
    - If GI upset occurs, no issues in giving the drug with food
    - Dry mouth may increase thirst and alter taste/pleasure of food
    - May be given with or without food
    - Alcohol may exacerbate CNS depressant effects

Trimethobenzamide (Tigan)
- Class: Antiemetic
- Mechanism of Action: Acts centrally in the chemoreceptor trigger zone by stopping emesis signals; also may have dopamine blocking activity
- Common Uses: Treatment of nausea/vomiting
- Memorable Side Effects: Diarrhea, injection site reaction and hypotension (IM), dizziness, sedation, EPS symptoms
- Clinical Pearls:
    - Use with caution in patients with movement disorders, like Parkinson's
- Monitoring: Kidney function, LFTs as clinically indicated
- Drug and Diet Considerations:
    - If vomiting is problematic, there is an injectable form
    - With or without food is acceptable
    - Alcohol intake may exacerbate CNS depressant activity

Trimethoprim (Trimpex)
- Class: Antibiotic

- Mechanism of Action: Inhibits dihydrofolate reductase which prevents formation of bacterial tetrahydrofolic acid, a necessary component for cell growth and reproduction
- Common Uses: Treatment of UTIs
- Memorable Side Effects: GI, rash, CNS changes, phototoxicity
- Clinical Pearls:
  - Often used in combination with sulfamethoxazole
  - Trimethoprim can increase risk for hyperkalemia in patients on ACEIs, ARBs, potassium supplements, and potassium sparing diuretics
- Monitoring: Potassium, renal function, LFTs, CBC as clinically indicated
- Drug and Diet Considerations:
  - Long term trimethoprim can reduce folic acid levels
  - Hyperkalemia can result on account of trimethoprim, be aware of any dietary changes that may impact potassium levels
  - May increase the risk for hypoglycemia in patients taking diabetes medications
  - May take with or without food

Trimethoprim/sulfamethoxazole (Bactrim)
- Class: Antibiotic
- Mechanism of Action: Sulfamethoxazole inhibits bacterial folic acid production, trimethoprim essentially does the same via a different mechanism
- Common Uses: Treatment of UTIs, upper respiratory infections (URIs) and PCP (common in HIV patients)
- Memorable Side Effects: GI, rash, CNS changes
- Clinical Pearls:
  - Very common treatment for UTI
  - Sulfa allergy is common in many patients, be aware and check allergy list
  - Major drug interaction with warfarin, may increase INR
  - Has some activity against MRSA
  - Trimethoprim can increase risk for hyperkalemia in patients on ACEIs, ARBs, potassium supplements, and potassium sparing diuretics
- Monitoring: Potassium, renal function, CBC as clinically indicated
- Drug and Diet Considerations:
  - Long term trimethoprim can reduce folic acid levels
  - Hyperkalemia can result on account of trimethoprim
  - Adequate hydration and taking the medication with water is important to reduce the risk of kidney stones
  - May increase the risk for hypoglycemia in patients taking diabetes medications
  - May take with or without food

Trospium (Sanctura)
- Class: Bladder anticholinergic
- Mechanism of Action: Blocks muscarinic receptors (anticholinergic medication) in the bladder which increases urine volume in the bladder and potentially decreases frequency/urge
- Common Uses: Treatment of overactive bladder and bladder spasms

- Memorable Side Effects: Anticholinergic effects possible (i.e. dry mouth, dry eyes, urinary retention, constipation)
- Clinical Pearls:
  - Anticholinergic effects
  - Trospium is less likely to cause anticholinergic effects than older bladder agents like oxybutynin as it is more selective for the bladder
  - Be sure to assess if the medication is working for incontinence/frequency
  - Keep an eye out for patients on diuretics and if frequency is the major issue, make sure that diuretics are at the minimum effective dose (not always possible to reduce diuretics with CHF history etc.)
  - Frequency can be especially problematic in patients who have an active social life as well as at night when trying to sleep
  - Trospium is least likely to penetrate CNS and cause confusion and other CNS side effects
- Monitoring: Renal function as clinically indicated, LFTs
- Drug and Diet Considerations:
  - Slows the motility of the GI tract which could increase the risk for constipation, maintain adequate fluids and non-constipating diet
  - Take with water, 1 hour before meals
  - Dry mouth may increase thirst and alter taste/pleasure of food

Umeclidinium (Incruse Ellipta)
- Class: Inhaled anticholinergic
- Mechanism of Action: Inhaled anticholinergic can open up airways and decrease secretions
- Common Uses: Treatment of COPD
- Memorable Side Effects: Dry mouth, cough, irritation to the lungs; usually well tolerated due to minimal systemic absorption
- Clinical Pearls:
  - Umeclidinium is primarily used for COPD, and because it has anticholinergic activity, it can help dry up the airways as well as open them up to allow for better breathing in patients who have think mucous/sputum
  - It is long acting and meant to be used as a controller medication
  - It will not provide acute relief from respiratory distress, not meant to be a rescue inhalation product
  - Often by using this medication in COPD, our goal is likely to improve respiratory status, but also to reduce the amount of as needed albuterol and/or albuterol/ipratropium (Duoneb or Combivent)
  - With the delivery device, it is imperative to assess if patients are able to adequately coordinate how to use the device as well as if they are able to inhale quickly and forcefully enough to get the drug into their lungs
  - Systemic anticholinergic effects are usually not a concern as systemic absorption is low
- Monitoring: FEV1, peak flow
- Drug and Diet Considerations:
  - Inhaled, local medication
  - Dry mouth may impact dietary/fluid intake

Umeclidinium and Vilanterol (Anoro Ellipta)

- Class: Inhaled anticholinergic and long acting beta-agonist
- Mechanism of Action: Provides anti-cholinergic effects through umeclidinium and stimulates beta-2 receptors leading to relaxation of smooth muscle and opening of airways
- Common Uses: Treatment of asthma and COPD
- Memorable Side Effects: Tachycardia, tremor, anxiousness, hypokalemia (rare), hyperglycemia (rare), dry mouth
- Clinical Pearls:
    - See Umeclidinium (Incruse Ellipta) for further information on this medication
- Monitoring: Frequency of use, FEV1, peak-flow, pulse, blood pressure, and potassium (usually only necessary in high dosages), glucose (rarely clinically significant
- Drug and Diet Considerations:
    - Assess potassium intake and blood levels of potassium if the patient is using a beta agonist frequently or has a history of hypokalemia
    - Be aware of caffeine intake in combination with a beta-agonist as it can have an additive effect on blood pressure and heart rate
    - Monitor diabetes patients for elevations in blood sugar
    - See Umeclidinium (Incruse Ellipta) for further information on this medication

Ursodiol (Actigall, Urso)

- Class: Gallstone dissolution drug
- Mechanism of Action: Dissolves cholesterol which can be an important component of gallstones
- Common Uses: Gallstone prevention and dissolution
- Memorable Side Effects: GI upset, change in bowel habits, dizziness
- Clinical Pearls:
    - Likely used if surgery is not appropriate or if patient is not a surgical candidate and if felt that cholesterol is a significant component of stones
    - Gallstones more common with increasing age, obesity, and diabetes
    - Be cautious in patients with liver disease
- Monitoring: LFTs
- Drug and Diet Considerations:
    - Given with food
    - Cholesterol based gallstones should prompt a cholesterol lowering diet

Valacyclovir (Valtrex)

- Class: Antiviral
- Mechanism of Action: Converted to acyclovir which inhibits DNA synthesis and viral replication
- Common Uses: Treatment of shingles, genital herpes and chicken pox
- Memorable Side Effects: GI most common, CNS side effects more likely in elderly and/or poor kidney function
- Clinical Pearls:

- o Typically for most viral infections (and bacterial for that matter), the sooner treatment is started once an infection is identified, the better
- o You can think of acyclovir and valacyclovir as the same...the big advantage of valacyclovir is that patients don't need to take it so many times per day
- o Monitor for GI side effects
- o LFTs will be more important if long term use is necessary
- o May need to reduce dose and/or have a heightened awareness for potential adverse effects in patients with poor kidney function
- Monitoring: Renal function, CBC, LFTs
- Drug and Diet Considerations:
  - o GI upset is possible, but not incredibly common
  - o It is important to maintain adequate hydration to prevent crystallization of the drug in the urine
  - o Can be given with or without food

Valsartan (Diovan)

- Class: Antihypertensive, ARB
- Mechanism of Action: Blocks the angiotensin 2 receptor which ends up preventing vasoconstriction and aldosterone release to ultimately lower blood pressure
- Common Uses: Treatment of hypertension and heart failure
- Memorable Side Effects: Hyperkalemia, exacerbate/worsen kidney function, low blood pressure
- Clinical Pearls:
  - o When you think of ARBs and ACE inhibitors, you can lump the side effects together as they are overall the same
  - o One major exception to the above rule is the side effect of cough; cough usually doesn't happen with ARBs, and in many patients, you will see patients who develop cough on an ACE inhibitor be transitioned to an ARB
  - o Kidney function changes and monitoring of potassium is critical when doses are changed or an ARB is initiated
  - o This worsening kidney function risk increases in patients who may be taking NSAIDs and/or diuretics
  - o As with any medication used to treat hypertension, we need to educate our patients to rise slowly when getting up to minimize risk of orthostatic (sometimes called postural) hypotension
- Monitoring: Renal function, potassium, blood pressure
- Drug and Diet Considerations:
  - o Be cautious and monitor potassium closely in patients with high dietary intake of potassium as this could contribute to hyperkalemia in combination with this medication
  - o Administer consistently with or without food

Vancomycin (Vancocin)

- Class: Antibiotic, glycopeptide
- Mechanism of Action: Inhibits bacterial cell wall synthesis
- Common Uses: Treatment of methicillin resistant Staphylococcus Aureus (MRSA), orally can be used to treat Clostridium difficile

- Memorable Side Effects: Hypotension, flushing, red man syndrome (rare), GI adverse effects when given orally
- Clinical Pearls:
  - Red man syndrome possible if infused too quickly
  - If red man syndrome happens, should be able to slow infusion rate to help treat
  - Trough concentration and kidney function may be important to help guide dosing
  - Drug of choice for MRSA
  - You should only see this medication taken orally to treat C. Diff; it has poor oral absorption into the blood circulation through the GI tract
- Monitoring: Renal function, drug concentrations (lab work is not essential for oral administration)
- Drug and Diet Considerations:
  - Oral administration can be taken with food

Vardenafil (Levitra, Staxyn)

- Class: PDE-5 inhibitor
- Mechanism of Action: Phosphodiesterase Type 5 inhibitor releases nitric oxide which is necessary for erection
- Common Uses: Treatment of erectile dysfunction and pulmonary arterial hypertension
- Memorable Side Effects: Low blood pressure, vision color changes (seeing blue tinges in vision), flushing, dizziness
- Clinical Pearls:
  - Originally developed as a blood pressure medication, caution patients about risk of low blood pressure
  - Drug interaction with systemic nitrate/nitroglycerin products, advise patients about potential interaction and elevated risk of low blood pressure
  - Be sure to assess if other medications may be contributing to sexual dysfunction, antidepressants like SSRIs are a classic example
- Monitoring: Blood pressure, heart rate
- Drug and Diet Considerations:
  - Can be given with or without food
  - Grapefruit juice can increase concentrations

Varenicline (Chantix)

- Class: Smoking cessation agent
- Mechanism of Action: Partial agonist at nicotine receptors, it blocks cravings and positive response from nicotine
- Common Uses: Smoking cessation
- Memorable Side Effects: Abnormal dreams, insomnia, GI, mental health concerns
- Clinical Pearls:
  - Abnormal behavioral and psych issues is a significant problem
  - Vivid or unusual dreams is a significant problem for patients
  - Boxed warning for depression/suicide risk
  - Intended to make smoking less rewarding/enjoyable
- Monitoring: No routine lab work Is necessary
- Drug and Diet Considerations:

- o   Give medication with food and water to help minimize GI upset
- o   Alcohol may exacerbate risk for psychiatric adverse effects
- o   With smoking cessation, many patients will report weight gain as being a barrier to quitting

Vasopressin (Vasostrict)
- Class: Vasoconstrictor
- Mechanism of Action: Causes an increase in cyclic AMP which causes multiple effects including vasoconstriction
- Common Uses: Treatment of vasodilation related shock
- Memorable Side Effects: Arrhythmia, MI, heart failure
- Clinical Pearls:
  - o   Vasoconstrictor used to increase BP in vasodilatory shock
  - o   Can impact sodium levels
  - o   BP/Pulse important to monitor
- Monitoring: Blood pressure, pulse, electrolytes (especially sodium), urine output
- Drug and Diet Considerations:
  - o   May cause water intoxication symptoms such as sedation, weakness, and headache

Venlafaxine (Effexor XR)
- Class: Antidepressant, SNRI
- Mechanism of Action: Selective serotonin and norepinephrine reuptake inhibitor (SNRI)
- Common Uses: Treatment of depression and off-label to treat neuropathic pain
- Memorable Side Effects: GI side effects, can exacerbate hypertension (usually at higher doses), CNS changes
- Clinical Pearls:
  - o   Has effects on both serotonin and norepinephrine
  - o   GI and central nervous system side effects (CNS) will likely be the most common
  - o   Decreased libido can be an issue for patients taking venlafaxine
  - o   Be careful with the risk of serotonin syndrome especially in patients on other serotonergic medications
  - o   Antidepressant effect may take weeks to work
- Monitoring: No routine lab work, but may check sodium, LFTs, blood pressure, or renal function if clinical concerns arise
- Drug and Diet Considerations:
  - o   Give with food
  - o   Adverse effects of nausea and dry mouth could impact nutrition, monitor if new concerns arise with initiation or dose escalation
  - o   Capsule can be open and sprinkled in applesauce
  - o   Alcohol can have negative added effects when used with venlafaxine

Verapamil (Calan)
- Class: Antihypertensive, calcium channel blocker
- Mechanism of Action: Blocks calcium channels resulting in vasodilation and cardiac relaxation

- Common Uses: Treatment of atrial fibrillation and hypertension
- Memorable Side Effects: Low pulse, low BP, constipation, edema
- Clinical Pearls:
  - Very important distinction: Verapamil and Diltiazem (non-dihydropyridine's) are the calcium channel blockers that act on the heart AND blood vessels; you will not see amlodipine and nifedipine used in atrial fibrillation, because their activity is primarily on the vessels. This also means that pulse monitoring will not be necessary with nifedipine and amlodipine
  - The higher you push the dose on these medications, the more likely you will see the side effect of edema. Keep an eye out for new requirement of diuretic prescriptions to treat the edema caused by the calcium channel blockers
  - Simvastatin is a very common medication that interacts with verapamil, leading to increased blood levels of simvastatin
  - Comes in multiple different formulations (long acting, short acting, etc.), make sure you have the right one
- Monitoring: Blood pressure, pulse, EKG, LFTs (as clinically indicated)
- Drug and Diet Considerations:
  - Give with or without food
  - May increase alcohol concentrations
  - Grapefruit juice can increase concentrations of the drug
  - Standard calcium supplementation typically will not impact the effectiveness of verapamil; excessive doses of calcium may have a higher likelihood of blunting the effects of the drug

Vinblastine (Vincasar)

- Class: Oncology agent, Vinca alkaloid
- Mechanism of Action: Vinca alkaloids bind tubulin and stops the production of microtubule formation which is necessary for cell replication and growth
- Common Uses: Treatment of a variety of different cancers
- Memorable Side Effects: Neuropathy, fatigue, hypertension, myelosuppression, hair loss, anorexia, constipation, elevated uric acid, ophthalmic and otic complications, pain, lung toxicity
- Clinical Pearls:
  - Boxed warning for the risk of extravasation
  - Benzyl alcohol may be a component of some dosage forms
- Monitoring: CBC, LFTs, uric acid, electrolytes (rare risk for hyponatremia)
- Drug and Diet Considerations:
  - Ensure adequate electrolyte intake, in particular if a patient is experiencing hyponatremia due to SIADH

Vincristine (Vincasar)

- Class: Oncology agent, Vinca alkaloid
- Mechanism of Action: Vinca alkaloids bind tubulin and stops the production of microtubule formation which is necessary for cell replication and growth
- Common Uses: Treatment of lymphomas, leukemias and various metastatic cancers
- Memorable Side Effects: Neuropathy, myelosuppression, hair loss, anorexia, constipation, elevated uric acid, ophthalmic and otic complications
- Clinical Pearls:
  - Boxed warning for the risk of extravasation

- o Peripheral neuropathy is often the dose-limiting side effect
- Monitoring: CBC, renal function, LFTs, uric acid, electrolytes (rare risk for hyponatremia)
- Drug and Diet Considerations:
  - o Ensure adequate electrolyte intake, in particular if a patient is experiencing hyponatremia due to SIADH

Vinorelbine (Navelbine)
- Class: Oncology agent, Vinca alkaloid
- Mechanism of Action: Vinca alkaloids bind tubulin and stops the production of microtubule formation which is necessary for cell replication and growth
- Common Uses: Treatment of a variety of different cancers
- Memorable Side Effects: Neuropathy, fatigue, hypertension, myelosuppression, hair loss, constipation, elevated LFTs, lung toxicity
- Clinical Pearls:
  - o Boxed warning for the risk of myelosuppression
- Monitoring: CBC, LFTs
- Drug and Diet Considerations:
  - o Ensure adequate electrolyte intake, in particular if a patient is experiencing hyponatremia due to SIADH

Vitamin A (Retinol)
- Class: Vitamin
- Mechanism of Action: Important vitamin in maintaining function of the eye, skin, and immune system
- Common Uses: Treatment of vitamin A deficiency
- Memorable Side Effects: Hypersensitivity reactions with IV formulation; CNS changes, hepatotoxicity and skin reactions may be signs of toxicity
- Clinical Pearls:
  - o Oral is the preferred route followed by IM if oral administration isn't acceptable
  - o Fat soluble
  - o RDA is 700-900 mcg for most adults
- Monitoring: Retinol levels may be considered in patients with likely deficiency or at risk for deficiency; <20 mcg/dL may indicate deficiency
- Drug and Diet Considerations:
  - o May be given with or without food
  - o Orlistat and mineral oil may reduce GI absorption
  - o Alcohol may reduce the liver's stores of vitamin A

Vitamin B12 (Cyanocobalamin)
- Class: Vitamin
- Mechanism of Action: Water soluble vitamin essential for many metabolic processes; also critical for red blood cell production
- Common Uses: Treatment of pernicious anemia, generalized B12 deficiency, intrinsic factor deficiency, malabsorption and drug induced deficiency
- Memorable Side Effects: Usually well tolerated; GI upset (oral) possible, but unlikely at normal dosages, injection discomfort (IM or deep SubQ)
- Clinical Pearls:

- - Symptoms of deficiency may include neuropathy, anemia, CNS changes such as confusion, depression, weakness, and mood changes (permanent CNS changes are possible with severe, prolonged B12 deficiency)
    - To release B12 from foods, gastric acid (low pH) is necessary
    - IM/deep SubQ administration is recommended for treatment of deficiency due to variable absorption with oral dosage forms
  - Monitoring: B12 levels, CBC (Elevated MCV can be indicative of B12 or folic acid deficiency); B12 deficiency is typically considered <200pg/mL
  - Drug and Diet Considerations:
    - Patients with alcohol use disorder may be at risk for numerous deficiencies and this would include B12
    - Elderly are at particular risk for low GI absorption due to a lack of intrinsic factor and a higher pH in their stomach
    - Metformin, colchicine, vitamin C, PPIs, and H2 blockers are common agents that may cause deficiency and necessitate need for replacement
    - Take vitamin C at least 2 hours after oral B12 supplement
    - 2.4 mcg is the recommended daily allowance (RDA) for a typical adult and is higher in pregnancy

Vitamin C (Ascorbic Acid)

- Class: Vitamin
- Mechanism of Action: Important cofactor and antioxidant for many enzymatic reactions; involved in the production of amino acids, hormones, carnitine, and collagen; also aids in iron absorption
- Common Uses: Improvement of wound healing, enhancement of iron absorption and management of scurvy
- Memorable Side Effects: Increases oxalate excretion through the urine which can increase the risk for oxalate stones, overall well tolerated
- Clinical Pearls:
  - Target RDA is in the range of 75-120 mg/day for most adults depending upon the population; pregnancy and breast-feeding typically require the upper end
  - Water soluble
  - Signs of deficiency include swollen, ulcerated or bleeding gums, skin discoloration, skin dryness, anemia, fatigue, bleeding
- Monitoring: Routine lab work is usually not necessary; may monitor renal function (patients at risk for renal stones) or CBC (those at risk for severe deficiency)
- Drug and Diet Considerations:
  - May be given with food
  - Must be dosed at the same time as iron if it is being used to enhance absorption of iron
  - Vitamin C may increase estrogen concentrations
  - Cyclosporine and amphetamine derivatives may have their concentration reduced

Vitamin D3 (Cholecalciferol)

- Class: Vitamin
- Mechanism of Action: Converted to active calcitriol which helps raise calcium and phosphate levels through increased gut absorption and renal resorption

- Common Uses: Treatment of osteoporosis, vitamin D deficiency and hypoparathyroidism
- Memorable Side Effects: Hypercalcemia and hyperphosphatemia in at risk patients; well tolerated in usual dosages, although, excessive intake could cause weakness, confusion, nausea, vomiting, weight changes and fatigue
- Clinical Pearls:
    - Target RDA is in the range of 800-2,000 IU/day for most adults depending upon the population, upper end for patients at risk for osteoporosis
    - Fat soluble
- Monitoring: 25-OH concentrations –(<30 nmol/L is likely considered deficient, however, there is no agreement on ideal level), calcium, phosphorus; lab work is typically not necessary in healthy patients
- Drug and Diet Considerations:
    - May be given with or without food
    - Orlistat and mineral oil may reduce GI absorption
    - Enzyme inducers such as phenytoin and carbamazepine may cause deficiency
    - Avoid aluminum hydroxide use with vitamin D as this may potentiate aluminum toxicity

Vitamin E (Alpha-tocopherol)
- Class: Vitamin
- Mechanism of Action: Helps prevent fatty acids and red blood cells from breakdown; antioxidant that binds free radicals
- Common Uses: Supplement
- Memorable Side Effects: Well tolerated at usual dosages; low potential to increase bleed risk at higher dosages
- Clinical Pearls:
    - Target RDA is in the range of 15-19 mg/day for most adults depending upon the population, pregnancy and breast-feeding typically require the upper end
    - Fat soluble
    - Approximately 1 mg is equal to 1.5-2.2 international units of vitamin E
- Monitoring: Routine lab work is usually not necessary
- Drug and Diet Considerations:
    - May be given with or without food
    - Use higher doses cautiously with anticoagulants and antiplatelet medications (i.e. aspirin, clopidogrel, warfarin, apixaban, etc.)
    - Orlistat and mineral oil may reduce GI absorption

Vitamin K (Phytonadione, Mephyton)
- Class: Vitamin
- Mechanism of Action: Important factor in the production of clotting factors 2, 7, 9, and 10
- Common Uses: Reversal of warfarin and vitamin K deficiency
- Memorable Side Effects: Skin reactions, dizziness, tachycardia, injection reaction
- Clinical Pearls:

- o Boxed warning on hypersensitivity reactions for injectable formulations (IV, IM) and because of this, oral administration is the safest administration route
- o Due to risk of hematoma with IM administration this route is generally avoided
- o Fat soluble
- o RDA is 90-120 mcg for most adults
- Monitoring: PT/INR
- Drug and Diet Considerations:
  - o May be given with or without food
  - o Orlistat and mineral oil may reduce GI absorption
  - o Alterations in dietary intake can alter warfarin's effectiveness; monitor INR closely

Warfarin (Coumadin, Jantoven)

- Class: Anticoagulant
- Mechanism of Action: Inhibition of clotting factors 2, 7, 9, and 10 – some folks remember this by the term "SNOT" seven, nine, '10', two
- Common Uses: Prevention of blood clots such as DVT and prevention of thromboembolic stroke from atrial fibrillation
- Common Side Effects: Bleeding, purple toe syndrome (rare)
- Clinical Pearls:
  - o Warfarin has a ton of drug interactions, most commonly with antibiotics (sulfamethoxazole/trimethoprim, metronidazole, levofloxacin, etc.); be sure physician is aware/reminded that patients are on warfarin when new medications are started or doses of medications might be changed
  - o Vitamin K is the antidote to too much warfarin; ideal way to give vitamin K is orally
  - o Many foods contain vitamin K (green leafy vegetables, etc.); diet changes can affect INR, consistency is the key!
  - o Younger patients may require doses > 10mg whereas elderly maybe need as little as 1-2 mg per day
  - o Usual goal range INR is 2-3; it is always important to have the goal INR range listed/addressed by the practitioner monitoring warfarin, this allows you to ask questions as to why the dose wasn't changed if the INR falls outside this range
  - o In patients who are at high risk for bleed (i.e. frequent falls, GI bleed history, etc.), a lower goal INR may be recommended
  - o Purple toe syndrome is rare but may happen if the patient is started on too high of an initial dose of warfarin
  - o Normal GI bacteria also produce vitamin K; changes in gut bacteria due to antibiotics can also impact the INR
- Monitoring: INR, CBC, bleed risk
- Drug and Diet Considerations:
  - o Variations in vitamin K intake will alter effectiveness
    - ▪ Higher intake = lower INR and increased risk of treatment failure
    - ▪ Reduced intake = higher INR and increased risk of bleed
    - ▪ Green leafy vegetables are the most common dietary source of vitamin K noted to have an impact

- o Acute alcohol intoxication may increase the bleed risk while chronic alcoholism may increase metabolism of the drug and cause lower INRs
- o Vitamin E, Omega-3 fatty acids, gingko, garlic, ginseng, turmeric, and fish oil supplements have been purported to have antiplatelet type activity which in theory could increase the risk of bleed – clinical significance is questionable; the most common resolution is to discontinue the supplements if they are not necessary
- o Cranberry juice and grapefruit juice may cause an increase in drug concentrations and subsequently increase INR

Zafirlukast (Accolate)
- Class: Leukotriene receptor blocker
- Mechanism of Action: Blocks leukotriene receptors which can help reduce inflammation
- Common Uses: Treatment of asthma
- Memorable Side Effects: Generally well tolerated; psychiatric or unusual behavior changes are rare, but possible
- Clinical Pearls:
    - o This medication is meant to control asthma, NOT provide acute relief with an exacerbation (albuterol is used for an asthma attack)
    - o Rare post-marketing case reports of neuropsychiatric problems including, abnormal behavior, aggression, or depression
- Monitoring: Asthma improvement/response
- Drug and Diet Considerations:
    - o Take on an empty stomach, 1 hour before or two hours after eating, as food will decrease bioavailability

Zaleplon (Sonata)
- Class: "Z" Drug, sedative
- Mechanism of Action: Enhances activity of GABA, an inhibitory neurotransmitter that causes sedation
- Common Uses: Treatment of insomnia
- Memorable Side Effects: Sedation, confusion, fall risk, dizziness, abnormal sleep behaviors (sleep walking, eating, etc.)
- Clinical Pearls:
    - o Often classified as a "Z" drug, medications like zaleplon are sedating; when medications are sedating we always have to be mindful of the morning after and make sure patients realize that driving and/or operating machinery can be extremely dangerous
    - o It is recommended to try to use these medications only for short term if possible
    - o Sleep hygiene and non-drug interventions are the preferred first line treatment for insomnia
    - o Before these types of medications are prescribed, keep an eye out for patients who may be on stimulating medications or medications that can contribute to insomnia and make sure that these are assessed prior to giving a sleep medication; classic examples include, methylphenidate, prednisone, too much levothyroxine, etc.
    - o Zaleplon is a controlled substance in the U.S. and carries a risk of addiction/dependence

- o Very similar effects to benzodiazepines, like lorazepam
- o Can greatly increase risk of falls especially in our elderly patients
- Monitoring: Routine lab monitoring typically isn't necessary unless clinically indicated
- Drug and Diet Considerations:
  - o Alcohol intake can have additive side effects of sedation, confusion, slurred speech, and other CNS depressant effects
  - o Significant food, large fat intake, may delay sedative effects

Zidovudine (Retrovir, AZT)

- Class: Antiretroviral, nucleoside reverse transcriptase inhibitor (NRTI)
- Mechanism of Action: Competes with natural substrates to inhibit reverse transcriptase; the HIV virus uses the enzyme reverse transcriptase to convert RNA into DNA
- Common Uses: HIV treatment
- Memorable Side Effects: Osteoporosis, GI adverse effects, fatigue, neuropathy; boxed warning for neutropenia and anemia, myopathy and lactic acidosis/fatty liver
- Clinical Pearls:
  - o IV dosage form available
- Monitoring: LFTs, HIV parameters such as viral load and CD4 count, CBC
- Drug and Diet Considerations:
  - o May be given with or without meals

Zinc

- Class: Mineral
- Mechanism of Action: Important mineral in proper immune system functioning; role in wound healing and smell/taste sensations
- Common Uses: Treatment of deficiency, improvement of wound healing and as an essential trace element in TPN; may be beneficial to shorten the duration of head colds, however, evidence is limited and controversial
- Memorable Side Effects: GI upset, metallic taste (oral)
- Clinical Pearls:
  - o Copper deficiency may result if IV zinc is given without copper
  - o RDA 8-12 mg/day for most adults, upper end for pregnancy and lactation
  - o Elemental zinc in salt forms: gluconate (14%), sulfate (23%), chloride (48%)
- Monitoring: Zinc, copper levels in patients on TPN
- Drug and Diet Considerations:
  - o May be given with or without food
  - o May bind and reduce concentrations of common antibiotics such as quinolones, certain cephalosporins, and tetracycline derivatives
  - o Bisphosphonates, baloxavir, and integrase inhibitors (HIV medications) may have concentrations reduced by zinc

Ziprasidone (Geodon)

- Class: Antipsychotic
- Mechanism of Action: Blocks dopamine receptors
- Common Uses: Treatment of schizophrenia, bipolar disorder and off-label to treat dementia-related behaviors like aggression, hallucinations and delusions

- Memorable Side Effects: Sedation, fall risk, orthostatic BP changes, EPS, metabolic syndrome
- Clinical Pearls:
    o Usually higher doses are required for younger patients with schizophrenia and/or bipolar disorder while lower doses can and should be used in the elderly
    o Remember with antipsychotic medications that they block dopamine and can exacerbate conditions where there is a shortage of dopamine like Parkinson's disorder (remember that we use dopamine to treat Parkinson's – i.e. carbidopa/levodopa or pramipexole)
    o Sedation, orthostatic hypotension, movement disorder side effects can all increase the risk of falls especially in our elderly patients
    o NMS (neuroleptic malignant syndrome) is a very rare but very serious complication with antipsychotic medications; a few symptoms of NMS include: fever, hyperreflexia, confusion, delirium, tremor
    o Antipsychotics increase risk of metabolic syndrome (diabetes, elevated lipids, weight gain etc.); it is important to periodically monitor for this, especially in younger patients with schizophrenia and/or bipolar disorder who may be likely to require long term use of higher doses
    o Anticholinergic effects are possible as well with antipsychotics, dry eyes, dry mouth, exacerbation of urinary retention (i.e. BPH), constipation (SLUD – can't salivate, lacrimate, urinate or defecate)
    o Antipsychotics can contribute to QTc prolongation, which can be especially problematic in patients who are already at risk (i.e. on antiarrhythmic medications)
- Monitoring: Weight, BMI, lipids, HbA1c, blood sugars, EKG as clinically appropriate, electrolytes (potassium and magnesium important if the patient is at risk for QTc prolongation)
- Drug and Diet Considerations:
    o Increased appetite and risk for metabolic syndrome
    o Increased blood sugars can result in our diabetes patients, monitor blood sugars closely with acute changes in the drug
    o Alcohol may exacerbate the CNS depressant effect
    o Give with food, at least 500 calories

Zoledronic Acid (Reclast, Zometa)
- Class: Bisphosphonate
- Mechanism of Action: Inhibits osteoclasts (osteoclasts break down bone)
- Common Uses: Treatment of osteoporosis, hypercalcemia and bone metastases
- Memorable Side Effects: Hypertension, hypocalcemia, fatigue, headache, infusion reactions, muscle pain, GI upset
- Clinical Pearls:
    o Osteonecrosis (destruction or dying) of the jaw is extremely rare; patients may be at increased risk if recently had an invasive dental procedure
- Monitoring: Bone mineral density, calcium, vitamin D levels, electrolytes, renal function (specific laboratory monitoring may depend upon the clinical use)

- Drug and Diet Considerations:
  - Ensure the patient has adequate vitamin D and calcium intake – at least 1,200 mg per day of calcium and 1,000 units of vitamin D in females with osteoporosis
  - Esophagitis and GI upset is possible which could cause changes in appetite and weight loss

Zolmitriptan (Zomig)
- Class: Anti-migraine, triptan
- Mechanism of Action: Serotonin 5HT agonist which causes vasoconstriction and reduction of inflammation associated with migraine
- Common Uses: Acute relief of migraine
- Memorable Side Effects: Dizziness, changes in CNS
- Clinical Pearls:
  - Meant for acute relief of migraine, not prophylaxis
  - Be sure to asses use, as frequent use may indicate that a controller medication like valproic acid, propranolol or topiramate, may need to be added to help prevent migraines
  - Often used with NSAIDs, like naproxen, in migraine treatment
  - Does have serotonin activity so it could potentially contribute to serotonin syndrome (higher risk in patients already on SSRIs, tramadol, etc.)
  - Nasal spray dosage form available
- Monitoring: Blood pressure, EKG when clinically indicated to assess risk for QTc prolongation
- Drug and Diet Considerations:
  - Given as needed for migraine, so administration at any point is fine with regards to food

Zolpidem (Ambien)
- Class: "Z" Drug, sedative
- Mechanism of Action: Enhances activity of GABA, an inhibitory neurotransmitter that causes sedation
- Common Uses: Treatment of insomnia
- Memorable Side Effects: Sedation, confusion, fall risk, dizziness, abnormal sleep behaviors (sleep walking, eating, etc.)
- Clinical Pearls:
  - Often classified as a "Z" drug, medications like zolpidem are sedating; when medications are sedating we always have to be mindful of the morning after and make sure patients realize that driving and/or operating machinery can be extremely dangerous
  - It is recommended to try to use these medications only for short term if possible
  - Sleep hygiene and non-drug interventions are the preferred first line treatment for insomnia
  - Before these types of medications are prescribed, keep an eye out for patients who may be on stimulating medications or medications that can contribute to insomnia and make sure that these are assessed prior to giving a sleep medication; classic examples include, methylphenidate, prednisone, too much levothyroxine, etc.
  - Zolpidem is a controlled substance in the U.S. and carries a risk of addiction/dependence
  - Very similar effects to benzodiazepines, like lorazepam

- - - o Can greatly increase risk of falls especially in our elderly patients
- Monitoring: Routine lab monitoring typically isn't necessary unless clinically indicated
- Drug and Diet Considerations:
  - o Alcohol intake can have additive side effects of sedation, confusion, slurred speech, and other CNS depressant effects
  - o Food may delay sedative effects

N

O

305

U

V

W

Printed in Great Britain
by Amazon